PEDIATRIC PICTORIAL
INTERROGATIVE RECKONER

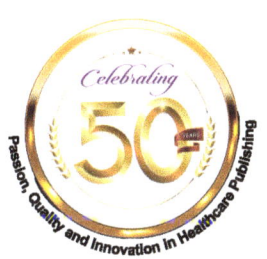

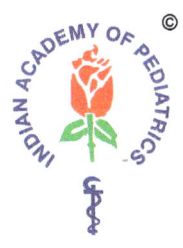

PEDIATRIC PICTORIAL INTERROGATIVE RECKONER

Editor-in-Chief

Ashok Kapse Md (Ped)
Professor and Head
Department of Pediatrics
Mahavir Superspecialty Hospital
Surat, Gujarat, India
Ex National Chairperson of Infectious Diseases Chapter of IAP

Academic Editor

G Sudhakar MD (Ped) Dch
Professor of Pediatrics (Retd)
Kurnool Medical College
Consultant Pediatrician
PG Teacher, Rainbow Hospitals
Kurnool, Kerela, India

Editor

Naveen Thacker MD (Ped) FIAP
Director
Deep Children Hospital and Research Center
Gandhidham, Gujarat, India

Forewords
Santosh T Soans
A Parthasarathy
Digant D Shastri

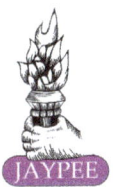

JAYPEE BROTHERS MEDICAL PUBLISHERS
The Health Sciences Publisher
New Delhi | London | Panama

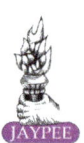

Jaypee Brothers Medical Publishers (P) Ltd

Headquarters
Jaypee Brothers Medical Publishers (P) Ltd
4838/24, Ansari Road, Daryaganj
New Delhi 110 002, India
Phone: +91-11-43574357
Fax: +91-11-43574314
Email: jaypee@jaypeebrothers.com

Overseas Offices

J.P. Medical Ltd
83 Victoria Street, London
SW1H 0HW (UK)
Phone: +44 20 3170 8910
Fax: +44 (0)20 3008 6180
Email: info@jpmedpub.com

Jaypee-Highlights Medical Publishers Inc
City of Knowledge, Bld. 235, 2nd Floor
Clayton, Panama City, Panama
Phone: +1 507-301-0496
Fax: +1 507-301-0499
Email: cservice@jphmedical.com

Jaypee Brothers Medical Publishers (P) Ltd
Bhotahity, Kathmandu, Nepal
Phone: +977-9741283608
Email: kathmandu@jaypeebrothers.com

Website: www.jaypeebrothers.com
Website: www.jaypeedigital.com

© 2019, Indian Academy of Pediatrics

The views and opinions expressed in this book are solely those of the original contributor(s)/author(s) and do not necessarily represent those of editor(s) of the book.

All rights reserved. No part of this publication may be reproduced, stored or transmitted in any form or by any means, electronic, mechanical, photocopying, recording or otherwise, without the prior permission in writing of the publishers.

All brand names and product names used in this book are trade names, service marks, trademarks or registered trademarks of their respective owners. The publisher is not associated with any product or vendor mentioned in this book.

Medical knowledge and practice change constantly. This book is designed to provide accurate, authoritative information about the subject matter in question. However, readers are advised to check the most current information available on procedures included and check information from the manufacturer of each product to be administered, to verify the recommended dose, formula, method and duration of administration, adverse effects and contraindications. It is the responsibility of the practitioner to take all appropriate safety precautions. Neither the publisher nor the author(s)/editor(s) assume any liability for any injury and/or damage to persons or property arising from or related to use of material in this book.

This book is sold on the understanding that the publisher is not engaged in providing professional medical services. If such advice or services are required, the services of a competent medical professional should be sought.

Every effort has been made where necessary to contact holders of copyright to obtain permission to reproduce copyright material. If any have been inadvertently overlooked, the publisher will be pleased to make the necessary arrangements at the first opportunity. The **CD/DVD-ROM** (if any) provided in the sealed envelope with this book is complimentary and free of cost. **Not meant for sale.**

Inquiries for bulk sales may be solicited at: jaypee@jaypeebrothers.com

Pediatric Pictorial Interrogative Reckoner

First Edition: **2019**

ISBN 978-93-5270-970-0

Dedication

This book is dedicated to our esteemed authors without whom this would not have been a reality. It was very kind of them to have spared time out of their busy schedules for this project.

Contributors

Abhay K Shah MD (Gold Medalist) DPed (UNI First) FIAP
Member ACVIP
Indian Academy of Pediatrics, 2018-19
Chairperson IAP ID Chapter 2015
Senior Consultant Pediatrician and Infectious
Diseases Specialist, Children Hospital
Ahmedabad, Gujarat, India

Alok Gupta MD (Ped) FIAP
Senior Consultant and Counselor
Pediatric Specialties Clinic, Former Assistant
Professor, Department of Pediatrics, Mahatma
Gandhi Medical College and Hospital
Jaipur, Rajasthan, India

Amar Shah MB MS MCh (Pediatric Surgery) MAMS FIAPS FRCS (Pediatric Surgery, England)
Neonatal and Pediatric Surgeon
Specialist Pediatric Endoscopic Surgery and
Urology, Director, Amardeep Multispecialty
Children Hospital and Research Center
Ahmedabad, Gujarat, India

Aniruddh Shah
MB MS FRCS (England) FRCS (Edinburgh)
Neonatal and Pediatric Surgeon
Specialist, Neonatal and Pediatric
Laparoscopic Surgery, Director
Amardeep Multispecialty Children Hospital
and Research Center, President
Indian Association of Pediatric Surgeons
(2008-2009), Chairman, Pediatric Endoscopic
Society of India (2009-2011)
Professor and Head
Department of Pediatric Surgery
Ahmedabad, Gujarat, India

Aniruddha Ghosh MD (Pediatrics)
Senior Resident
Institute of Child Health
Kolkata, West Bengal, India

Ankit Kumar Parmar MD FNB FIAP
Consultant Pediatric Hematologist Oncologist
Healing Hands Clinic and Day Care
Surat, Gujarat, India

Anoop Verma MD FIAP FIAMS FCGP FPNC FPAI
Consulting Pediatrician
Swapnil Institute of Child Health
Indian Academy of Pediatrics
Neurology Chapter of IAP
Raipur, Chhattisgarh, India

Aroon Narendra Trivedi MS (General Surgery)
MCh (Pediatric and Neonatal Surgery) DNB (Pediatric and Neonatal Surgery) MNAMS
Pediatric and Neonatal Urologist and Surgeon
Surat Pediatric Association Charitable Trust
Apple Superspecialty Hospital
Fellow Indian Society of Pediatric Urology
Member of Indian Medical Association
Member of Indian Association of Pediatric
Surgeons, Member of Indian Academy of
Pediatrics, Surat, Gujarat, India

Arun Shah MD DCH FRCP (London) FIAP
Consultant Pediatrician
Muzaffarpur Bihar, India
President IAP Bihar 2018
EB Member CIAP 2012, 2019

Ashok Banga MD (Ped)
Consultant Pediatrician and Director
Chirayu and Astha Hospitals
Gwalior, Madhya Pradesh, India

Ashok Kapse MD
Professor and Head
Department of Pediatrics
Mahavir Superspecialty Hospital
Surat, Gujarat, India

Atul Kulkarni MD (Ped)
Assistant Professor
Ashwani Rural Medical College
Solapur, Maharashtra, India

Bakul Jayant Parekh
MD DCH (Mumbai University) FIAP
Professor and CEO
BPCH Children's Hospital and Tertiary Care Unit, Bakul Parekh Children's Hospital
President Elect, CIAP 2019
Mumbai, Maharashtra, India

Bankim Parekh MD (Pediatrics)
Private Practitioner
Vraj Children Hospital
Vadodara, Gujarat, India

Barnali Bhattacharya MD
Consultant Pediatrics
Children's Clinic
Pune, Maharashtra, India

Chetan Trivedi MD (Pediatrics) DPed
Consultant Pediatrician and Neonatologist
Ex ID Consultant UN Mehta Institute of Cardiology, Neha Children Hospital and Neonatal Center
Ahmedabad, Gujarat, India

Chintan Bhatt MBBS DCH DNB Pediatrics Fellowship in Pediatric Cardiology (FNB)
Pediatric Cardiologist
Shri BD Mehta Mahavir Heart Institute
The Little Heart - Center for Congenital Heart Disease, Surat, Gujarat, India

Chirag Bhalvani MBBS MS (Orthopedics) Fellow Pediatric Orthopedics
Consultant Pediatric Orthopedic Surgeon
SAACHI Children Hospital
Surat, Gujarat, India

Darshan Vinodchandra Chauhan MD (Ped)
Consultant Pediatrician and Neonatologist
Param NICU and Children Hospital
Param Children Hospital, Param Baby Care Hospital, Param Child Care Hospital
Surat, Gujarat, India

Deval Arora MDS (Pedodontics)
Senior Lecturer
Department of Pedodontics, Sardar Patel Dental Institute of Medical Sciences
Lucknow, Uttar Pradesh, India

Dhanya Dharmapalan MD PG Dip in PID (Oxford)
Consultant in Pediatric Infectious Diseases
Apollo Hospitals
Mumbai, Maharashtra, India

Fagun Shah MD (Pediatrics) Post-Doctoral Fellowship in Pediatric Nephrology
Consultant Pediatric Nephrologist
Child's Kidney Care Center
Surat, Gujarat, India

Himanshu P Tadvi MD (Pediatrics) IDPCCM
Pediatrician and Pediatric Intensivist
PICU, SAACHI Children Hospital and Mahavir Hospital, SAACHI Children Hospital
Surat, Gujarat, India

Jagdish Chinnappa MD
Cluster Head, Bengaluru Region
Manipal Hospital
Bengaluru, Karnataka, India

Ketan Shah MD Ped
CEO, Ketan Children Hospital
Surat, Gujarat, India

Kewal Kishore Arora MD FIAP
Assistant Professor and Senior Consulting Pediatrician, Sri Aurobindo Medical College and Postgraduate Institute
Visiting Consultant Pediatrician
Medical Center, RR Center of Advanced Technologies
Indore, Gujarat, India

Kosha Gajera MD (Ped)
Consultant Pediatric Gastroenterologist
SAACHI Children Hospital
Child Gastro Care
Surat, Gujarat, India

M Indra Shekhar Rao
MD (Ped) DCH NEO (USA) FIAP FNNF
Director, Navodaya Hospital
Secunderabad, Professor
Department of Pediatrics NMC
Former Chairperson, ID Chapter/Neonatology Chapter, IAP
Hyderabad, Telangana, India

Contributors

Manish Jain MS MCh
Consultant Pediatric Surgeon and Director
SAACHI Children Hospital
Surat, Gujarat, India

Meenakshi Girish MD DNB FRCPCH
Associate Professor
Department of Pediatrics
NKP Salve Institute of Medical Sciences
Nagpur, Maharashtra, India

Mehul Gosai MBBS DPed MD
Associate Professor
Department of Pediatrics
Government Medical College
Bhavnagar, Gujarat, India

Mohit Vohra
DNB (Pediatrics) MBA (Hospital Administration)
Senior Consultant and Head
Department of Pediatrics, CKS Hospitals
Jaipur, Rajasthan, India

Mukul Tiwari MD DCH FIAP
Director, Apex Nursing Home, Chairperson
Medicolegal Group, IAP 2015-17
Zonal Chairman, Indian Medico Legal & Ethics
Association, President, Adolescent Health
Academy, State Coordinator, Medicine and
Law Program, IMA
Gwalior, Madhya Pradesh, India

Narayanappa D MD FIAP
Professor, Department of Pediatrics
JSS Medical College, JSS Academy of Higher
Education and Research
Mysuru, Karnataka, India

Narendra Rathi MD DNB FIAP
Consultant Pediatrician, Smile Institute of
Child Health, Akola, Maharashtra, India

Naveen Thacker MD(Ped) FIAP
Director, Deep Children Hospital and Research
Center, Gandhidham, Gujarat, India

Nigam Prakash Narain
MD DCH PhD MRCP (UK) FRCPCH
Former Professor and Head
Department of Pediatrics
Patna Medical College, Member of IAP, NNF,
IMA, Patna, Bihar, India

Nirav Buch
MD (Pediatrics) FNB (Pediatric Hematology and Oncology)
Consultant Pediatric Hematologist and
Oncologist, Advait Clinic
Lions Cancer Hospital, Surat, Gujarat, India

Piyali Bhattacharya DCH MD (Ped) FIAP
Consultant Pediatrician
Sanjay Gandhi Postgraduate Institute of
Medical Sciences
Lucknow, Uttar Pradesh, India

Pramod Jog MD (Ped) DNB (Ped) FIAP
Professor, Department of Pediatrics
DY Patil Medical College
Consultant Pediatrician, Jog Children's Clinic
Medipoint Hospital, Jehangir Hospital
Deenanath Mangeshkar Hospital
Pune, Maharashtra, India
Standing Committee Member, IAP
(International Pediatric Association), Steering
Committee Member, GAVI (CSO), Ex-President,
IAP, Chief Editor, Times of Pediatrics

Rajani HS MBBS DCH DNB
Assistant Professor
Department of Pediatrics, JSS Medical College
and Hospital, Mysuru, Karnataka, India

Rakesh Bhargav MBBS MS FICS DIP Ped Surg (London)
Senior Consultant and Head
Department of Pediatric and Neonatal
Surgery, Jaipur Golden and Sant Parmanand
Hospitals, New Delhi, India

Rashmi Nagaraj
MBBS DNB Pediatrics MA Psychology in Child Mental Health
Assistant Professor, Department of Pediatrics
JSS Medical College, JSS Academy of Higher
Education and Research
Mysuru, Karnataka, India

Ritabrata Kundu MD (Ped) FIAP
Professor
Department of Pediatrics, Institute of Child
Health, Kolkata, West Bengal, India

Ritesh Sukharamwala MBBS MD Pediatrics
Fellowship in Pediatric Cardiology (RGUHS)
Pediatric Cardiologist
Shri BD Mehta Mahavir Heart Institute
The Little Heart - Center for Congenital Heart
Disease, Surat, Gujarat, India

Ritesh Shah MD (Ped)
Consultant Pediatric Neurophysician
SAACHI Children Hospital, Child Neurology
and Epilepsy Center, Surat, Gujarat, India

S Balasubramanian MD DCH FRCS CP (UK)
Medical Director and Head, Department of
Pediatrics, Kanchi Kamakoti CHILDS Trust
Hospital, Chennai, Tamil Nadu, India

Sanjay Bafna MD (Pediatrics) European Diploma in Pediatric Respiratory Medicine
Head and Senior Consultant
Department of Pediatrics and Pediatric Critical
Care, Pediatric Pulmonologist
Jehangir Apollo Hospital
Pune, Maharashtra, India

Siddhartha R Nayak MS MCh
Pediatric Surgeon, Balvishva Hospital
Vadodara, Gujarat, India

Sumanth Amperayani DCH DNB
Junior Consultant
Department of Pediatrics
Kanchi Kamakoti CHILDS Trust Hospital
Chennai, Tamil Nadu, India

Swati Mulye MD
Professor, Department of Pediatrics
Sri Aurobindo Medical College and
Postgraduate Institute
Indore, Gujarat, India

Uma Siddhartha Nayak MBBS DPed MD (Ped)
Professor and Head
Department of Pediatrics, Parul Institute of
Medical sciences and Research (PIMSR) and
Parul Sevashram Hospital (PSH)
Baroda, Gujarat, India

Upendra Kinjawadekar MD DCH
Consultant Pediatrician and Neonatologist
Kamalesh Mother and Child Hospital
Navi Mumbai, Maharashtra, India

Upendra Chaudhari
MD (Pediatrics)
Assistant Professor
Department of Pediatrics, Government
Medical College and New Civil Hospital,
Member, Indian Academy of Pediatrics
Surat Pediatric Association Charitable Trust
Indian Medical Association
Surat, Gujarat, India

Usha Banga MD (Ped)
Consultant Pediatrician and Director
Astha and Prayas Hospitals
Gwalior, Madhya Pradesh, India

Vasant Khalatkar MD (Ped) FIAP PG Dip in Ped Infectious Diseases
Consultant Pediatrician
Guide for DCH, Khalatkar Hospital and Colors
Children Hospital for Critical Care
Nagpur, Maharashtra, India

Vijay Shah MD (Pediatrics)
Professor and Head
Department of Pediatrics, Government
Medical College and New Civil Hospital
Member, Indian Academy Of Pediatrics
Surat Pediatric Association Charitable Trust
Indian Medical Association
Adolescent Health Academy
Rotary Club of Surat West, Surat, Gujarat, India

Vipin Goyal MD DCH
Consultant Pediatrician and Neonatologist
Kamalesh Mother and Child Hospital
Navi Mumbai, Maharashtra, India

Vishal Gajimwar MD (Ped)
Assistant Professor
Department of pediatrics
Government Medical College
Nagpur, Maharashtra, India

FOREWORD

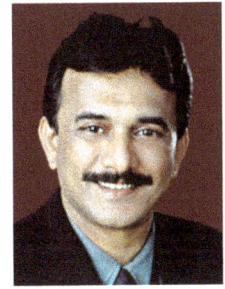

I am delighted to know that *Pediatric Pictorial Interrogative Reckoner* has been compiled under the editorial stewardship of Dr Ashok Kapse, Dr G Sudhakar and Dr Naveen Thacker with an astonishing 97 chapters contributed by as many as 59 authors. This is a remarkable and commendable achievement. When I first requested them, both readily agreed and I am happy to say that they have brought it out before time. I wish to congratulate all colleagues involved in this monumental effort.

Pediatric Pictorial Interrogative Reckoner, as its very name suggests, is a path breaking venture to understand pediatrics in a creative, innovative and engaging format. It is an old saying that 'a picture is worth a thousand words'. Pictures carve out everlasting images in our memory. What we see, we rarely forget. Liberal use of pictures to convey the narrative makes the absorption of knowledge economical and efficient for the busy pediatrician. Hence, I am sure this book will find the ready acceptance it so richly deserves.

Sharing of knowledge and expertise is a foundational tenet of modern medicine. The 28,000 members of the Indian Academy of Pediatrics (IAP) are an unimaginably huge and diverse resource base for harvesting the knowledge to be shared. By participating in academic projects like these, practicing pediatricians can elevate themselves to the next level in the profession. Authoring of authoritative articles and helming of literary projects with editorial vision is the need of the hour as it leads to the creation of a large body of reference material which pediatric community needs to enhance its clinical proficiency. I hope this book will inspire more colleagues to consider exploring academic ventures in the future.

Since inception, the IAP's cherished objective has been to focus on academics. We have seen from experience that whenever this focus on academics has reduced, there has been a corresponding decrease in our stature as an institution of relevance. I am glad that we are constantly blessed with ever increasing number of doctors who are willing to dedicate themselves to academic causes and kept our movement alive and thriving. May their tribe increase.

I wish the reader an enlightening academic experience.

Santosh T Soans
President
Indian Academy of Pediatrics

FOREWORD

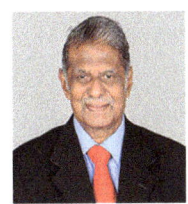

Dr Ashok Kapse, Dr G Sudhakar, and Dr Naveen Thacker, all are leading IAP faces and known for their academic expertise. This book is an example of their expertise, 59 renowned authors who are luminaries in their own field of specialization have contributed 97 pictorial interactive topics in a reader-friendly concise manner signifying practical aspects. The editorial board under the stewardship of Dr Kapse has done a laudable job in the production of this desktop reference treatise. They deserve all praise and congratulations. It is my good fortune that editors gave me an opportunity to go through this book and learn the latest and new information.

It is rightly said that we learn to unlearn only to relearn and thus continue to learn.

This book is a classical example of this maxim. I am sure medical students', postgraduates, faculty members and practitioners both pediatric and family medicine will find this book useful for their day-to-day learning, teaching and practice. I wish the publication large acceptance and huge readership. I once again congratulate the editors, authors as well as the publication house.

A Parthasarathy
National President IAP 1997
Regional Adviser Association of Pediatric Societies of
South East Asia Region 1997-1999. International Associate Editor
American Academy of Pediatrics (AAP) Publication Atlas of
Pediatrics in Tropical Countries. Founder Editor of
several IAP books and Parthas series of private books

FOREWORD

It is a privilege for me to write the foreword for the book titled *Pediatric Pictorial Interrogative Reckoner*.

"The eye cannot see what the mind does not know" was a quotation that my teachers often used to recall during my medical student days, to emphasize the fact that without study and acquisition of knowledge one would miss many clinical signs and clues, which would be unbecoming of a medical practitioner. But the other side of the coin is that the visual impression surely can be of help in diagnosing many clinical conditions. 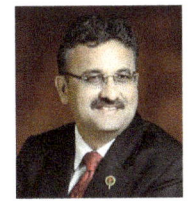 The book *Pediatric Pictorial Interrogative Reckoner* can be of help in diagnosing uncommon presentation of common clinical conditions and common presentation of uncommon condition.

This book is a collection of pictorial display of various clinical conditions which can provide as insight in the clinical analysis and rational management. I have a firm conviction that the Indian Academy of Pediatrics has a great pool of intellect, talent, and knowledge. This book exemplifies my belief. 59 authors contributing 97 chapters show how great resources IAP have. Beautiful images of common to exceptional conditions and an interrogative format ensure easy reading, on the whole book guarantees a fun-filled learning. All the authors deserve hearty compliments for a commendable work. Taking out time to conduct this academic activity out of their busy clinical practice is worthy of highest praises. Editorial team of Dr Ashok Kapse, Dr G Sudhakar, and Dr Naveen Thacker merits special greetings. Their professional approach ensured that the book got completed well within such a short time limit given to them.

Friends, the book is out, go grab it; my hearty wishes for enjoyable learning. I am sure, within short span it will gain popularity amongst PG students, practicing doctors and teaching faculties.

Digant D Shastri
IAP President, 2019

PREFACE

Around mid-September our esteemed IAP Presidents Dr Santosh Soans and Dr Digant Shastri approached us to edit a book based on clinical images. IAP wished to launch the book during the Pedicon 2019. It was a Herculean task, but we accepted the challenge as we had confidence that our fellow pediatricians would extend a helping hand in this endeavor.

A Chinese proverb goes "A picture is worth a thousand words". Images make a lasting impact on the human mind and we wanted to encash on this capability of the mind to learn medical education. We selected authors who have an extensive collection of clinical images.

Indian Academy of Pediatrics (IAP) does have a few picture-based books, but this book is different and unique in its format. It is in a question answer form which makes it easy and interesting to understand and remember, even answering patients' and parents' queries become easy.

While compiling the book we felt the need for an appropriate title. After some brainstorming, we came up with the title *Pediatric Pictorial Interogative Reckoner* (PPIR). Dr Soans accepted the change very graciously and we are very thankful about it.

The 97 chapters of the book contributed by 59 authors with a wide range of useful subjects. This book will be of great assistance to the practicing pediatricians to solve common to not-so-common conditions and at the same time educate and placate parents' concerns and anxieties.

Editing the work of such highly accomplished authors has been a very enriching experience for us. We extend our gratitude to them.

We would like to take this opportunity to express our thanks to Dr Santosh Soans and Dr Digant Shastri for giving us the freedom to edit the book but at the same time extending their helping hand whenever needed. Our heartfelt thanks to Dr Parthasarathy Sir for his blessings.

Last but not least, we would like to appreciate the soft, pleasant yet firm nudge from Miss Nedup Denka Bhutia, the book developer from Jaypee Brothers Medical Publishers, New Delhi, which prodded us to finish before time.

Ashok Kapse
G Sudhakar
Naveen Thacker

ACKNOWLEDGMENTS

Sincere thanks to IAP and its Presidents Dr Santosh Soans and Dr Digant Shastri for entrusting us with this prestigious project of editing *Pediatric Pictorial Interrogative Reckoner*. Their trust was a catalyst for us to complete this task in time.

Interacting with all the authors of such high caliber was in itself a once in a lifetime experience. Please accept our humble gratitude.

We would also like to appreciate our dear friend Lata Mathur for coming up with an apt title for the book which was accepted unanimously.

Jaypee Brothers Medical Publishers, New Delhi and Miss Nedup Denka Bhutia (Development Editor) need a special mention as they supported and encouraged us through the whole process. Thank you Miss Nedup Bhutia for your friendly but firm goading.

CONTENTS

1. **Acanthosis Nigricans** — 1
   Mehul Gosai

2. **Adolescent Gynecomastia** — 4
   Mukul Tiwari

3. **Amniotic Band Syndrome** — 7
   Narayanappa D, Rashmi Nagaraj

4. **Amniotic Band Syndrome** — 11
   Mehul Gosai

5. **Ankyloglossia** — 13
   Manish Jain

6. **Anteriorly Displaced Anus** — 15
   Chetan Trivedi

7. **Ataxia Telangiectasia** — 18
   Narayanappa D, Rajani HS

8. **Bernard-Soulier Syndrome** — 26
   Ankit Kumar Parmar

9. **Carotenemia** — 29
   Ashok Kapse

10. **Rectal or Colonic Polyp** — 32
    Kosha Gajera

11. **Choledochal Cyst** — 34
    Alok Gupta, Mohit Vhora

12. **Congenital Adrenocortical Hyperplasia** — 36
    Kewal Kishore Arora, Swati Mulye

13. **Congenital Diaphragmatic Hernia** — 40
    Siddhartha R Nayak

14. **Congenital Dislocation of Knee** — 45
    Chirag Bhalvani

15. **Congenital Duodenal Atresia** — 48
    Rakesh Bhargav

16. **Congenital Dyserythropoietic Anemia Type 1** — 51
    Pramod Jog

17. **Congenital Esotropia** — 54
    Barnali Bhattacharya

18. Chest X-rays in Congenital Heart Disease ... 56
    Ritesh Sukharamwala

19. Congenital Hydrocephalus ... 62
    Darshan Vinodchandra Chauhan

20. Congenital Hypothyroidism ... 66
    Nigam Prakash Narain

21. Congenital Rubella Syndrome ... 68
    Darshan Vinodchandra Chauhan

22. Congenital Varicella Syndrome ... 71
    Darshan Vinodchandra Chauhan

23. Dental Caries ... 74
    Piyali Bhattacharya, Deval Arora

24. Dermatitis Herpetiformis ... 78
    Kosha Gajera

25. Desquamating Rash ... 81
    M Indra Shekhar Rao

26. Duchenne Muscular Dystrophy ... 85
    Piyali Bhattacharya

27. Ectodermal Dysplasia ... 89
    Piyali Bhattacharya

28. Empyema Thoracis ... 92
    Aroon Narendra Trivedi

29. Erb's Palsy ... 99
    Chetan Trivedi

30. Eruptive Xanthomatosis ... 103
    Ashok Kapse

31. Erythema Infectiosum ... 105
    Atul Kulkarni

32. Erythema Multiforme ... 107
    Ashok Kapse

33. Erythema Nodosum ... 110
    Bakul Jayant Parekh

34. Erythema Nodosum 2 ... 113
    Aniruddha Ghosh, Ritabrata Kundu

35. Fanconi Anemia ... 115
    Nirav Buch

36. Foreign Body in Bronchus ... 118
    Aroon Narendra Trivedi

37. **Febrile Urticaria** 123
Vasant Khalatkar

38. **Forehead Hematoma: Unveiling as "Child Abuse"** 126
Uma Siddhartha Nayak

39. **Gastroesophageal Reflux Disease** 133
Bankim Parekh

40. **Griscelli Syndrome** 136
Ankit Kumar Parmar

41. **Hair on End Appearance** 139
Ashok Kapse

42. **Henoch-Schonlein Purpura** 141
Nigam Prakash Narain

43. **Hepatic Abscess** 143
Dhanya Dharmapalan

44. **Herpes Simplex Infection** 146
Aniruddha Ghosh, Ritabrata Kundu

45. **Herpes Zoster Infection** 151
Aniruddha Ghosh, Ritabrata Kundu

46. **Hereditary Angioedema** 154
Ashok Banga, Usha Banga

47. **Hereditary Methemoglobinemia** 157
Sanjay Bafna

48. **Hand–Foot–Mouth Disease** 160
Ketan Shah

49. **Hunter's Disease** 163
Jagdish Chinnappa

50. **Hydrocele** 165
Amar Shah, Aniruddh Shah

51. **Hypospadias** 168
Amar Shah, Aniruddh Shah

52. **Infantile Hemangioma** 171
Upendra Kinjawadekar, Vipin Goyal

53. **Infective Endocarditis** 174
Ritesh Sukharamwala, Chintan Bhatt

54. **Iron Deficiency Anemia** 178
Nirav Buch

55. **Lamellar Ichthyosis** 182
Vijay Shah, Upendra Chaudhari

56.	**Lymphangioma** Aniruddh Shah, Amar Shah	186
57.	**Microtia** Jagdish Chinnappa	188
58.	**Mitral Stenosis** Kewal Kishore Arora, Swati Mulye	189
59.	**Molluscum Contagiosum** Vijay Shah, Upendra Chaudhari	193
60.	**Moyamoya Disease** Alok Gupta, Mohit Vhora	195
61.	**Mucormycosis** Vishal Gajimwar, Vasant Khalatkar	197
62.	**Necrotizing Fasciitis** Atul Kulkarni	201
63.	**Neonatal Post-pyrexial Hyperpigmentation** M Indra Shekhar Rao	204
64.	**Neonatal Purpura Fulminans** Narendra Rathi	206
65.	**Nephrotic Syndrome** Fagun Shah	208
66.	**Neurocysticercosis** Ritesh Shah	212
67.	**Neurofibromatosis** Vijay Shah, Upendra Chaudhari	216
68.	**Nutritional Rickets** Meenakshi Girish	219
69.	**Phimosis** Aniruddh Shah, Amar Shah	225
70.	**Post Kala-Azar Dermal Leishmaniasis** Arun Shah	227
71.	**Pulled Elbow** Chetan Trivedi	231
72.	**Purpura Fulminans** Mehul Gosai	234
73.	**Renal Osteodystrophy** Fagun Shah	237
74.	**Renal Tubular Disorders** Fagun Shah	240

75.	**Rickettsial Fever** *Atul Kulkarni*	242
76.	**Roseola Infantum** *Bakul Jayant Parekh*	248
77.	**Spina Bifida** *Mehul Gosai*	250
78.	**Sacral Agenesis** *Pramod Jog*	253
79.	**Scarlet Fever** *Aniruddha Ghosh, Ritabrata Kundu*	256
80.	**Scarlet Fever** *S Balasubramanian, Sumanth Amparayani*	259
81	**Staphylococcal Scalding Skin Syndrome** *Kewal Kishore Arora, Swati Mulye*	264
82.	**Sturge–Weber Syndrome** *Ritesh Shah*	267
83.	**Systemic Lupus Erythematosus** *Anoop Verma*	269
84.	**Tuberculous Lymphadenitis with Sinus** *Abhay K Shah*	271
85.	**Torsion Testis** *Manish Jain*	275
86.	**Trichobezoar** *Manish Jain*	277
87.	**Tuberous Sclerosis** *Kewal Kishore Arora, Swati Mulye*	279
88.	**Tuberous Sclerosis Complex** *Ritesh Shah*	284
89.	**Hair Tuft at the Lumbosacral Spine** *Alok Gupta, Mohit Vhora*	288
90.	**Turbinate Hypertrophy** *Jagdish Chinnappa*	290
91.	**Turner Syndrome** *Alok Gupta, Mohit Vhora*	291
92.	**Umbilical Hernia** *Aniruddh Shah, Amar Shah*	295
93.	**Urticaria Multiforme** *Ashok Kapse, Himanshu P Tadvi*	297

94. **Vesicoureteric Reflux** 299
Fagun Shah

95. **Varicella Zoster** 305
Anoop Verma

96. **Cardiac Causes of Stridor and Dysphagia** 307
Ritesh Sukharamwala, Chintan Bhatt

97. **Waardenburg Syndrome** 310
Narayanappa D, Rashmi Nagaraj

Index 315

Acanthosis Nigricans

Chapter 1

Mehul Gosai

CASE STUDY

A 14-year-old boy presented to the outpatient department with complaints of excessive thirst and appetite, and loss of weight for 2 months' duration. On examination, the patient had dark patches over the nape of the neck (Fig. 1). The finding is known as Acanthosis Nigricans.

On investigation, the patient had elevated spot sugar which was confirmed by the plasma random sugar test. Hemoglobin A1c (HbA1c) levels were elevated which was suggestive of poor glucose control for the last 3 months. Renal and retinal examinations were normal.

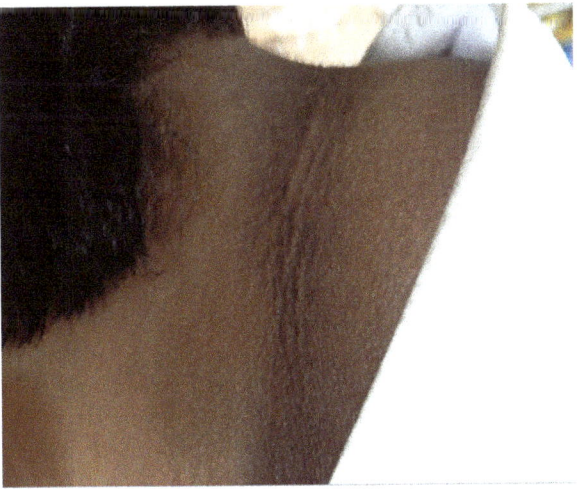

Fig. 1: Case of acanthosis nigricans.

1. **What is acanthosis nigricans?**
   Acanthosis nigricans is a skin condition characterized by areas of dark, velvety discoloration in body folds and creases. The affected skin can become thickened.

2. **What is the pathophysiology of acanthosis nigricans?**
   Acanthosis nigricans is most likely caused by factors that stimulate epidermal keratinocyte and dermal fibroblast proliferation. In the benign form of acanthosis nigricans, the factor is probably insulin or an insulin-like growth factor (IGF) that incites the epidermal cell propagation. Other proposed mediators include other tyrosine kinase receptors [epidermal growth factor receptor (EGFR) or fibroblast growth factor receptor (FGFR)].

3. **What are the causes of acanthosis nigricans?**
   The definitive cause for acanthosis nigricans has not yet been ascertained. The most common cause is diabetes mellitus and insulin resistance. In rare cases, acanthosis nigricans can be caused by adrenal gland disorders, such as Addison's disease, disorders of the pituitary gland, low levels of thyroid hormones and high doses of niacin.

4. **Which clinical history findings are characteristic of acanthosis nigricans?**
   Patients usually present with an asymptomatic area of darkening and thickening of the skin. Pruritus occasionally may be present. Lesions begin as hyperpigmented macules and patches, and progress to palpable plaques. In approximately, one-third of the cases of malignant acanthosis nigricans, patients present with skin changes before any signs of cancer. In another one third of the cases, the lesions of acanthosis nigricans arise simultaneously with the neoplasm. In the remaining one third of cases, the skin findings manifest sometime after the diagnosis of cancer. Malignant acanthosis nigricans has been reported to appear abruptly and exuberantly and may be associated with a higher rate of pruritus.

5. **Which physical findings are characteristic of acanthosis nigricans?**
   Skin tags are often found in and around the affected areas. Occasionally, lesions of acanthosis nigricans may be present on the mucous membranes of the oral cavity, nasal and laryngeal mucosa, and esophagus. The areola of the nipple also may be affected. Eye involvement, including papillomatous lesions on the eyelids and conjunctiva, may occur. Nail changes, such as leukonychia and hyperkeratosis, have been reported.

6. **What laboratory investigations should be done in acanthosis nigricans?**
   Screen for diabetes with a glycosylated hemoglobin level or glucose tolerance test. Screen for insulin resistance; screening test for plasma insulin level, which will be high in those with insulin resistance. This is the most sensitive test to detect insulin resistance because many children do not yet have overt diabetes mellitus and an abnormal glycosylated hemoglobin level, but they do have a high plasma insulin level. When there is abrupt development of acanthosis nigricans, screening for malignancy should be done.

7. **What are the differential diagnoses of acanthosis nigricans?**
   - Atopic dermatitis
   - Becker melanosis
   - Candidiasis
   - Dermatologic manifestations of pellagra
   - Erythrasma
   - Giant melanocytic nevi
   - Ichthyosis hystrix
   - Linear epidermal nevus
   - Parapsoriasis en plaque
   - Pemphigus vegetans
   - Reticulate pigmented anomaly

- Seborrheic keratosis
- Tinea corporis.

8. **What is the role of skin biopsy in acanthosis nigricans?**
   Skin biopsy may be useful if clinical diagnosis is not easily made. Histological examination reveals hyperkeratosis, papillomatosis, with minimal or no acanthosis or hyperpigmentation. The dermal papillae project upward as finger-like projections, with occasional thinning of the adjacent epidermis. Pseudohorn cysts may be present. Mucosal acanthosis nigricans reveals epithelial hyperkeratosis and papillomatosis along with parakeratosis.

9. **What are the types of acanthosis nigricans?**
   - Obesity-associated acanthosis nigricans
   - Syndromic acanthosis nigricans
   - Acral acanthosis nigricans
   - Unilateral acanthosis nigricans
   - Generalized acanthosis nigricans
   - Familial acanthosis nigricans
   - Drug-induced acanthosis nigricans
   - Malignant acanthosis nigricans
   - Mixed-type acanthosis nigricans.

10. **What is the sexual predilection of acanthosis nigricans?**
    The incidence of acanthosis nigricans is equal for men and women. Acanthosis nigricans has no known sex predilection.

11. **What is the treatment of acanthosis nigricans?**
    No treatment of choice exists for acanthosis nigricans. The goal of therapy is to correct the underlying disease process. Treatment of the lesions of acanthosis nigricans is for cosmetic reasons only. Correction of hyperinsulinemia often reduces the burden of hyperkeratotic lesions. Likewise, weight reduction in obesity-associated acanthosis nigricans may result in resolution of the dermatosis. Topical medications that have been effective in some cases of acanthosis nigricans include keratolytics (e.g., topical tretinoin 0.05%, ammonium lactate 12% cream or a combination of the two) and triple-combination depigmenting cream (tretinoin 0.05%; hydroquinone 4%; fluocinolone acetonide 0.01%) nightly with daily sunscreen. Calcipotriol, podophyllin, urea, adapalene and salicylic acid have also been reported with variable results. Oral agents that have shown some benefits include etretinate, isotretinoin, metformin and dietary fish oils. Octreotide showed sustained improvement in one patient with insulin resistance 6 months after completing the course.

12. **What are the complications of acanthosis nigricans?**
    Complications vary depending on the etiology of acanthosis nigricans. Appearance of acanthosis nigricans during childhood usually is associated with a benign condition.

13. **What is the prognosis of acanthosis nigricans?**
    The prognosis for patients with malignant acanthosis nigricans is often poor. Patients with the benign form of acanthosis nigricans experience very few, if any, complications of their skin lesions.

14. **What are all the dietary modifications that should be done in acanthosis nigricans?**
    Weight loss and glycemic control are essential for those with obesity-related acanthosis nigricans or hyperinsulinemic states.

Adolescent Gynecomastia

Chapter 2

Mukul Tiwari

CASE STUDY

Rajesh, a 13-year-old boy, presented in the clinic with bilateral enlargement of breasts which started about a year ago and is now static. He is shy to unbutton his shirt in front of his friends when he goes to picnics and outings. His parents are worried about the adverse psychological effect this is causing to his self-esteem.

There has been no complaint of pain or discharge from the nipples. There was no history of mumps or trauma to the testicles. The father gave a similar history of gynecomastia in his teens which lasted for a year and a half (Fig. 1).

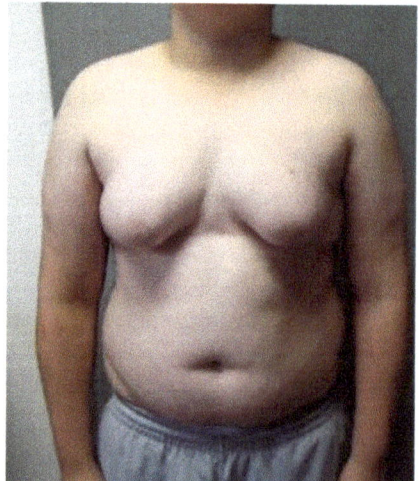

Fig. 1: Case of adolescent gynecomastia.

POSITIVE POINTS IN CLINICAL EXAMINATION

The boy was in Tanner stage 4. He appeared reasonably intelligent. There was no nipple discharge or axillary lymphadenopathy. On breast examination, the boy was found to have true gynecomastia which can be differentiated from pseudogynecomastia by having the patient lie on his back with his hands resting behind his head. The examiner places his thumbs on each side of the breast, and attempts to join them. In true gynecomastia, glandular tissue is felt which is symmetrical to the nipple–areolar complex. The boy's testicles were normal in size and consistency. There were no nodules or asymmetry. There were no signs of feminization, including typical body hair distribution and eunuchoid habitus. There were no stigmata of chronic liver disease, thyroid disease or renal disease.

1. **What is adolescent gynecomastia?**
   Physiological adolescent gynecomastia is benign enlargement of the male breast. It results from proliferation of the glandular tissue of the breast. It presents as a rubbery or firm mass behind the nipples. Physiological gynecomastia is usually bilateral but can be unilateral. It results from an altered estrogen–androgen balance, with estrogen predominance. It can occur with normal estrogen levels also, due to increased breast sensitivity to a normal circulating estrogen level. Here the stimulatory effect of estrogen dominates over inhibitory effect of androgen resulting in imbalance. Estrogens have the effect of causing increased vascularity, ductal hyperplasia and proliferation of the periductal fibroblasts. Histologically, the male breast looks similar to female breast tissue. Pseudogynecomastia is deposition of fat behind breast nodule without real growth of glandular tissue.

2. **What is the prevalence rate of adolescent gynecomastia?**
   Prevalence rate of benign pubertal gynecomastia ranges from 4% to 69%. Pubertal gynecomastia usually starts around 10–12 years and generally regresses within 18 months. Persistence beyond 18 years is not common.

3. **What is the main differential diagnosis of gynecomastia?**
   Gynecomastia should be differentiated from pseudogynecomastia (lipomastia), which is characterized by fat deposition without glandular proliferation.

4. **What causes adolescent gynecomastia?**
   Since the gynecomastia was bilateral, the following conditions, which lead to bilateral gynecomastia, are to be considered:
   - Obesity
   - Hypogonadism
   - Cirrhosis
   - Adrenal carcinoma (see Adrenal gland symptoms)
   - Hepatic carcinoma
   - Hypothyroidism
   - Klinefelter's syndrome
   - Pituitary tumor
   - Reifenstein's syndrome
   - Testicular cancer
   - Hemodialysis
   - Testicular irradiation
   - Drugs: ethylstilbestrol, estramustine, chlorotrianisene, Marijuana, heroin phenothiazine
   - Tricyclic antidepressants

5. **What are the necessary investigations?**
   In patients who are clinically diagnosed as having physiologic gynecomastia, no further evaluation is required. Further evaluation is necessary in patients who have breast size

greater than 5 cm, a lump that is tender, progressive, recent or of unknown duration, if there are signs of malignancy, if the physical examination reveals abnormality of sex organs, thyroid, renal, hepatic disorders. The following investigations are required:
- Liver, kidney and thyroid tests should be performed if the physical examination points towards liver failure, kidney failure or hyperthyroidism.
- If examination of breast tissue suggests malignancy, a biopsy should be performed.
- Mammogram if malignancy is suspected upon clinical examination.
- A fine-needle aspiration or breast biopsy if the case merits.
- Serum testosterone, estradiol, luteinizing hormone (LH) and beta-human chorionic gonadotropin (β-HCG) should be measured. An elevated β-HCG or a markedly elevated serum estradiol suggests neoplasm and a testicular ultrasound should be advised. A low testosterone level, with an elevated LH and normal to high estrogen level indicates primary hypogonadism. Low testosterone, low LH and normal estradiol levels indicate secondary hypogonadism, and hypothalamic or pituitary causes should be looked for. If testosterone, LH and estradiol levels are all elevated, then the diagnosis of androgen resistance should be entertained.
- If the history and physical examinations point towards Klinefelter's syndrome, then a karyotype should be performed.

6. **What was the final diagnosis in this case?**

The case was clinically diagnosed as having physiological gynecomastia on the basis of the following—age of onset, bilateral, no signs of liver, kidney or thyroid disorder, normal secondary sex characters, etc. Physiological (asymptomatic; pubertal) gynecomastia does not require further tests and should be re-evaluated in 6 months.

Amniotic Band Syndrome

Chapter 3

Narayanappa D, Rashmi Nagaraj

CASE STUDY

A 2-year-old girl born to a non-consanguineous couple, presented with the history of fever of 3 weeks' duration, deformity of right lower limb, and pain and swelling of the same since 1 week. On examination, she was found to have multiple deformities of the limbs (Figs. 1A to D) including constriction bands over the right wrist and right thigh, syndactyly of the right ring and middle fingers, hypoplastic right little finger, rudimentary toes on the left side and absence of right leg and foot (due to congenital amputation) replaced by a rudimentary stump, which was infected and swollen due to an abscess. However, she was found to have normal intelligence. Her younger male sibling was said to be normal. In view of the above clinical features, she was diagnosed to have the severe form (Grade 4) of amniotic band syndrome.

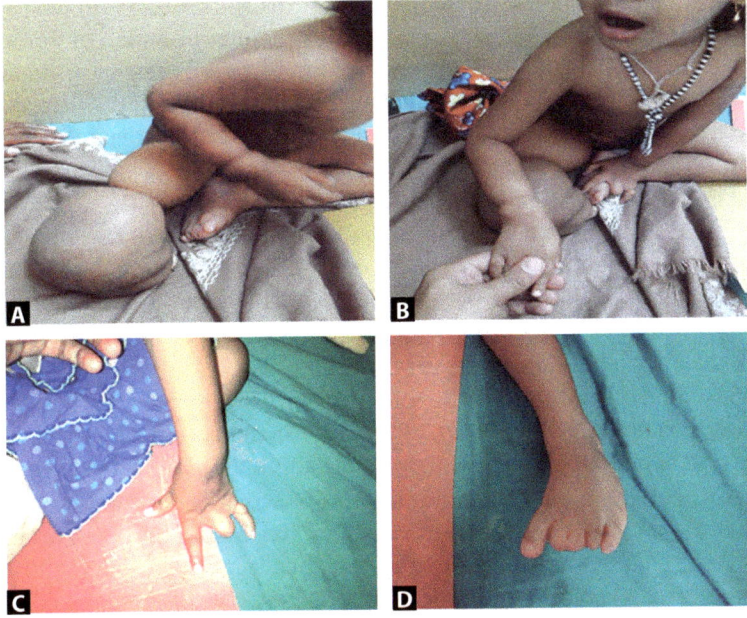

Figs. 1A to D: Examples of amniotic band syndrome.

1. **What is amniotic band syndrome?**
   Amniotic band syndrome (ABS) is a set of congenital malformations attributed to amniotic bands that entangle fetal parts during intrauterine life, which results in a broad spectrum of anatomic disturbances—ranging from minor constriction rings and lymphedema of the digits to complex, bizarre multiple congenital anomalies, incompatible with life.

2. **What are the other names for ABS?**
   Amniotic band sequence, congenital constriction band syndrome and amniotic band disruption.

3. **What is the mode of inheritance?**
   It is a congenital sporadic disorder, the frequency of occurrence ranging from 1:1200 to 1:15,000 births.

4. **What causes ABS?**
   Amnion is a membrane that surrounds the baby in utero. If it ruptures, strands of amnion can end up floating in the amniotic sac and can attach to the baby's developing body parts and cause injury. If untreated, the bands become tighter around the body part they are attached to, leading to amputation, severe deformity of limbs, webbed toes or fingers, or severe defects of the head, face or spine. Many pediatricians and researchers agree that it starts with the rupture of the amnion (a thin sac that forms around the fetus that protects it) early in pregnancy. Bands of amnion then encircle parts of the fetus' body. The rupture of the amnion appears to be random and is not related to anything the mother did or did not do during pregnancy. Teratogenic drugs such as methadone may play a role.

5. **What are the theories which explain the presence of amniotic bands?**
   These malformations were first described by Streeter, who proposed the presence of amniotic bands as a result of the theory of germplasm (intrinsic theory). Even though there are many theories to explain the presence of amniotic bands, the most accepted theory is the one developed by Richard Torpin (extrinsic model) who postulated rupture or infection as an initial event, with a decidual reaction, formation of fibrous cords with progressive separation of the cord and recollection of the amniotic sac producing transient oligohydramnios. These mesodermal flanges trap and strangle limbs, fingers or other fetal organs. The results of the deformation, amputation or disruption depend on the gestational age at which the rupture occurred.

6. **What are the different types of amniotic band syndrome?**
   Amniotic band syndrome may present in many different forms. For example, it may cause only a minor groove or indentation in one of the limbs; or it may cause syndactyly of multiple digits on the hand or foot with multiple bands or constriction rings on multiple digits; or amputations of digits or larger parts of the limbs.

7. **What are the clinical manifestations of ABS?**
   The manifestations of amniotic band syndrome range from constriction rings of the thorax, extremities, and head, to syndactyly, amputations, and spontaneous abortion. Seventy-seven percent of patients present with multiple anomalies.

8. **Are there other problems that occur commonly with amniotic band syndrome?**
   The most common problems that are associated with amniotic band syndrome are cleft lip/palate and clubfoot. Associated anomalies may occur in approximately 40–60% of cases. Usually, there are no abnormalities of the internal organs.

9. **How do we explain the variability in the severity of manifestations in ABS?**
   The variability in defect and severity has been attributed to differences in timing of the amniotic rupture. Early rupture, within the first 45 days of gestation, leads to the most severe defects, including central nervous system and skull defects, facial clefts, cleft lip and palate, limb anomalies and major visceral defects. Early compression may also result in incomplete separation of the digits (syndactyly) or extra finger rays (polydactyly). When an amniotic rupture occurs after 12 weeks of gestation, constriction of isolated limb parts may occur more frequently than central nervous anomalies or clefts.

10. **What are the different degrees of severity of ABS?**
    Varying degrees have been described depending on the level of injury as follows:
    - Grade 1 involves the subcutaneous cellular tissue
    - Grade 2 extends to the fascia
    - Grade 3 extends to the fascia and requires release
    - Grade 4 is described when amputation has occurred.

11. **How is ABS diagnosed?**
    ABS can be diagnosed prenatally by ultrasound, which can sometimes show amniotic bands, but more often malformations consistent with ABS, as well as oligohydramnios and reduction of fetal movements. The diagnosis can be made as early as 12 gestational weeks. In the second trimester of gestation, most of the ABS defects could be seen during routine ultrasound examinations.
    The most important ultrasound diagnostic criteria are visible amniotic bands, constriction rings on extremities and irregular amputations of fingers and/or toes with terminal syndactyly. Mild defects, however, are less likely to be diagnosed prenatally, and however, are seen after birth.
    Latest ultrasound techniques—three-dimensional and four-dimensional ultrasounds contribute to more sensitive prenatal diagnostics of ABS, and in complicated cases, fetal magnetic resonance can be helpful.

12. **What are the differential diagnoses of ABS?**
    Differential diagnosis must be made with other causes of amputation or congenital limb absence. Some of them include the following:
    - Michelin tire baby syndrome which is characterized by abnormal limb enlargement with folds rather than constriction.
    - Fetal varicella syndrome which is the result of maternal infection between 13 and 20 weeks of gestation. Fetal involvement with varicella (the risk is approximately 2%) usually presents with localized absence of skin, usually on limbs, due to intrauterine ulceration, dermatomal scar, papular lesions resembling connective tissue nevus, limb or digital hypoplasia associated with ocular and central nervous system (CNS) abnormalities.

    There are many genetic syndromes that cause reduction of the size of the extremities.
    - Holt-Oram syndrome—agenesis or hypoplasia of radius and thumb.
    - VATER/VACTERL association (Vertebral defects, Anal defects, Cardiac, Tracheoesophageal fistula, Esophageal atresia, Renal anomalies, Limb defects).
    - Unilateral hypomelia syndrome or caudal regression syndrome often appears in children of diabetic mothers in which there is a decrease in femoral length but not a distal amputation.

13. **What is the management of ABS?**

    Therapy of ABS is mostly surgical, with an individual approach to every single case. It is mostly multidisciplinary involving plastic surgeon, orthopedic surgeon, orthodontist, ophthalmologist and neurosurgeon, not to forget the pediatrician.

    Timing of repair and surgical planning are important in improving its functional outcome. The most accepted method of treatment for constriction bands is excision of the ring and staged Z-plasty with fairly large flaps. In addition, excision of the ring and a single-stage multiple Z-plasty repair have also been described. These techniques have been described for constriction band defects in the more common locations of the upper or lower limbs, trunks or digits.

    Of late, there have been some attempts of prenatal ABS treatment which involves fetoscopic laser cutting of amniotic bands, before the occurrence of malformations as a result of compression caused by them.

    Termination of pregnancy may be advised if fetal anomalies seem to be incompatible with life.

14. **What is the risk of recurrence of ABS?**

    It is important to note that ABS is sporadic, with no recurrence in siblings or children even if one parent is affected. However, there are some reports of amniotic band syndrome among families with collagen disorders, such as the Ehler-Danlos syndrome.

15. **What is the prognosis?**

    Prognosis is variable depending upon the grade of severity.

Amniotic Band Syndrome

Chapter 4

Mehul Gosai

1. **What is the other name for amniotic band syndrome?**
   Streeter dysplasia
2. **What is the pathophysiology of amniotic band syndrome?**
   Incomplete obliteration of the extracoelomic space renders the amnion fragile and subject to spontaneous or traumatic rupture. After the rupture, a transient oligohydramnios occurs due to extravasation of amniotic fluid. The decrease in space also allows the resultant floating amniotic bands to easily encircle a developing body part.
3. **What are the etiologies of amniotic band syndrome?**
   The intrinsic and extrinsic causes are as follows:
   Intrinsic: Disruptive event occurs during blastogenesis, leading to an intrinsic germ plasm defect. This causes the soft tissue to slough. External healing of the slough leads to the constricting rings and the resultant localized developmental defects.
   Extrinsic: Intrauterine trauma leads to premature rupture of the membranes, and strands of residual membranes could encircle the digits and cause amniotic band syndrome.
4. **What is the epidemiology of amniotic band syndrome?**
   There is an incidence of one case per 10,000–15,000 population.
5. **What are the common conditions associated with amniotic band syndrome?**
   The common conditions associated with amniotic band syndrome include constricting rings, acrosyndactyly, amputations of the extremities of neonates, encephalocele, cleft lip or palate, renal abnormalities, cardiac defects, hemihypertrophy, anterolateral bowing of the tibia, tibial pseudarthrosis, and leg-length discrepancy.
6. **What are the common sites in the body involved in amniotic band syndrome?**
   On the extremities, the distal portion is most often involved.
7. **What is Patterson's classification in amniotic band syndrome?**
   Extremity deformities in amniotic band syndrome are classified into Patterson's four types, as follows (Fig. 1):
   - Type I—Simple ring constriction
   - Type II—Ring constriction accompanied by fusion of the distal bony parts, with or without lymphedema
   - Type III—Ring constrictions accompanied by fusion of soft-tissue parts
   - Type IV—Intrauterine amputations

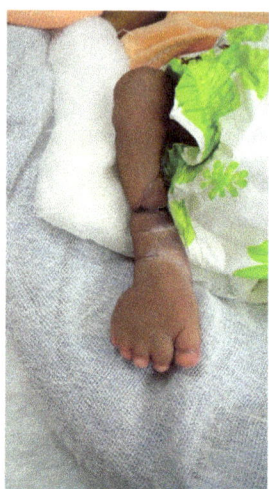

Fig. 1: Ring constriction in amniotic band syndrome (Type II Patterson's classification).

8. **How is ultrasonography useful in amniotic band syndrome?**
   Serial antenatal ultrasonograms can show the gross lack of formation, such as anencephaly or intrauterine amputations.

9. **What are all the medical treatments available for amniotic band syndrome?**
   No medical treatment exists for the condition. Avoidance of certain drugs that can lead to spontaneous rupture of membranes, such as cocaine and mifepristone, may help decrease the potential risk.

10. **What are all the surgical treatments available for amniotic band syndrome?**
    Due to tight constrictions on the digits or extremities, urgent surgical treatment often is necessary for patients with vascular compromise. Surgery also is indicated for patients with syndactyly or acrosyndactyly that compromises hand function.

11. **What are all the complications of amniotic band syndrome?**
    The complications include severe lymphatic or venous congestion at the time of birth due to tight bands. This congestion may lead to necrosis and gangrene, neurovascular compromise caused by the release of the entire band at one sitting or lack of attention to the superficial level of the attenuated nerves and vessels.

12. **What is the prognosis of amniotic band syndrome?**
    All patients with amniotic band syndrome should be monitored regularly until skeletal maturity because of the potential for recurrence of the rings and for secondary contractures that may develop.

Ankyloglossia

Chapter 5

Manish Jain

CASE STUDY

A 3-year-old child presented by parents for concern about limited movement of tongue and some speech development issues. On examination, the child was found to have an ankyloglossia (tongue tie) (Fig. 1).

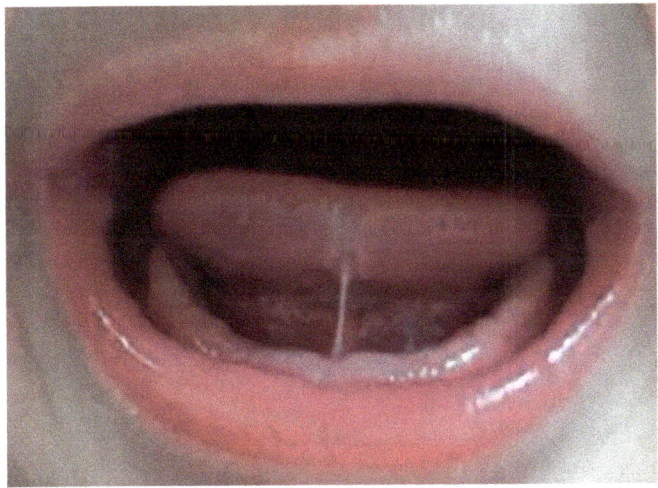

Fig. 1: Case of ankyloglossia.

1. **What is ankyloglossia?**
   This congenital condition is characterized by an abnormally short, thickened, tight lingual frenulum or an anterior attachment of the lingual frenulum which restrict the mobility of tongue.
2. **What are the clinical implications of this condition?**
   It variably causes reduced anterior tongue mobility and is associated with functional limitations in breastfeeding, swallowing, articulation, orthodontic problems, including malocclusion, open bite and separation of lower incisors; mechanical problems related to oral clearance; and psychological issues.

3. **Are these findings found in all children?**
   No, any particular child may have none, any, some or rarely all of these findings.
4. **What is the treatment?**
   Surgery should be considered at any age depending on the patient's history of speech, feeding or mechanical/social difficulties but conventionally surgery is performed after 1 year of age.
5. **Does surgery correct all clinical issues?**
   It may not correct or rectify all issues but it definitely helps in many of them, including improvement in speech.

Anteriorly Displaced Anus

Chapter 6

Chetan Trivedi

CASE STUDY

A 15-month-old female presented with complaint of constipation since 4 months of age.

1. **Can we see something abnormal in the pic (Fig. 1)?/Can we find any abnormality in the position of anus?**

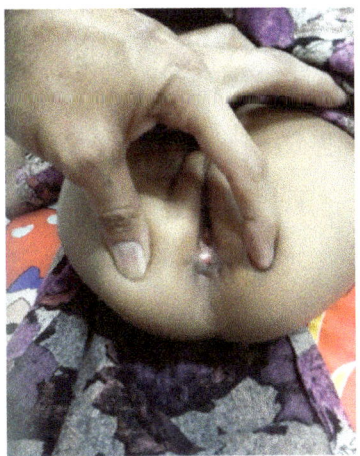

Fig. 1: Anteriorly displaced anus.

It is an anteriorly displaced anus.

2. **What is anterior displacement of anus?**
   Anterior displacement of the anus (ADA) is recognized as a common congenital developmental abnormality of anorectal region.

3. **How to diagnose and confirm diagnosis of ADA?**
   - Physical examination: In previous studies, the diagnosis of ADA is usually relied on inspection; therefore, the incidences widely vary, according to physician experience. We can suspect anteriorly displaced anus by physical examination only.
   - Quantitative measurements using anal position index (API).

4. What is API?

Anal position index is the ratio of anal–fourchette distance to coccyx–fourchette distance for females and the ratio of anal–scrotum distance (Fig. 2A) to coccyx–scrotum distance (Fig. 2B) for males. API less than 0.46 in boys and less than 0.34 in girls is indicative of ADA. Reisner et al. had first reported a simple and reliable method to determine the normal position of the anus; this parameter has been called anogenital (anal position) (Fig. 3) index by Bar-Moar and Eiton.

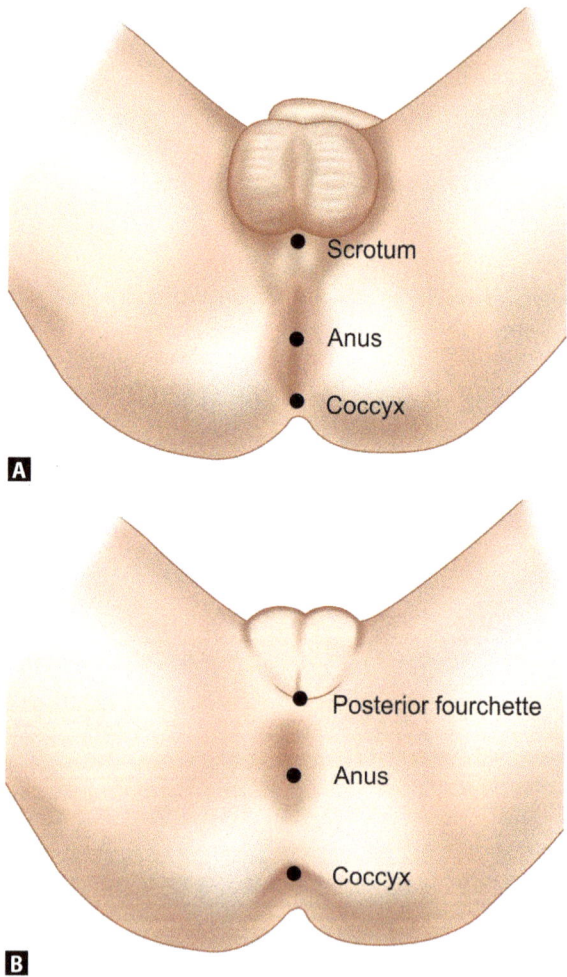

Figs. 2A and B: (A) API in males; (B) API in females.

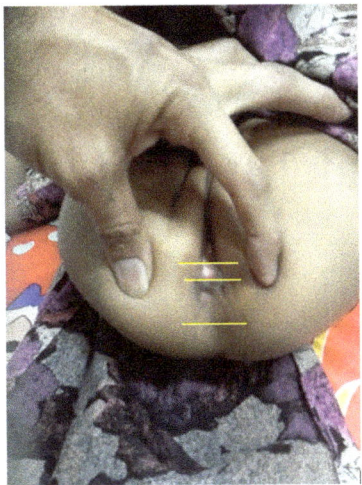

Fig. 3: Calculation of anal position index.

5. **What is the significance of ADA?**
   Clinical presentation of ADA is usually consistent with early onset of constipation since birth or at the time of weaning from breastfeeding. According to the study by Leape and Romenofsky, ADA is accounted in more than one third of patients examined in consultation for chronic constipation. However, the more recent cross-sectional studies fail to demonstrate a direct association between ADA and constipation.

6. **Can constipation be caused in the index case?**
   The etiology of constipation in childhood may be multifactorial. In most children, constipation is functional, without objective evidence of pathological condition. Otherwise, the congenital abnormality of anus position is considered a possible cause of constipation, especially in infancy and early childhood.

7. **How to manage a case of ADA with constipation?**
   Symptomatic therapy with laxative administration is usually adequate in mild cases. On the other hand, posterior anoplasty with or without sphincterotomy to remove the deranged lower loop of the external sphincter is recommended as a procedure of choice in severe cases. However, the surgical operation is generally not indicated in the majority of infancy constipation associated with ADA. A prominent posterior rectal shelf and an anal dimple posterior to the anus are the most common characteristics reported in patients requiring surgical treatment.

Ataxia Telangiectasia

Chapter 7

Narayanappa D, Rajani HS

CASE STUDY

An 18-year-old girl, born to second degree consanguineously married couple, apparently normal except for recurrent infections in the first 5 years of life, presented with reddish discoloration of both eyes since 12 years, involuntary movements of hands since 11 years, unsteady gait and slowing of speech since 8 years, hair loss since 3 years and increased frequency of micturition since 1 month. Perinatal history was uneventful with normal developmental milestones till the age of 5 years and had recurrent respiratory tract infections, diarrhea and pyoderma in the first 5 years of life. On examination, she looked grossly wasted with weight less than third centile and stunted with height below third centile. Vital signs were within normal limits. Hairs were thin and sparse with patchy areas of baldness. Telangiectasia were evident on bulbar conjunctiva of both eyes and hyperpigmentation of skin around eyes with synophrys was noted (Fig. 1). Acanthosis nigricans at nape of the neck (Fig. 2), café au lait spots, cubitus valgus and genu valgus deformity on standing (knock-knees), and plantar flexion with contractures at both ankle joints were present. On neurological examination, cerebellar signs like wide-based ataxic stepping gait, bilateral nystagmus, staccato speech, intention tremor, dysdiadochokinesia, dysmetria and past pointing were noted. Investigations revealed grossly elevated alpha fetoprotein, decreased levels of immunoglobulin A (IgA) and immunoglobulin E (IgE) levels, and mild cerebellar atrophy of cerebellar vermis more than cerebellar hemisphere on magnetic resonance imaging (MRI). The brainstem evoked response audiometry (BERA) was suggestive of right ear sensorineural hearing loss. Fasting blood sugar was high with hemoglobin A1c (HbA1c)–12.6 and C-peptide level was low.

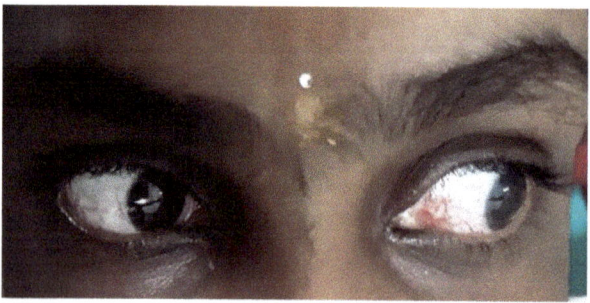
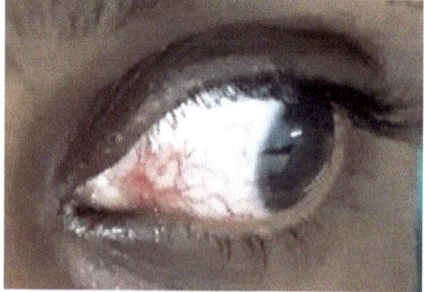

Fig. 1: Telangiectasia on bulbar conjunctiva and synophrys.

A diagnosis of ataxia telangiectasia with type 2 diabetes mellitus was made based on clinical manifestations and laboratory investigations. She has a younger male sibling who is normal. None of the other family members had similar features. Genetic studies could not be done due to financial constraints.

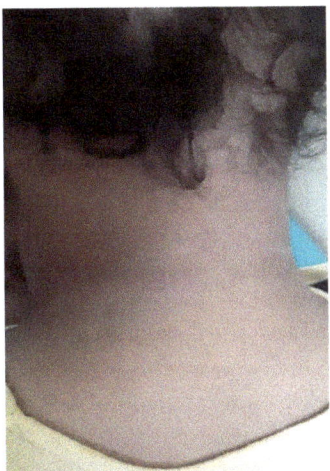

Fig. 2: Acanthosis nigricans and sparse hair.

1. **What is ataxia telangiectasia?**
   Ataxia telangiectasia (A-T) is an autosomal recessive disorder primarily characterized by cerebellar degeneration, telangiectasia, immunodeficiency, cancer susceptibility and radiation sensitivity. A-T is often referred to as a genome instability or deoxyribonucleic acid (DNA) damage response syndrome.

2. **What is the background of ataxia telangiectasia?**
   Elena Boder and Robert P Sedgwick, in 1957, described a familial syndrome of progressive cerebellar ataxia, oculocutaneous telangiectasia and frequent pulmonary infection, and coined the term ataxia telangiectasia or A-T. It is also referred to as Louis-Bar syndrome, cerebello-oculocutaneous telangiectasia and immunodeficiency with ataxia telangiectasia.

3. **What is its frequency?**
   The worldwide prevalence of A-T is estimated to be between 1 in 40,000 and 1 in 100,000 live births.

4. **What are the most frequent clinical signs of ataxia telangiectasia?**
   The principal features are as follows:
   1. *Progressive truncal ataxia* that begins during the first year. In infants, choreoathetosis develops instead of, or in addition to, ataxia. The ataxia begins as clumsiness and progresses so slowly that cerebral palsy is often the erroneous diagnosis.
   2. *Oculomotor apraxia* is present in 90% of the patients but may be mild at first and overlooked.
   3. *Intellectual development* is normal at first but often lags with time. One third of the children ultimately function in the mildly retarded range.

4. *Telangiectasia* usually develops after 2 years of age and sometimes as late as age 10. It first appears on the bulbar conjunctivae, giving the eyes a bloodshot appearance. Similar telangiectasia appears on the upper half of the ears, on the flexor surfaces of the limbs and in a butterfly distribution on the face. Sun exposure or irritation exacerbates the telangiectasia.
5. *Recurrent sinopulmonary infection* is one of the more serious features of the disease and reflects an underlying immunodeficiency.

5. **What are the other manifestations of A-T?**
Poor growth, premature aging, alopecia areata, delayed pubertal development and gonadal dysgenesis, ballistic, retropulsive or jerky movements, sensory and motor neuropathy, brain telangiectasia (observed by MRI), restrictive lung disease, elevated cholesterol and triglyceride levels, glucose intolerance and diabetes (4%), liver abnormalities (e.g., fatty liver; non-alcoholic cirrhosis; elevated serum transaminases), malignancies (there is an increased incidence for both lymphoid and solid tumors), osteoporosis/osteopenia and low vitamin D levels, postural scoliosis and progressive foot deformities, gastroesophageal reflux (especially if reflux was an issue in infanthood), early menopause and depression.

6. **When does the telangiectasia become evident?**
Telangiectasia usually develops after 2 years of age and sometimes as late as age 10; sometimes may not appear at all.

7. **What are the sites of telangiectasia?**
It first appears on the bulbar conjunctivae, giving the eyes a bloodshot appearance. Similar telangiectasia appears on the upper half of the ears, on the flexor surfaces of the limbs, roof of the mouth and in a butterfly distribution on the face. Sun exposure or irritation exacerbates the telangiectasia. It can also arise in bladder, brain and also in liver and lungs.

8. **What are the types of ataxia telangiectasia?**
The classic A-T and mild forms of A-T are as follows:

Classic form:
- Neurological manifestations are typically observed during the toddler years resulting in wheelchair dependency around the age of 10.
- Immunodeficiency—Roughly two thirds of people with classic A-T suffer from some type of immunodeficiency and/or lymphopenia.
- Pulmonary disease—Relatively common
- Cancer—Although malignancies in these individuals tend to occur at a younger age and are often lymphoid in nature, cancers in older individuals do occur and include both hematopoietic and non-hematopoietic malignancies.

Mild variant form (Fig. 3):
- Neurological manifestations—Individuals have more mild neurological deficits in childhood with slower age-related neurodegeneration. The predominant neurological symptoms or symptoms to present first may be myoclonus, dystonia, choreoathetosis or tremor with ataxia appearing later. Oculomotor apraxia may also appear later or not at all.
- Immunodeficiencies do occur, but are less common.
- Pulmonary disease is less common.
- Malignancies tend to appear later in life and include a higher proportion of non-hematopoietic cancers. The diagnosis of cancer can precede the diagnosis of A-T.

Ataxia Telangiectasia

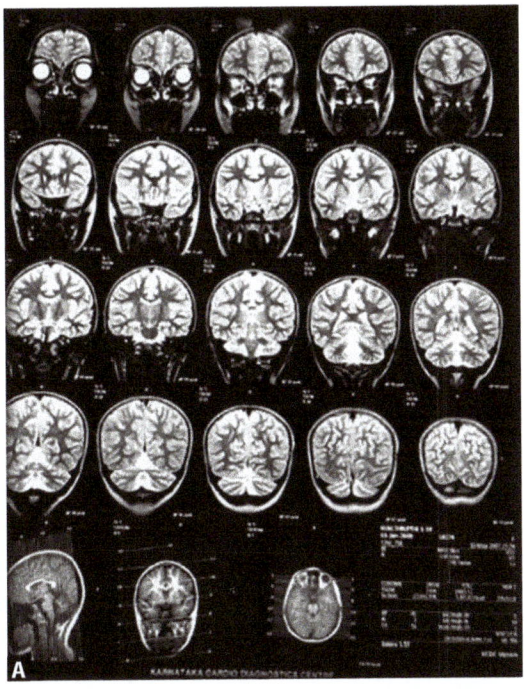

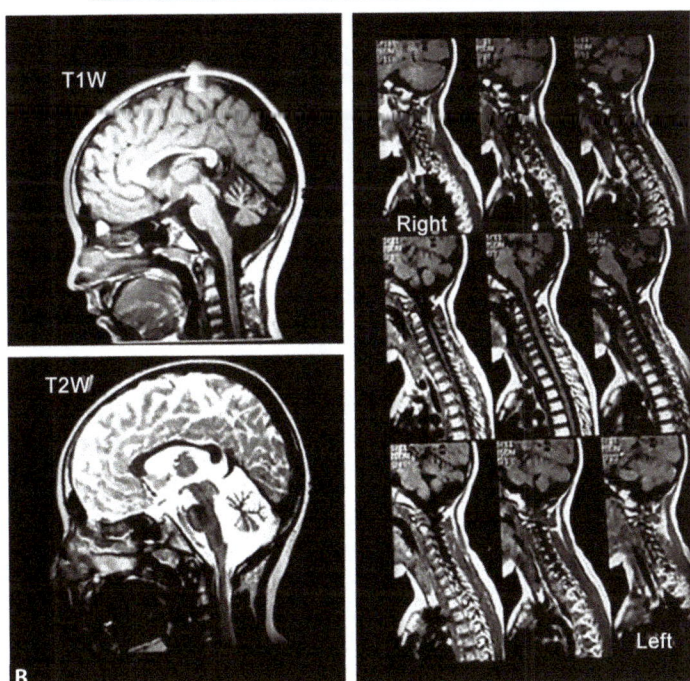

Figs. 3A and B

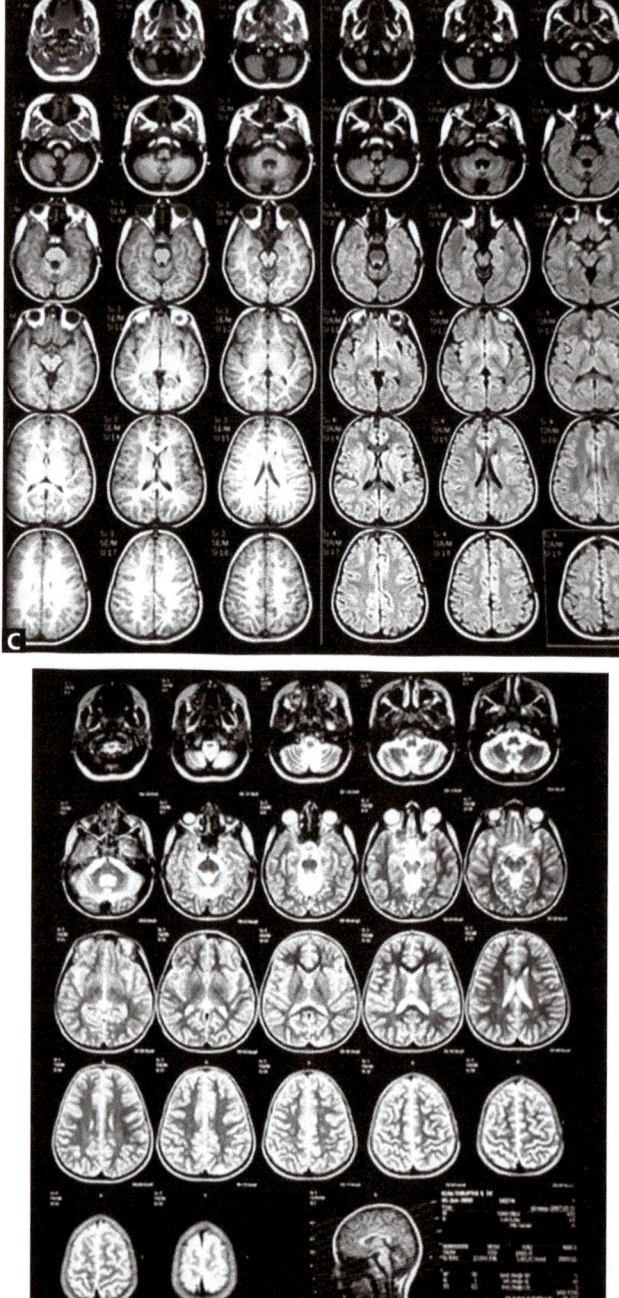

Figs. 3C and D

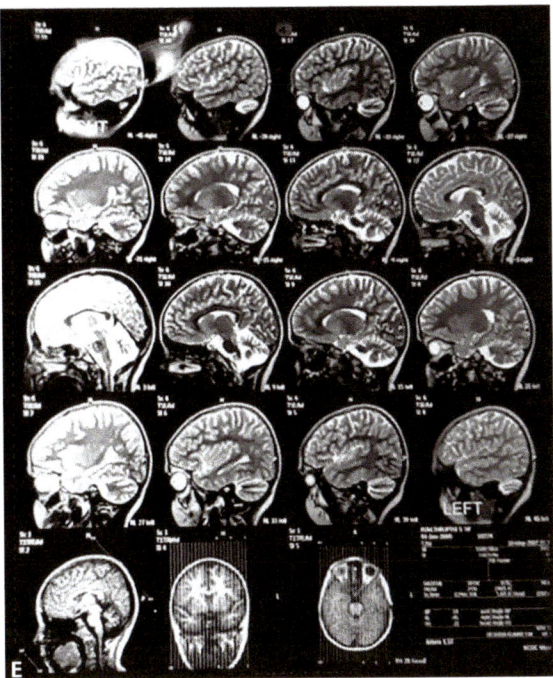

Figs. 3A to E: Magnetic resonance imaging (MRI) showing mild cerebellar atrophy.

9. **What are the characteristic eye abnormalities in A-T?**

   The telangiectasia does not affect vision and visual acuity is normal in A-T. However, control of eye movement and visual fixation is often impaired affecting functions that require fast, accurate eye movements from point to point (e.g., reading).

   Abnormal eye movements associated with A-T include: oculomotor apraxia, nystagmus (including horizontal nystagmus in primary gaze, nystagmus on lateral gaze, post-rotary nystagmus and periodic alternating nystagmus), hypometric saccades and saccadic intrusions, convergence/accommodation and vestibulo-ocular (VOR) abnormalities. Strabismus is common. There may be difficulty in coordinating eye position and *shaping the lens to see objects clearly at close distances.*

10. **What are the immunological abnormalities in A-T?**
    - The synthesis of antibodies and certain immunoglobulin subclasses is disturbed because of disorders of B-cell and helper T-cell function.
    - Approximately, 80% have decreased serum IgA, IgE or immunoglobulin G (IgG). Especially characteristic is a selective deficiency of the IgG2 subclass.
    - Serum and salivary IgA is absent in 70–80% of children, and IgE is absent or diminished in 80–90%. The immunoglobulin (IgM) concentration may be elevated in few as a compensation for the IgA deficiency.
    - Failure to make antibodies in response to vaccines or infections, andlymphopenia, especially affecting T-lymphocytes.
    - There are reduced numbers of new B cells leaving the bone marrow and new T cells leaving the thymus decreased proportions of naive B and T cells, andreduced antigen receptor repertoire.

- The thymus has an embryonic appearance, and α-fetoprotein concentration is elevated in 90% of patients.

11. **What is the risk of developing malignancy in A-T and what are the malignancies associated with A-T?**

    The risk of developing malignancy is around 25–38%. Most are lymphoma and lymphocytic leukemia. Cancers of solid organs, such the stomach, esophagus, liver, parotid gland, thyroid, skin, breast and lung can also be seen.

12. **What are the laboratory abnormalities in A-T?**
    - Elevated and slowly increasing serum alpha-fetoprotein levels after 2 years of age
    - Low serum levels of immunoglobulins (IgA, IgG, IgG subclasses and IgE) and lymphopenia (particularly affecting T-lymphocytes)
    - Spontaneous and X-ray induced chromosomal breaks and rearrangements in cultured lymphocytes and fibroblasts
    - Reduced survival of cultured lymphocytes and fibroblasts after exposure to ionizing radiation
    - Cerebellar atrophy detected by MR.

13. **What is the inheritance pattern in A-T?**

    Ataxia telangiectasia is inherited as an autosomal recessive trait.

14. **Which gene is associated with A-T?**

    The disease gene that causes ataxia telangiectasia, known as the ataxia telangiectasia mutated (ATM) gene, is located on the long arm (q) of chromosome 11 (11q22.3). The *ATM* gene encodes a protein that plays a role in regulating cell division after DNA damage. The protein, which is known as ATM for "A-T mutated," is an enzyme (protein kinase) that normally responds to DNA damage by triggering the accumulation of a protein (p53) that prevents cells from dividing (tumor suppressor protein). However, in individuals with ataxia telangiectasia, abnormal changes (mutations) of the ATM gene cause an absence or defect of the ATM protein and delayed accumulation of the p53 protein. As a result, cells with DNA damage continue dividing (replicating) without appropriate repair of their DNA, causing an increased risk of cancer development.

15. **Is antenatal diagnosis available?**

    Antenatal diagnosis can be performed if the pathological ATM mutations in that family have been identified in an affected child. In the absence of identifying mutations, antenatal diagnosis can be made by haplotype analysis if an unambiguous diagnosis of the affected child has been made through clinical and laboratory findings and/or ATM protein analysis.

16. **What is the treatment approach in A-T?**

    Treatment of the neurologic problems associated with A-T is symptomatic and supportive, as there are no treatments known to slow or stop the neurodegeneration.

    Physical, occupational and speech therapies as well as exercise may help maintain function but will not slow the course of neurodegeneration. However, other manifestations of A-T, e.g., immunodeficiency, pulmonary disease, failure to thrive and diabetes can be treated effectively. Treat all infections vigorously. Intravenous antibiotics are sometimes required for what would otherwise be a trivial sinusitis in a normal child.

    Patients with A-T are exquisitely sensitive to radiation, which produces cellular and chromosomal damage. Radiation may be a precipitant in the development of neoplasia. Therefore, despite the frequency of Sino pulmonary infections minimize radiation exposure.

For respiratory infections, therapy with an antibiotic drug, postural drainage (with the head lower than the rest of the body) of the bronchial tubes and lungs, and gamma globulin injections in some cases may be effective.

Avoidance of undue exposure to sunlight may help control spread and severity of dilated blood vessels (telangiectasia).

Vitamin E therapy has, in some cases, been reported to provide temporary relief of some symptoms.

17. **What is the role of a pediatrician in treating children with A-T?**

    Suspect the diagnosis in infants with a combination of ataxia, recurrent Sino pulmonary infections and oculomotor apraxia. As the child gets older, the addition of telangiectasia to the other clinical features makes the diagnosis a certainty. Genetic counselling can help family members of a patient with A-T.

18. **What is the life expectancy in A-T?**

    Historically, individuals with A-T succumbed to their disease in childhood or the teenage years. However, the average life expectancy for individuals with A-T has improved, and continues to improve, with advances in care. In 2006, the average life expectancy was reported to be approximately 25 years.

    The two most common causes of death are chronic lung disease (about one-third of cases) and cancer (about one-third of cases).

19. **What are the vaccine recommendations for A-T?**
    - If a person with A-T does not need gamma globulin replacement therapy, he/she should receive all standard childhood vaccines, including the live vaccines for measles, mumps, rubella and varicella-zoster viruses.
    - The individual with A-T and all household members should receive the influenza (flu) vaccine every fall.
    - People with A-T who are less than 2 years old should receive three doses of a pneumococcal conjugate vaccine given at 2-month intervals.
    - People older than 2 years who have not previously been immunized with pneumococcal conjugate vaccine should receive two doses of pneumococcal conjugate vaccine.
    - At least 6 months after the last pneumococcal conjugate vaccine has been given, and after the child is at least 2 years old, the 23-valent pneumococcal vaccine should be administered. Immunization with the 23-valent pneumococcal vaccine should be repeated approximately every 5 years after the first dose.

20. **What are the common differential diagnosis?**

    The three most common disorders that are sometimes confused with A-T are as follows:
    - Cerebral palsy
    - Congenital ocular motor apraxia
    - Friedreich's ataxia

    Each of these can be distinguished from A-T by neurologic exam and clinical history.

Bernard-Soulier Syndrome

Chapter 8

Ankit Kumar Parmar

CASE STUDY

The first case is of a 6-year-old male child, born of third degree consanguineous marriage who presented with multiple episodes of epistaxis and bluish discoloration of skin after trivial injury since 1 year.

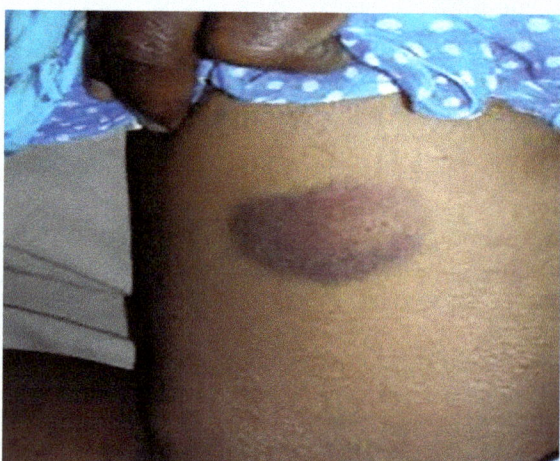

Fig. 1: Bernard-Soulier Syndrome.

In the past, the patient had blood in stools at day 7 of life and hematemesis at 2 years of age. On examination, there was pallor with no organomegaly. On investigation, the patient was found to have thrombocytopenia. Platelet count ranged between 30,000 and 50,000/mm^3. The patient was mistakenly diagnosed as idiopathic thrombocytopenic purpura (ITP) outside and given multiple trials of steroids, intravenous immunoglobulin (IVIG), but was not responsive. On PS, giant platelets without platelet-clumps were observed. Hence, he was investigated for a functional platelet disorder.

On platelet flow cytometry, glycoprotein (GP) receptors measured GP Ib = 0.05% and GP IX = 0.19%. This confirmed the diagnosis of Bernard-Soulier syndrome.

1. **What is Bernard-Soulier syndrome?**
   Bernard-Soulier syndrome is a platelet function disorder caused by an abnormality in the genes for GP Ib/IX/V. Bernard-Soulier syndrome is a platelet function disorder caused by an abnormality in the genes for GP Ib/IX/V. Because this receptor is absent or is not working properly, platelets do not stick to the injured blood vessel wall the way they should, and it is difficult for the normal blood clot to form.

2. **What is the genetic transmission pattern of Bernard-Soulier syndrome?**
   Bernard-Soulier syndrome is an autosomal recessive disorder, meaning that both parents must carry an abnormal gene and pass that abnormal gene on to their child.

3. **What are the clinical manifestations of this disease?**
   - Easy bruising
   - Nose bleeds
   - Bleeding from gums
   - Heavy or prolonged menstrual bleeding (menorrhagia) or bleeding after childbirth
   - Abnormal bleeding after surgery, circumcision or dental work
   - Rarely, vomiting blood or passing blood in stool due to bleeding from the gut (gastrointestinal hemorrhage).

4. **How to differentiate Bernard-Soulier syndrome with ITP?**
   - Prolonged and frequent history of bleeding not correlating with platelet counts.
   - Positive family history if present can provide important clue to the diagnosis of BSS.
   - No response to IVIG, steroid, etc. used for ITP.
   - Increased red blood cell (RBC) counts (giant platelets mistakenly counted as RBC on complete blood count (CBC) by machine) and typical giant platelets as shown in the Figures 1 and 2 can help to differentiate.

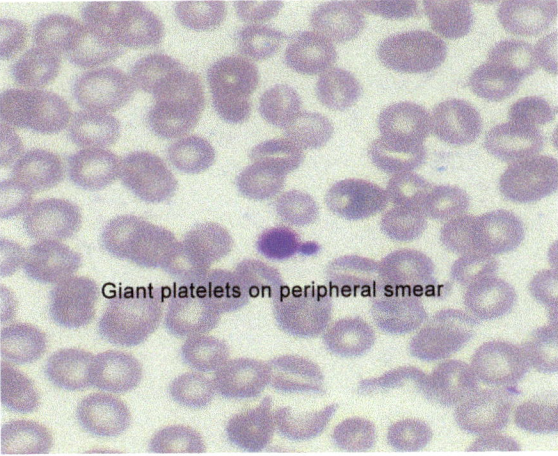

Fig. 2: Giant platelets on peripheral smear.

5. **How to diagnose Bernard-Soulier syndrome?**
   - Platelet counts on CBC will be low.
   - The bleeding time is longer than normal.
   - Platelets appear larger than normal under a microscope.

- Platelets do not clump together normally in the presence of ristocetin (a substance that normally promotes platelet aggregation).
- GP Ib/IX/V receptors on platelets are not detectable in blood samples using a test flow cytometry.

6. **How to treat a child with Bernard-Soulier Syndrome?**
    - General measures include educating the patients about their bleeding diathesis and the importance of avoiding even relatively minor trauma and advising them against the use of antiplatelet medications such as NSAIDs, blood thinners, etc.
    - Adequate dental hygiene should be maintained to prevent gingival disease and to minimize dental procedures.
    - Iron deficiency may result from chronic gingival bleeding or menorrhagia and should be treated.
    - People with mild BSS can sometimes be treated with desmopressin for minor bleeding.
    - Birth control pills may help some women with BSS, who have very heavy periods.
    - For severe bleeding, people with BSS may be given platelets transfusion.
    - Recombinant factor VIIa (NovoSeven) has been used to treat severe bleeding in people with BSS.

Carotenemia

Chapter 9

Ashok Kapse

CASE STUDY

An 18-month-old female child presented with increasing yellowish discoloration of body. Discoloration was more marked on face sole and palms, and strikingly, sclera was white. The child had no other complaint, and physical examination was essentially normal (Figs. 1 to 3).

The child's liver function tests were normal. A high serum carotene level of 475 ug/dL clinched the diagnosis as carotenemia.

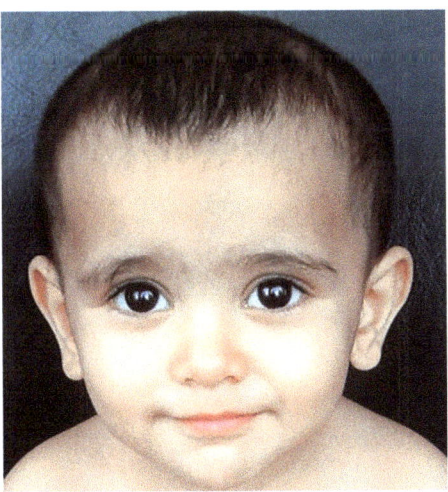

Fig. 1: Yellow discoloration of face.

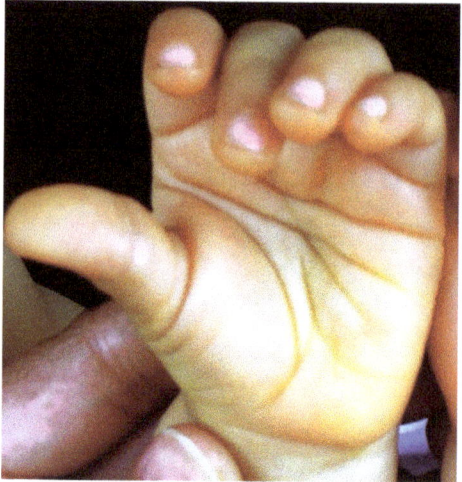

Fig. 2: Discoloration on palms.

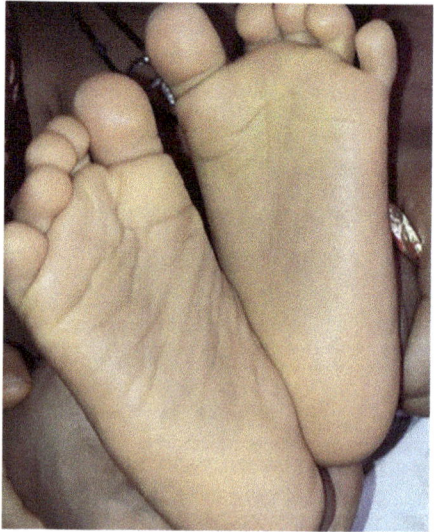

Fig. 3: Discoloration on sole.

1. **What is carotenemia?**
   Carotenemia is clinically characterized by a yellow discoloration of the skin (xanthoderma), due in turn to elevated beta-carotene levels in the blood. The condition was originally described as xanthosis diabetica in 1904 by von Noorden.

2. **What is carotene?**
   Carotenes are pigments of plant origin and are responsible for the yellow and orange color of fruits and vegetables. They act as antioxidants, affect cell growth regulation and modulate gene expression and immune response. Carotene derived from plant foods is the primary source of dietary vitamin A (retinol). Ingested carotenes, enclosed as crystals or amorphous solids within vegetable cells, are converted to vitamin A in the mucosal cells of the small intestine.

Cooking, pureeing or mashing fruits and vegetables ruptures cell membranes, thereby increasing the bioavailability of carotene for absorption. Consumption of mashed or pureed food, which is common in infants, may account for an increased incidence of diet-induced carotenemia in them. Carotenemia is more common in vegetarians.

3. **Which body parts acquire yellow discoloration?**
Yellow pigmentation often appears first on the tip of the nose, and carotenoids maximally accumulate in areas with an abundance of sweat glands, such as the nasolabial folds, palms and soles; therefore, these areas are more highly pigmented. Yellow coloration is easily appreciated in light complexioned persons, however, discoloration may not be easily evident in dark complexioned people.

4. **What is the etiology?**
Carotenemia is usually seen in infants and young children; mothers, in a false belief, may induce the condition by over feeding children with fruit and vegetable juices, particularly carrots.

5. **How to differentiate it from jaundice?**
Carotenemia is usually confused with jaundice; normal untainted sclera is the principal differentiating point from jaundice.

6. **What are the other differentials?**
Excess ingestion or percutaneous absorption of chemicals—e.g., quinacrine, mepacrine, dinitrophenol, saffron, tetryl, picric acid and canthaxanthin—can cause yellowish discoloration.
- *Lycopenemia:*
Orange-yellow skin discoloration could also occur from the ingestion of large amounts of tomatoes or other fruits containing lycopene.
- *Systemic diseases:*
The systemic diseases are diabetes mellitus, hypothyroidism, anorexia nervosa, liver disease, kidney disease and inborn errors of metabolism. Familial conditions could also be associated with carotenemia.

7. **Can carotenemia cause hypervitaminosis A?**
Vitamin A is formed from carotene. Elevation of serum carotene levels correspondingly accompanies an increase in serum vitamin A levels; however, hypervitaminosis A is not observed, for the reason that conversion of carotenoids to vitamin A is tightly regulated.

8. **What laboratory findings confirm the diagnosis?**
Normal liver function tests and a high serum carotene levels (ranging between 250 and 500 µg/dL) confirm the diagnosis.

9. **How is carotenemia treated?**
Dietary carotenemia is a benign condition and does not need any treatment. To allay parental anxiety, the child can be given a carotene-deficient diet. With elimination of the intake of carotene-rich foods, serum carotene levels drop within a week and the yellow discoloration of the skin gradually disappears over several weeks to months.

Rectal or Colonic Polyp

Chapter 10

Kosha Gajera

CASE STUDY

A 4-year-old boy with the complaint of bleeding per rectum for 4 months, which is intermittent, painless, bright red and in drops. No constipation, fever, vomiting, abdominal pain, weight loss, anorexia or loose stools (Figs. 1A and B).

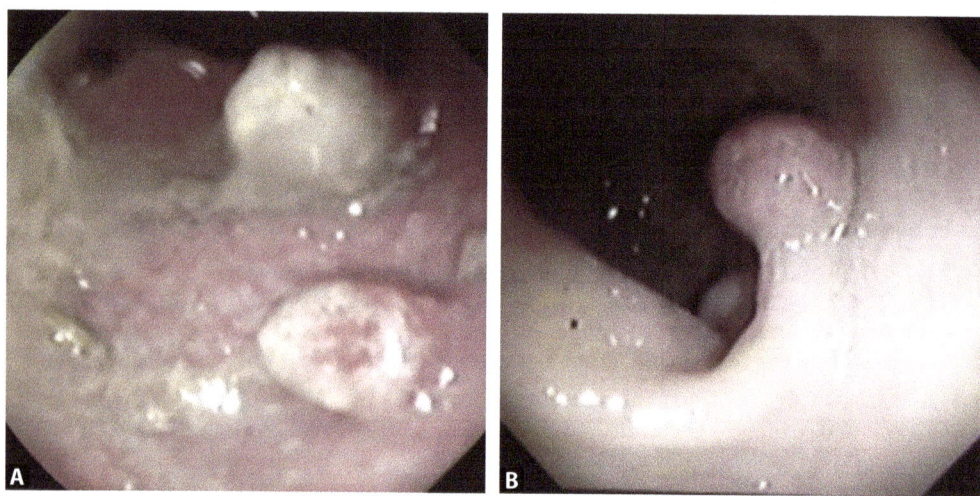

Figs. 1A and B: Case of colonic polyp.

On examination: Pallor +; no organomegaly.
Growth: Normal.
Per rectal examination: Normal.
On colonoscopy, single polyp was seen in sigmoid colon, which was removed.

1. **What is the common type of polyp in children?**
   The most common type of polyp encountered in pediatric gastroenterology is the isolated juvenile polyp. The term "juvenile" refers to the type of polyp and not the age of onset of the polyp.

2. **How colonic polyps present?**
   The most frequent presentation is painless rectal bleeding. Other presentations include a prolapsing rectal mass (frequently mislabeled as a rectal prolapse) or mucopurulent stools.

3. **What are the characteristic features of juvenile polyps?**
   Approximately 50% of the children with juvenile polyps have more than one polyp, with the majority being left-sided colon. Polyps measure 1–3 cm in size, with 90% being pedunculated.

4. **What is the histopathology of typical juvenile polyp?**
   The typical juvenile polyp has a distinctive cystic architecture, mucus-filled glands, a prominent lamina propria and dense infiltration with inflammatory cells.

5. **What is the age of presentation?**
   Juvenile polyps are most frequently diagnosed in the first 10 years of life, with a peak age of diagnosis between 2 and 5 years of age.

6. **What is the risk of developing colorectal cancer (CRC)?**
   Solitary juvenile polyps carry no risk of intestinal cancer. The number of juvenile polyps is important because more than five polyps may carry implications for risk of CRC.

7. **How it is managed?**
   Colonoscopy with snare polypectomy and histological review is sufficient for management of isolated juvenile polyps. When there is a family history of juvenile polyps or when multiple polyps are found, the possibility of juvenile polyposis syndrome (JPS) is raised and a different management strategy is necessary.

8. **What is JPS and how does it present?**
   JPS is an autosomal dominant condition characterized by multiple (more than five) juvenile polyps throughout the colon and sometimes in the whole gastrointestinal (GI) tract. Patients usually present late in childhood or in early adolescence with rectal bleeding. Children (including infants) present with failure to thrive, anemia, hypoalbuminemia and abdominal pain secondary to large numbers of polyps throughout the GI tract. It carries 50% risk of developing cancer.

9. **What are the common genetic mutations for JPS?**
   SMAD4 or BMPR1A has been identified in 40–60% of patients with juvenile polyposis.

Choledochal Cyst

Chapter 11

Alok Gupta, Mohit Vhora

ULTRASONOGRAPHY FINDINGS

Massive dilatation of common bile duct (CBD) more than 7 mm. Along with massive dilatation of intrahepatic biliary radicals (IHBR) in ultrasound as depicted in Figure 1 in an infant presenting with recurrent bouts of pain abdomen with distension of abdomen is diagnostic of choledochal cyst.

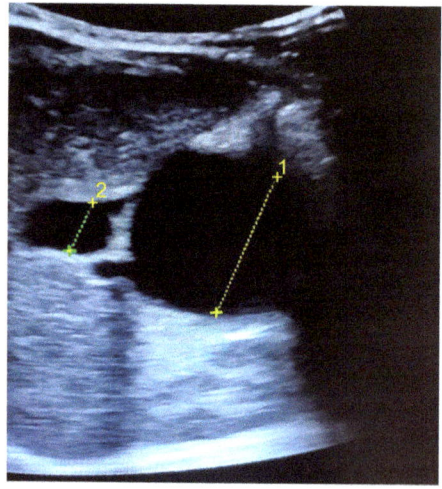

Fig. 1: USG showing choledochal cyst [1—common bile duct (dilated); 2—IHBR (dilated)].

1. **What are the symptoms of choledochal cyst?**
   Infants with choledochal cyst can present with the following symptoms:
   i. Jaundice and acoholic stools
   ii. Palpable mass in the right upper quadrant of the abdomen, with hepatomegaly.

   The clinical manifestations in older children and adults are variable. Children diagnosed with choledochal cysts after infancy typically present with intermittent biliary obstruction or recurrent bouts.

2. **What are the complications of choledochal cyst?**
   The complications include hepatic abscesses, cirrhosis, portal hypertension, recurrent pancreatitis, and cholelithiasis.
3. **What is the investigation of choice of choledochal cyst?**
   The test of choice for the diagnosis of a choledochal cyst is abdominal ultrasonography.
4. **What other investigations can be useful in managing choledochal cyst?**
   The abdominal computed tomography (CT) scanning and magnetic resonance imaging (MRI) help to delineate the anatomy of the lesion and the surrounding structures. It can also assist in defining the presence and extent of intrahepatic ductal involvement. Magnetic resonance cholangiopancreatography (MRCP) is done for defining anomalous pancreato-biliary junctions and pancreato-biliary anomalies.
5. **What is the treatment of choice for choledochal cyst?**
   The treatment of choice for choledochal cyst is complete excision of the involved portion of the extrahepatic bile duct, with construction of a biliary-enteric anastomosis to restore continuity with the gastrointestinal tract.
   Patients who present with cholangitis should be treated with broad-spectrum antibiotic therapy directed against common biliary pathogens, such as *Escherichia coli* and *Klebsiella* species, in addition to other supportive measures, such as volume resuscitation.

Congenital Adrenocortical Hyperplasia

Chapter 12

Kewal Kishore Arora, Swati Mulye

CASE STUDY

Master M A was admitted at SAIMS Indore with the history of recurrent vomiting and failure to gain weight from 22nd postnatal day. The child was born to a 23-year-old primigravida mother out of third-degree consanguineous marriage in Muslim community with no significant antenatal history. Antenatal ultrasonography at 7th month of gestation was suggestive of oligohydramnios for which treatment was given. There was no history of similar disorder or unexplained fetal loss and/or genital ambiguity in the families of either parent. The baby was delivered vaginally at term without any adverse perinatal event with birthweight of 2.8 kg and he was started on exclusive breastfeeding.

The baby was admitted in a hospital on 22nd paroxysmal nocturnal dyspnea (PND) with severe dehydration and hyponatremic seizures in the form of eyelid myoclonia. Investigations done there were suggestive of negative septic screen with hyponatremia and hyperkalemia. The child was treated for dehydration and electrolyte imbalance and was discharged after 8 days of admission. The child was started on spoon feeding with formula milk as he was not able to take breast milk and was referred to us with the complaint of not gaining weight and persistent recurrent vomiting on regular follow-up visit at the previous hospital.

At the time of admission at our hospital, the baby was in severe dehydration with shock with altered sensorium in the form of lethargy. Slight hyperpigmentation was noted at the nipples and scrotum, the baby was given initial normal saline boluses followed by deficit and maintenance fluid correction along with other supportive treatment. He was started on antibiotic cover for possible meningitis and sepsis/gastroenteritis (Figs. 1A and B).

Investigations were suggestive of normal blood sugar level, severe hyponatremia, severe hyperkalemia and metabolic acidosis.

Accordingly, he was started on fluid therapy with targeted rehydration with increase in serum sodium by 8 mEq/L over 24 hours along with the management of hyperkalemia.

In view of recurrent documented hyponatremia and hyperkalemia with metabolic acidosis, possibility of salt losing congenital adrenal hyperplasia (CAH) was considered and after taking blood samples, the patient was started on the management of adrenal crisis (hydrocortisone 15 mg/met square/day in two divided doses and fludrocortisone 0.2 mg daily in two divided doses along with monitoring of vital signs for tachycardia, hypertension. Correction of hyponatremia and measures to reduce hyperkalemia were also started simultaneously as per standard protocol. Fluid resuscitation was continued for 3 days till hydration corrected and electrolytes normalized. Breastfeeding and spoon feeding were initiated as the baby's general condition improved.

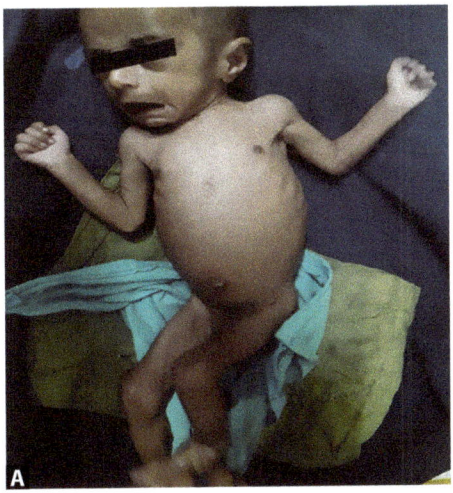
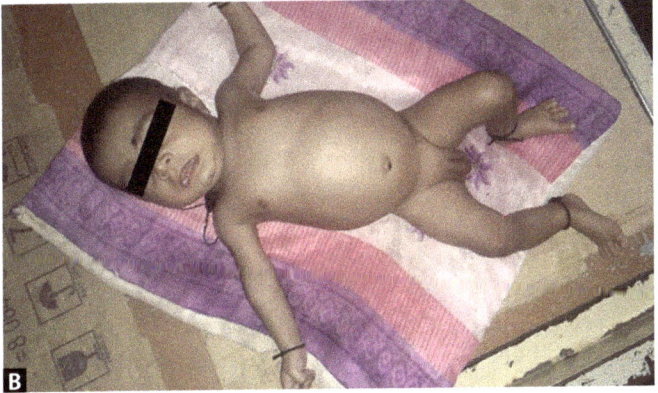

Figs. 1A and B: Cases of congenital adrenocortical hyperplasia.

Screening for sepsis and blood culture did not reveal any evidence of sepsis. Unstimulated serum 17-OH Progesterone 37 ng/mL (normal <0.5–1.86 ng/mL). As the child was accepting breast feeds and spoon feeds well, gaining weight regularly, vaccinated appropriately for age, the child was discharged from the hospital with the advice of regular follow-ups. Proper counseling regarding the disease to the parents was given. On subsequent follow-up, the baby showed remarkable improvement in general condition.

1. **What is CAH?**
   CAH is a group of *rare* inherited condition caused by mutations in genes that code for enzymes involved in making steroid hormones in the adrenal glands. The most common enzyme defect, *21-hydroxylase deficiency*, leads to excess amounts of male hormones being produced by the adrenal glands. Congenital adrenal hyperplasia, also called CAH, is a group of genetic disorders in which the two adrenal glands do not work properly. People inherit one gene that causes this disorder from each of their parents, an autosomal *recessive* genetic disorder (mutation of chromosome 6 results in 21-hydroxylase enzyme impairment). Commoner in consanguineous marriage.

2. **What causes CAH (Basic Defect)?**
   A group of heritable disorders associated with an inability or reduced ability to produce cortisol. The disease begins early in gestation and leads to disease that is manifest at birth or later. Without cortisol, no negative feedback and so, excessive secretion of corticotropin-releasing hormone (CRH) from hypothalamus and adrenocorticotropic hormone (ACTH) from anterior pituitary occurs. Continued secretion of ACTH causes unremitting stimulation of the adrenal cortex, leading to hyperplasia.

3. **What are the various types of CAH?**
   Types of CAH:
   - In most cases, adrenal hyperplasia also involves a deficiency in *aldosterone*, which results in mild to severe loss of body sodium.
   - In some, it also involves overproduction of *adrenal androgens*, which, in affected females, results in prenatal virilization with an ambiguous or male external genitalia at birth.
   - CAH due to 21-hydroxylase deficiency

   Greater than 90% of the cases of CAH are the result of deficiency in the enzyme steroid 21-hydroxylase. Absolute or partial deficiency in this enzyme leads to two problems: deficiency in production of cortisol and aldosterone.

4. **What is the incidence of CAH 21-Hydroxylase deficiency?**
   One of every 15,000 births. there are three primary forms:
   - *Simple virilizing form:* 25%—Excess prenatal production of androgens resulting in masculinization in females as "ambiguous genitalia" or appears male. Males are usually normal at birth. Linear growth is accelerated, but epiphyses fuse early leading to short stature subsequently.
   - *Salt-wasting form:* 75%—Resulting from inadequate aldosterone, leading to electrolyte and water imbalance; "adrenal crisis" at 1–4 weeks (nonspecific signs: poor appetite, vomiting and failure to grow).
   - *Non-classical form:* Mild—usually manifest as androgen excess later in life.

5. **What are the other rare forms?**
   Others rare forms are:
   - 11β-hydroxylase deficiency (3–5%, 1 in 100,000)
   - 17α-hydroxylase deficiency/C17 lyase deficiency (1%)
   - Hydroxysteroid dehydrogenase deficiency (1%)

6. **What are the clinical manifestations?**
   The clinical manifestations are:
   - Cortisol deficiency—hypoglycemia, inability to withstand stress, vasomotor collapse, hyperpigmentation, apneic spells, muscle weakness and fatigue
   - Aldosterone deficiency—hyponatremia, hyperkalemia, vomiting, urinary sodium wasting, salt craving, acidosis, failure to thrive, volume depletion, hypotension, dehydration, shock and diarrhea
   - Androgen excess—ambiguous genitalia, virilization of external genitalia, hirsutism, early appearance of pubic hair, penile enlargement, excessive height gain and skeletal advance
   - Late onset CAH—normal genitalia, has acne, hirsutism, irregular menses or amenorrhea.

7. **How CAH is diagnosed?**
   - By karyotyping (determine sex chromosome), abdominal ultrasound—to detect presence of uterus, cervix and vagina, serum 17-hydroxyprogesterone are basic tests

- To diagnose CAH, high index of suspicion is must; it can be diagnosed even by prenatal screening
- 21-hydroxylase deficiency is first suspected in a newborn infant with "ambiguous genitalia"
- Elevated blood levels of 17-hydroxyprogesterone, and ultrasonography (USG) aids in rapid diagnosis
- Differentiation of true hermaphrodite, pseudo hermaphrodite and sex chromosome abnormalities is simple as none has high 17-hydroxyprogesterone
- Biochemical diagnostic studies—elevated serum 17-OHP (0.25 mg IV bolus of ACTH after 60 min).

8. How to manage a case of CAH?

Management consists of large replacement. All forms require glucocorticoid replacement therapy, to alleviate glucocorticoid deficiency; this also provides negative feedback to suppress ACTH secretion and prevent continued adrenal stimulation. As a result, excessive 17-hydroxyprogesterone is not available as a substrate for excessive androgen production. Glucocorticoids (oral hydrocortisone) 13–18 mg/m^2/24 hours in three divided doses. Further monitoring of serum concentration of adrenal precursors (17-OHP) is required and linear growth and skeletal age assessment should be followed. During stressful state, i.e., febrile illnesses or surgery, three times higher dose is required. In severe emergency, intramuscular or subcutaneous glucocorticoid is required.

Patients with the salt-wasting form also need mineralocorticoid therapy. Mineralocorticoid therapy (fludrocortisone) at a dose of 0.1–0.2 mg/day with sodium chloride supplement of 1–2 g daily is required with monitoring of serum sodium and potassium, plasma renin activity levels.

Surgical correction of ambiguous genitalia by 1–2 years of age so as to have normal development of gender identity.

Prenatal treatment of mother with glucocorticoids can prevent/reduce the virilizing effects of fetal 21-hydroxylase deficiency (previous afflicted babies; AR inheritance).

CYP21 genotyping can be performed in a family with history of CAH.

Treatment with dexamethasone to suppress fetal ACTH-induced androgen production can reduce/eliminate ambiguity of external genitalia in affected female fetuses.

9. What are the possible complications in either sex?

In female patients, suboptimal breast enlargement, late menarche, amenorrhea, irregular menses, even reduced insulin sensitivity and polycystic ovarian syndrome can be seen. In males, oligospermia and testicular tumor has been seen as complication.

10. What is adrenal crisis?

It is a potentially life-threatening condition; when the adrenal is prevented from producing normal amounts of its vital hormones, symptoms and signs of adrenal crisis are varied and non-specific. In infancy, these include lethargy, vomiting, poor appetite and failure to thrive. In older children, chronic fatigue, headache, gastrointestinal symptoms, salt-craving and excess skin pigmentation may be noted. The underlying problems include low blood sugar, low blood sodium, dehydration and low blood pressure, all predisposing the individual to heart failure and shock (collapse).

Congenital Diaphragmatic Hernia

Chapter 13

Siddhartha R Nayak

INTRODUCTION

Congenital diaphragmatic hernia (CDH) is one of the most common non-cardiac fetal intrathoracic anomalies.

CASE STUDY

A newborn child—female, 2.2 kg born by cesarean section was referred immediately. Fortunately, it was antenatally diagnosed by maternal ultrasonography at 27 weeks of gestation; so the entire team of neonatologist, pediatric anesthetist and pediatric surgeon was ready. The neonate had only mild respiratory distress. Investigations done were—chest X-ray (Fig. 1), hematological profile, echocardiography and X-ray abdomen with pelvis (standing). She underwent operation successfully at the age of 8 hours for a Bochdalek hernia (Fig. 2); contents of the hernia were the liver and small bowel loops (Fig. 4). Postoperative recovery was uneventful; she did not require mechanical ventilator. The child was discharged after 9 days. A follow-up at 8 months she is doing well.

Left congenital diaphragmatic hernia (CDH) chest X-ray: Preoperative.

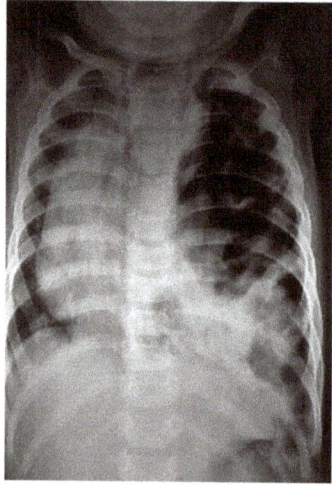

Fig. 1: Shows herniated contents; and mediastinal shift.

CONGENITAL DIAPHRAGMATIC HERNIA

- A congenital diaphragmatic hernia is due to the abnormal development of the diaphragm while the fetus is forming. A defect in the diaphragm of the fetus allows one or more of their abdominal organs to move into the chest and occupy the space where their lungs should be. As a result, the lungs cannot develop properly. In majority of the cases, this affects only one lung. The most common defect is through left-sided patent pleuroperitoneal canal or (Fig. 2) *foramen of Bochdalek*. A hernia through the foramen of Morgagni is uncommon, and one into pericardium is very rare.

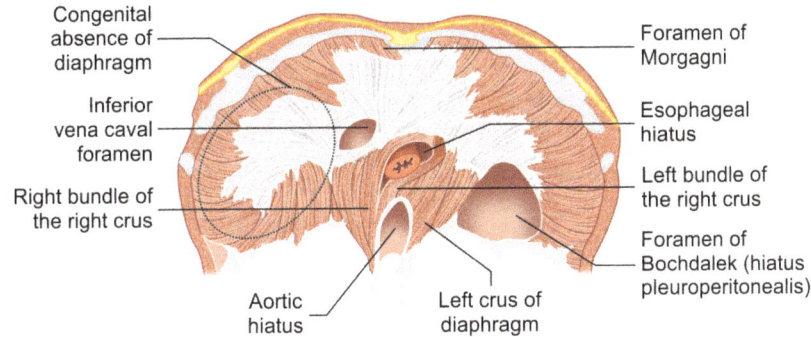

Fig. 2: Surgical anatomy.

- Eighty percent are left-sided and 20% are right-sided.
- An acquired diaphragmatic hernia (ADH) is usually the result of a blunt or penetrating injury. Traffic accidents and falls cause the majority of blunt injuries. Surgery on the abdomen or chest may also cause accidental damage to diaphragm.
- CDH: Incidence—1 in 2,000 to 5,000.
  1. **What are the associated anomalies?**
     - *Associated anomaly:* 10–50%
     - Polyhydramnios in 80% of pregnancy associated with CDH
     - *Associated anomaly:* While a CDH can occur as an isolated condition, associated anomalies are relatively common and include:
       - *Pulmonary hypoplasia:* also a complication
       - Bronchopulmonary sequestration
       - *Aneuploidy:* can be present in up to 50% of cases.
       - Trisomy 13
       - Trisomy 18
       - Trisomy 21
       - Trisomy 21
       - *Turner syndrome:* monosomy X
       - Pallister-Killian syndrome: tetrasomy 12p
       - Fryns syndrome
       - Cornelia de Lange syndrome
       - Congenital cardiac anomalies: 24%. Patent ductus arteriosus (PDA) is common
       - Neural tube defects
       - Anencephaly
       - Gastrointestinal tract (GIT): Malrotation of the bowels.

2. **How antenatal diagnosis is done?**
   Prenatal diagnosis: Ultrasound (US) is accurate in 40–90%. The mean gestational age at discovery is 24 weeks. A prenatal magnetic resonance imaging (MRI) is performed for pulmonary hypoplasia. It is used to determine the liver position in relation to the diaphragm. It may also be used to access the volume to determine pulmonary hypoplasia. Fetal karyotyping is very important. Chromosomal anomaly is present in about 25% of cases. Once diagnosis of CDH is confirmed, echocardiography and both renal and cranial US scans should be obtained.

3. **What are the clinical symptoms and signs?**
   - Clinical symptoms: Respiratory distress/cyanosis/tachypnea/tachycardia/decrease breathe sounds on chest/bowel sounds in the chest.
   - Marked cyanosis and dyspnea is caused by compression of the lung on the same side and by the herniated abdominal contents and by mediastinal shift and compression of the opposite lung.
   - Clinical signs: Scaphoid abdomen.
   - Anterior post bulge of the chest.

4. **What are the laboratory tests?**
   - Arterial blood gas (ABG) measurements: To assess for pH, partial pressure of carbon dioxide ($PaCO_2$), and partial pressure of oxygen (PaO_2)
   - Serum lactate may be helpful for assessing for circulatory insufficiency or severe hypoxemia associated with tissue hypoxia
   - Chromosome studies, including microarray analysis
   - Levels of serum electrolytes, ionized calcium and glucose.

5. **What is the differential diagnosis?**
   Differential diagnosis:
   - Cystic adenomatoid malformation
   - Bronchogenic cyst
   - Tumors and neurenteric cyst.

6. **What are the prognostic criteria?**
   Prognostic criteria:
   - Liver herniation into pleural cavity
   - Early diagnosis before 25 weeks of gestation
   - Low lung-to-head ratio (LHR)
   - With these criteria postoperative prognosis is poor.

   Lung-to-head ratio: Measurement of the contralateral fetal lung area to head circumference ratio (LHR), using two-dimensional (2D) US imaging, as a predictor of outcome. If it is less than 1, then it is poor prognosis.

7. **What are the newer therapies?**
   - Extracorporeal Membrane Oxygenation: Extracorporeal membrane oxygenation (ECMO) has been deployed to treat respiratory failure and pulmonary hypertensive crisis in CDH following failure of conventional therapies.
   - The role of antenatal corticosteroid therapy to enhance the fetal lung remains undetermined.

8. **How do we manage CDH?**
   Preoperative X-ray shows herniated contents and mediastinal shift.
   CDH is a "Physiologic" emergency of the first order.
   Management:
   - Endotracheal tube and nasogastric tube
   - Oxygen—warmth
   - Blood
   - Intravenous fluid
   - *Position:* Head up and side of hernia in a dependent position
   - Mechanical ventilator may be needed preoperative, and postoperative occasionally
   - *Resuscitation by bag and face-mask ventilation:* Contraindicated (to avoid distension of stomach and intestine in thorax).

9. **What is the surgical modality?**
   The abdominal approach is preferred (Figs. 3 to 5). Abdominal cavity is opened, defect in diaphragm is defined and abdominal contents are reduced gently. A catheter is passed retrograde through the ninth intercostal space into the pleural cavity. Then defect is closed. The intestines are inspected for malrotation.

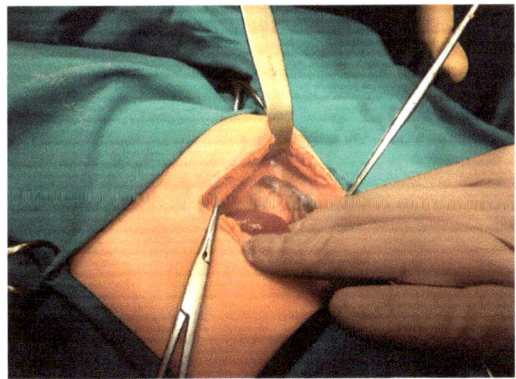

Fig. 3: Peritoneal cavity opened, herniated contains examined.

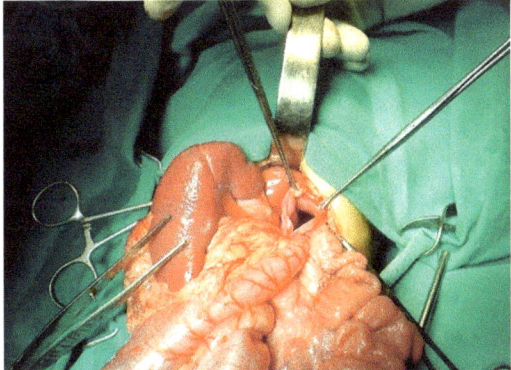

Fig. 4: Herniated contains were left lobe liver and bowel loops. Contents reduced and left diaphragmatic defect defined.

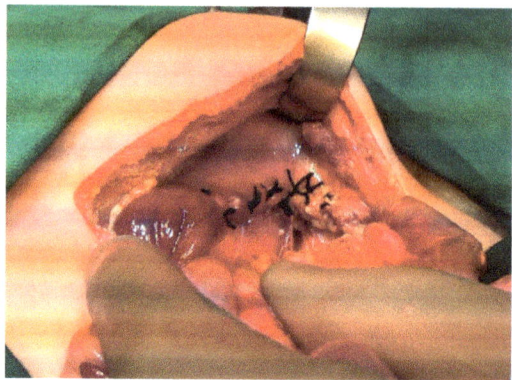

Fig. 5. Defect repaired.

Postoperative: Infant is nursed in incubator. Oxygen may be necessary. In many cases, indwelling nasotracheal tube and mechanical ventilator may be required.

10. **What is the survival rate?**
    Mortality—overall survival in India is around 70%.
    CDH is commonly associated with *high* mortality due to associated lung hypoplasia, pulmonary hypertension and coexistent anomalies.

11. **What is antenatal fetal surgical intervention?**
    Future: Fetal medicine
    Fetal surgical intervention is at experimental stage based on experiments on lamb (Fig. 6). Fetal tracheal occlusion is done with balloon between 22 and 27 weeks' gestation.

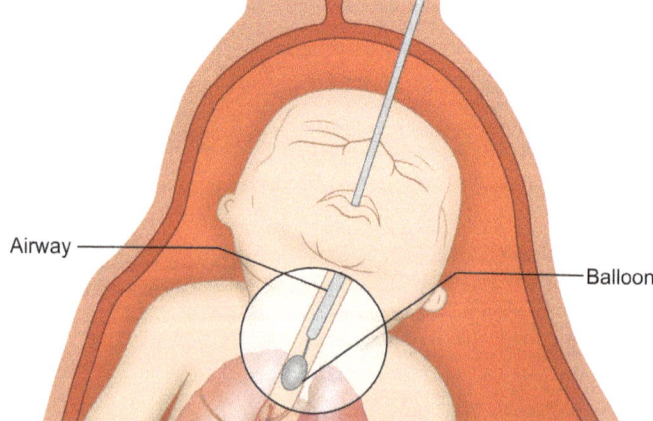

Fig. 6: Future: fetal medicine

It is presumed that tracheal occlusion accelerates the fetal lung growth. However, still more trials are needed. Fetoscopic endoluminal tracheal occlusion (FETO) is a fetal procedure that may improve outcomes in babies with severe cases of CDH diagnosed antenatally. FETO is a procedure to reversibly block the trachea of the fetus with a latex balloon.

Congenital Dislocation of Knee

Chapter 14

Chirag Bhalvani

1. **This 4-days old female has hyperextended knees (Fig. 1). Diagnosis?**

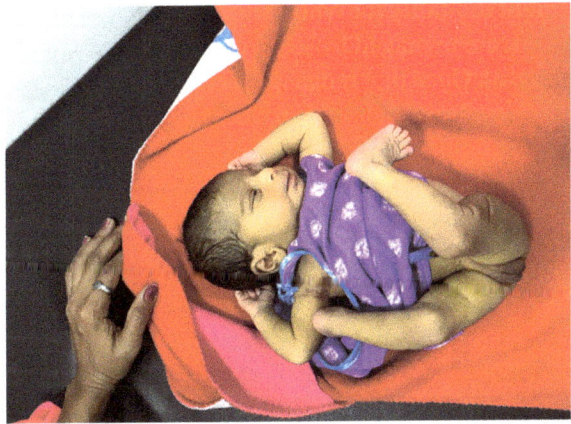

Fig. 1: Bilateral dislocated knees (hyperextended knees).

Congenital dislocation of knee (CDK) (bilateral hyperextended knee).

2. **Which other associated conditions should be looked for in these cases?**
Children presenting with these conditions should also be screened for DDH (developmental dysplasia of hip) and syndromes like arthrogryposis multiplex congenita, Larsen's syndrome, etc.

3. **How is CDK classified?**
There could be three types of CDK.
- Type I and II are the one where the knee can be flexed beyond neutral (Fig. 2).
- Type III is the one in which the knee remains hyperextended and cannot be flexed to neutral. These are usually associated with syndromic children.

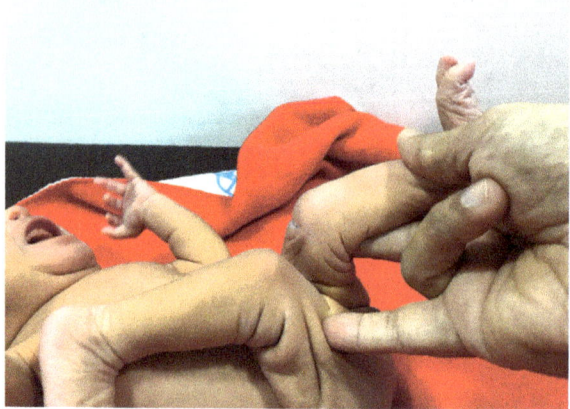

Fig. 2: Reducibility of left knee.

4. **What is the treatment modality for type I and II CDK?**
   The type I and II CDK are managed by serial casting till a range beyond 90° of flexion of knee is achieved (Fig. 3). Once that range is achieved, the child is put in a Pavlik Harness (Fig. 4) to maintain knee flexion, for up to 6 weeks (Fig. 5).

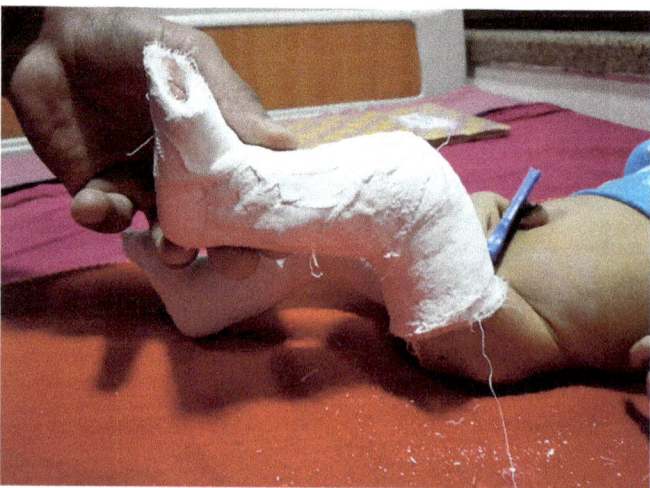

Fig. 3: Cast in maximally corrected position.

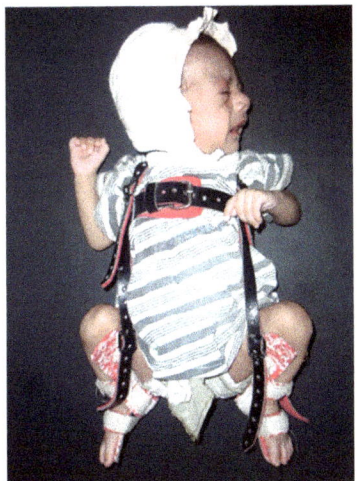

Fig. 4: Child in Pavlik harness.

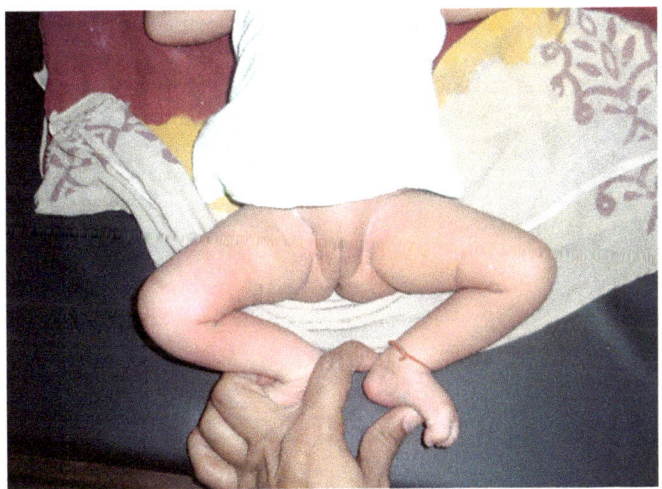

Fig. 5: Fully corrected knee.

5. **What is done for the Type III CDK?**
   These children usually require surgical lengthening (mostly V-Y plasty) of the quadriceps followed by prolonged splinting.

Congenital Duodenal Atresia

Chapter 15

Rakesh Bhargav

CASE STUDY

A 1.4 kg, 34-week, male had LSCS for polyhydramnios and fetal distress. The patient's APGAR score was normal, he cried at birth, was active, had patent anus and nasogastric tube (NGT) could be passed, and had bilious fluid.

On antenatal ultrasound mother had polyhydramnios. Post-natally plain X-ray abdomen showed typical double bubble appearence (Fig. 1). Level III ultrasound evaluation did not show any other anomalies.

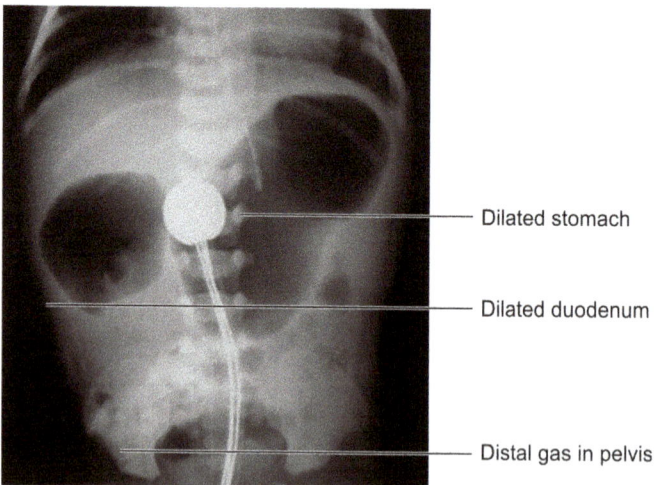

Fig. 1: Plain X-ray abdomen showing dilated stomach and duodenum (double bubble appearance).

1. **What is the probable diagnosis?**
   Strong possibility of congenital duodenal atresia (Fig. 2) and needs evaluation.
2. **What are the types**
   Classification and types of duodenal obstruction:
   Extrinsic: Annular pancreas, malrotation and volvulus

Intrinsic: Complete or incomplete
Type: Atresia with hole, but bowel continuity maintained. Can be simple, fenestrated or elongated (windsock type)
Type II: Solid cord between two segments
Type III: Total discontinuity between two segments

3. **How will you proceed with further management?**
   No feeding and keep NGT patent and decompress stomach. Maintain intravenous fluids and add ongoing bilious losses with Ringer's as volume replacement 2-4 hourly. Nursing monitoring and care for preterm, including strict temperature regulation and intake output.

4. **What examination findings you expect?**
   Examine neonate, mostly normal preterm findings. Abdominal distension or visible peristalsis seen if baby has been fed or NGT aspiration has been delayed. Peristalsis is from left to right, disappearing on emptying stomach. Look for associated anomalies. Trisomy 21 is seen in 30%. VACTERAL association: Vertebral 2-3%, Anorectal (malrotation 20-30%), Congenital heart 20%, Tracheoesophageal fistula 10%, Renal 9% and Limb anomalies.
   Look for features of Trisomy 21, and if so, need parental counseling. Cardiac murmur, lung aeration, lump in abdomen, jaundice are other important findings. Specially look for areation of both lungs to rule out aspiration of vomit. Jaundice as may have associated biliary duct anomalies.
   All have dehydration and electrolyte imbalance due to loss of bile.
   Always look for dehydration and acidosis.

5. **What investigation will you do?**
   Complete blood counts including blood group. Hemogram and blood grouping as needed for operation. Routine and microscopic urine exam with specific gravity liver function test (LFT), kidney function test (KFT), electrolytes and blood gases
   X-ray abdomen erect is very important and informative. Always include whole chest and abdomen. X-ray should be done. At birth baby crys and swallows air that distends intestinal tract. It takes about 6 hours for gas to reach distally till rectum. So, plain X-ray evaluation should be done after 8–10 hours after birth. Empty stomach and inject 20 mL air via NGT and the take erect film.
   Do ECHO and USG to rule out other congenital abnormalities.

6. **What are the findings on X-ray abdomen?**
   Always look for bony cage, position of diaphragm, heart enlargement, aeration of both lungs and abdomen bowel gas pattern. Look for dilated stomach and duodenum (more marked with air contrast) giving "double bubble appearance," (Fig. 1) which is diagnostic for duodenal atresia. Distal gas shadows distally denotes atresia with hole.

7. **What are the differentials?**
   Differential diagnoses are annular atresia, band obstruction, malrotatin with mid gut volvulus. other causes on upper intestinal obstruction like malrotation and volvulus.

8. **What are important preoperative precautions.?**
   Preoperation:
   Always a semi-elective operation on stable baby unless mid gut volvulus is suspected
   NGT and central line as prolonged postoperative ileus, correct nutritional status and electrolytes
   Blood grouping (mother's sample needed). Vitamin K and antibiotics

9. **What are common operative problems?**
   Operation: Duodeno-duodenostomy.
   Problems at operation: Proximal duodenum hugely dilated and distal very small caliber, so difficult anastomosis and also reason for leak (Fig. 2). Dilated proximal segment does not function well so need to plicate/resect partially. Prolonged return of effective peristalsis from overdistended duodenum to collapsed distal bowel. Anomalies of bile ducts. Malrotation is always there and has to be corrected.

   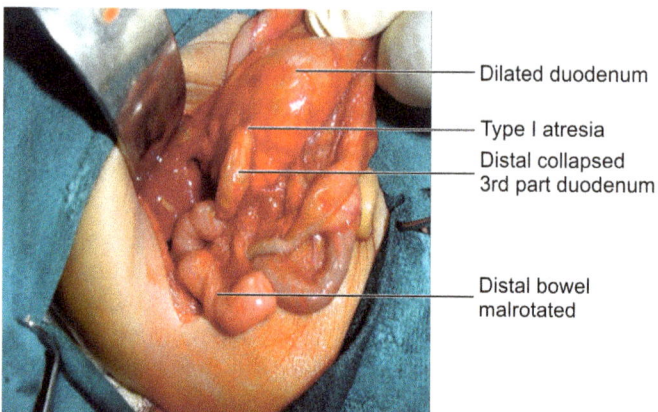

   Fig. 2: Intraoperative image showing duodenal atresia.

10. **What are the complications?**
    Postoperative management and complications:
    Prolonged duodenogastric reflux needing NGT aspiration, replacement of ongoing losses in addition to maintenance fluids and total parenteral nutrition (TPN). Usually it takes 2–3 weeks before significant feed to commence.
    Short term: Anastomotic leak and wound infection
    Long term: Adhesion and anastomotic stenosis

11. **How is the prognosis?**
    Duodenal atresia is resected and dilated upper duodenum anastomosed to small distal duodenum in dependent position. May need reducing size of proximal duodenum before anastomosis (Doudeno-denostomy).
    Effective peristalsis delayed so problems of leak, infection and nutrition. TPN integral to management and prognosis.
    Overall outlook very favorable due to advanced monitoring, central line, TPN and operative techniques.
    Survival: 95–98%
    Mortality is mainly due to associated conditions.

Congenital Dyserythropoietic Anemia Type 1

Chapter 16

Pramod Jog

CASE STUDY

6-year-old male child, first baby of a non-consanguineous marriage brought by grandmother for progressively increasing pallor and history of recurrent blood transfusions since 2 months of age. Baby developed hyperbilirubinemia within 2 hours of postnatal life which required exchange transfusion.

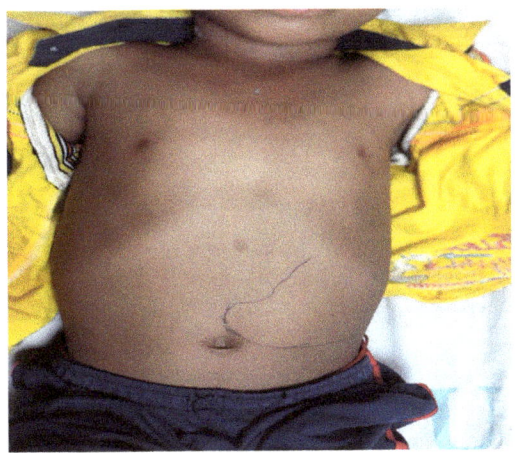

Fig. 1: Splenomegaly

History of recurrent transfusions since 2 years of age (Fig. 1).
- Pyruvate Kinase levels: Normal
- Glucose-6-phosphate dehydrogenase (G6PD) levels: Normal
- Hemoglobin (Hb) electrophoresis: Normal
- Flow cytometry: Normal
- Bone Marrow: Erythroid hyperplasia, megaloblastosis with binucleated polychromatic erythroblasts with thin chromatin ridges.

1. **What is this?**
   Congenital dyserythropoietic anemia (CDA) type 1.
2. **What is the etiology?**
   - Autosomal recessive disorder due to mutation in Codanin 1/CDAN 1 gene on chromosome 15q15.1.3.
   - Gene codes for Codanin 1 which expedites histone assembly into chromatin and regulates cell cycle.
3. **What are the clinical features?**
   - Mostly present in neonatal period or early childhood with anemia related symptoms, hepatosplenomegaly and jaundice.
   - Patient might show signs of extramedullary hematopoiesis, iron overload, and cholelithiasis.
   - Bone marrow aspirate shows erythroid hyperplasia, megaloblastosis, and basophilic stippling. Binucleated and more rarely multinucleated polychromatophilic erythroblasts are also appreciated. Incompletely divided cells with thin chromatin bridges (Fig. 3) in between nuclei are highly specific for type 1CDA.
   - Electron Microscopy—erythroblasts with a characteristic "Swiss cheese" heterochromatin pattern (Fig. 2).

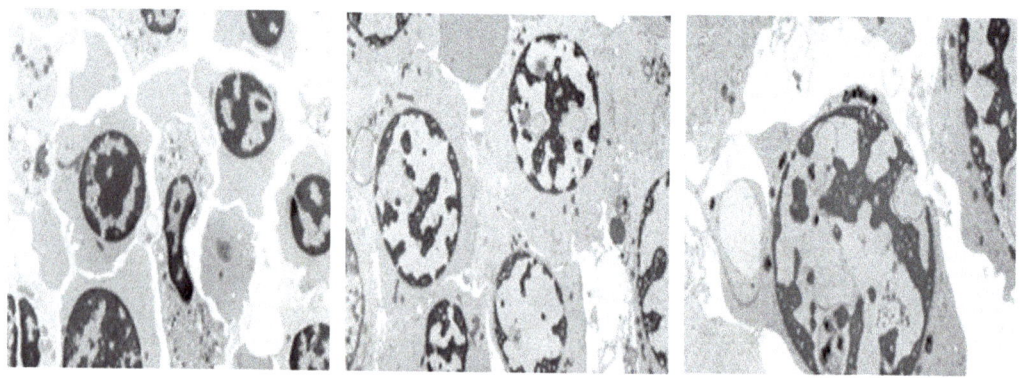

Fig. 2: "Swiss cheese" heterochromatin pattern.

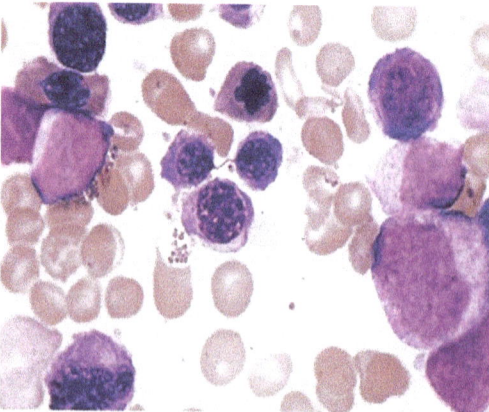

Fig. 3: Chromatin bridges.

4. **What is the differential diagnosis?**
   - Hereditary spherocytosis
   - Hereditary elliptocytosis
   - Pyruvate kinase deficiency
   - Glucose-6-phosphate dehydrogenase (G6PD) deficiency
   - Hemolytic disease of newborn
   - Thalassemia major
   - Triosephosphate isomerase deficiency
   - Aldolase deficiency
   - Phosphofructokinase deficiency.

5. **How do you treat it?**
   - Treatment is primarily supportive, 50% of newborns will require exchange transfusion.
   - Hemosiderosis will require iron chelation.
   - Cholecystectomy for cholelithiasis.
   - Interferon-alpha (IFN-α) has been tried for some cases and has proven to reduce transfusion requirement and splenomegaly.
   - Allogenic bone marrow transplantation with a human leukocyte antigen (HLA) matched donor is curative in severe cases.

Congenital Esotropia

Chapter 17

Barnali Bhattacharya

CASE STUDY

A 5-month-old child is brought to the pediatrician, with complaints of "eyes not looking straight (Figs. 1A and B)."

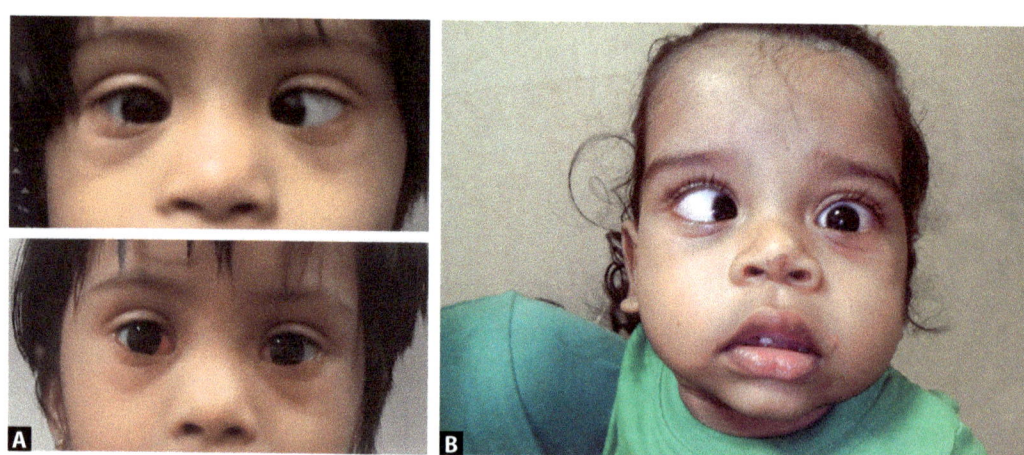

Figs. 1A and B: Case of congenital esotropia.

1. **What is congenital esotropia?**
   It is a squint, or strabismus. If the eyes are deviated towards the nose, then it is called esotropia, and if away from the nose, then it is called exotropia.
2. **What is the best time to refer these children? Do I need to refer immediately, or can I wait for the child to wait to turn one year?**
   It is best to refer immediately, because the squint may just be a presenting symptom of something more sinister, like a congenital cataract, retinoblastoma, high refractive error and retinal dystrophies. Treatment such as congenital cataract needs to be done at the earliest.

3. **Do I need to do any blood tests or investigations before referring?**
   No blood tests are required, but a simple red glow examination would give very valuable insights. A red glow can be tested by a direct ophthalmoscope. A pen ophthalmoscope, like an otoscope, can be a very useful tool to a pediatrician. Shine the ophthalmoscope in the eye, to note the red glow. The red glow is the reflection of the red retina, and is also the reason we get red reflex in flash cameras.
   A white or yellow glow can give you indication on congenital cataract, or late stages of retinopathy of prematurity and retinoblastomas, retinal colobomas, or even ocular albinism. Websites like *knowthglow.org* were started with the idea of educating the general public and pediatricians about early signs of eye diseases in children.

4. **Can this be hereditary?**
   Yes, it can be. You can ask for family history of the same.

5. **Any other birth history that I need to ask?**
   A detailed family history, birth history of prematurity, seizures, any perinatal insults and hospitalizations will be taken by the ophthalmologist.

6. **Why is it caused?**
   There are many hypotheses as to why a congenital or infantile squint occurs, but none of them are due to maternal poor nutrition or maternal infection. Thus, it is important to explain that no blame should be attributed, and also no precautionary measures can be taken for subsequent pregnancies.

7. **Can it be corrected with spectacles?**
   If the cause of the esotropia is because of high hypermetropia (plus number) along with squint, then it might be a case of accommodative esotropia. But not all esotropia are because of accommodative hypermetropia. In other words, not all squints are because of refractive error.

Chest X-rays in Congenital Heart Disease

Chapter 18

Ritesh Sukharamwala

1. **How to calculate cardiothoracic ratio on chest X-ray?**
   The cardiothoracic ratio (CTR) is equal to the transverse cardiac diameter (TCD) divided by the transthoracic diameter (TTD) measured at the inner border of the ninth rib (CTR = TCD/TTD). The normal values of CTR in an adult are 0.41–0.5 (Fig. 1). The upper limit of normal CTR in infants is 0.55, and 0.60 in neonates. A TCD greater than 15 cm is significant irrespective of normal CTR. An increase of >2 cm of TCD is significant if previous chest X-ray is available. An expiratory film and enlarged thymus shadow lead to pseudocardiomegaly.

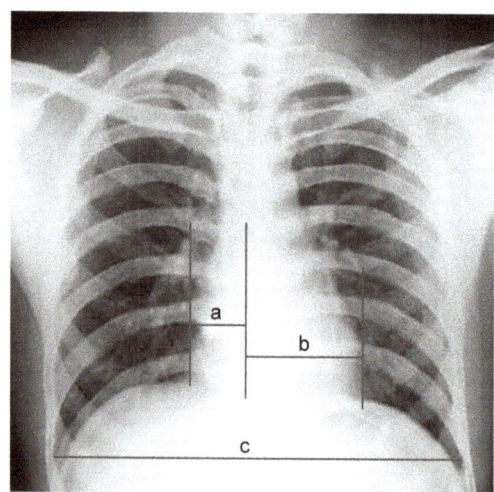

Fig. 1: CT ratio.

2. **How to identify thymic shadow on chest X-ray?**
   It is seen during the first few years of life in chest X-ray and should not be mistaken for mediastinal widening or cardiomegaly. As it is a soft organ, lateral margins appear wavy due to indentation of rib cage (Figs. 2A to C).

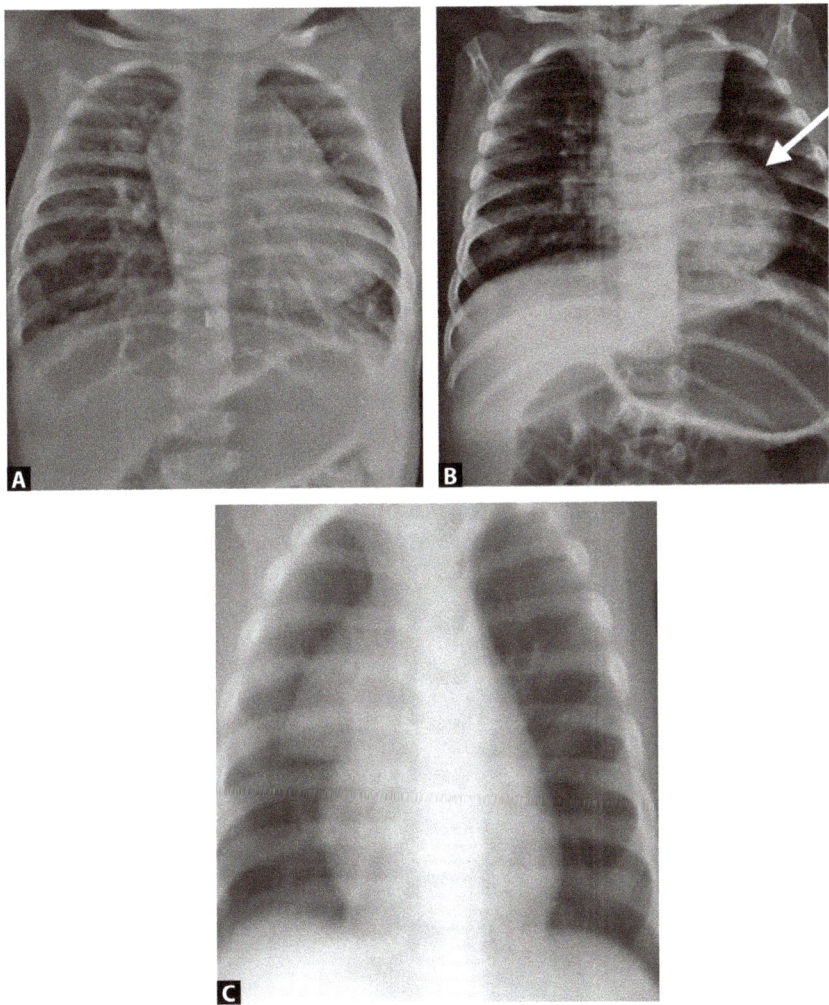

Figs. 2A to C: Thymic shadow.

3. **How is chest X-ray useful to differentiate various congenital heart disease (CHD)?**
   Pulmonary vascularity and cardiac size on X-ray can give clue to pathophysiology of heart disease in a case of suspected CHD. CHDs have either increased, decreased or normal pulmonary blood flow physiology. Left-to-right shunts will have increased pulmonary blood flow; hence, chest X-ray will show pulmonary plethora with cardiomegaly. Pulmonary stenosis with ventricular septal defect (VSD) physiology will have decreased pulmonary blood flow; hence, chest X-ray will show pulmonary oligemia with normal size heart. Certain CHDs have characteristics tale-tell X-ray feature.
4. **Which CHDs are Having Typical Tale-Tell X-ray Features?**
   Common CHDs which are having characteristic X-ray features are:
   - *Transposition of great arteries (TGA):* Egg on side appearance with narrow mediastinal shadow (Figs. 3 and 4)

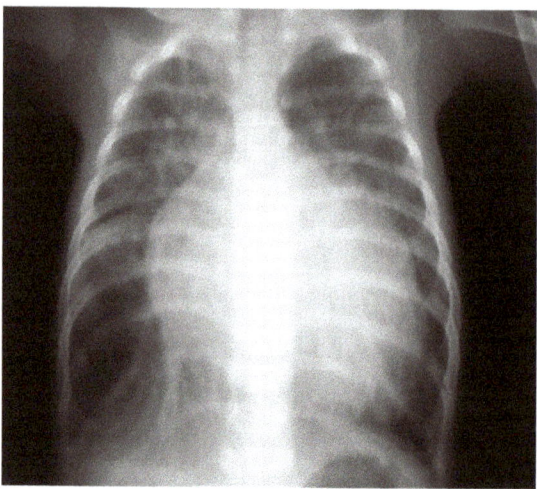

Fig. 3: Cardiomegaly with narrow pedicle – classical chest X-ray of TGA.

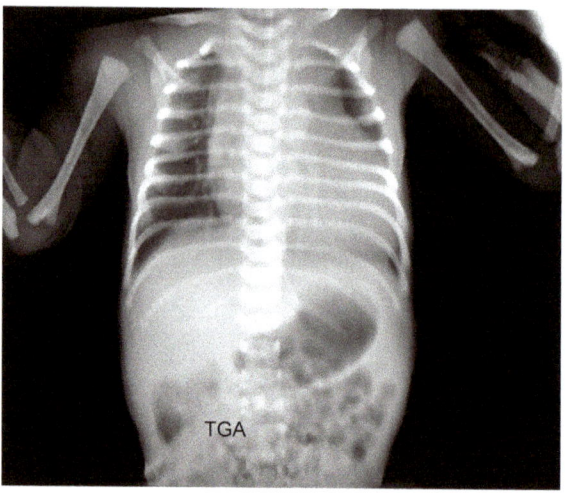

Fig. 4: TGA without narrow mediastinal pedicle.

- *Tetralogy of Fallot (TOF):* Boot-shaped heart with pulmonary oligemia (Fig. 5)
- *Neonatal Ebstein anomaly:* Cardiomegaly with box-shaped heart with pulmonary oligemia (Fig. 6)
- *Supracardiac total anomalous pulmonary venous return:* Snowman silhouette (Fig. 7)
- *Coarctation of aorta:* Rib notching (↖↗) and figure of "3" formed by dilatation above and below coarctation site (older children) (Fig. 8)

However, it is not necessary that all cases with the above-mentioned disease will have characteristic X-ray findings (e.g., not all TGAs will have egg on side appearance.

Chest X-rays in Congenital Heart Disease

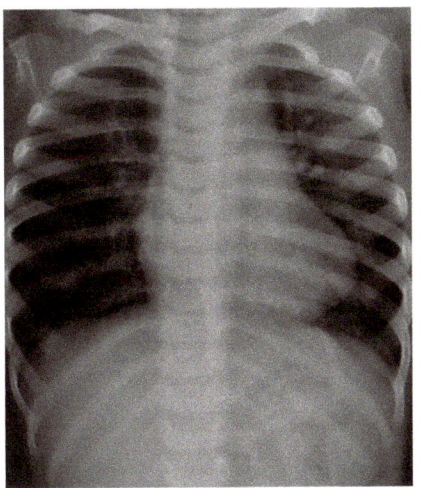

Fig. 5: Boot shaped heart with pulmonary oligemia–a case of TOF.

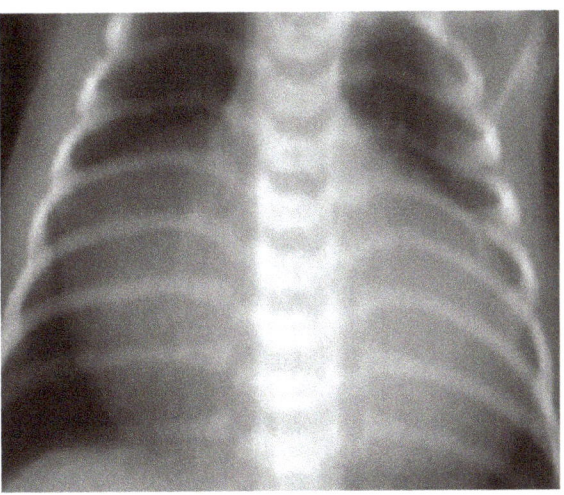

Fig. 6: Huge heart occupying almost total thoracic diameter–neonate with Ebstein Anomaly.

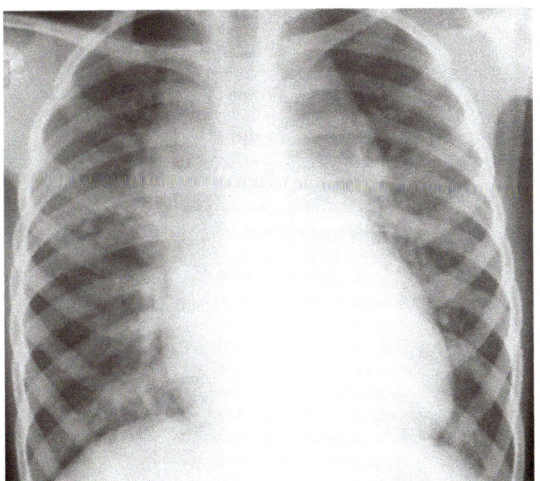

Fig. 7: Snowman shaped heart in TAPVC.

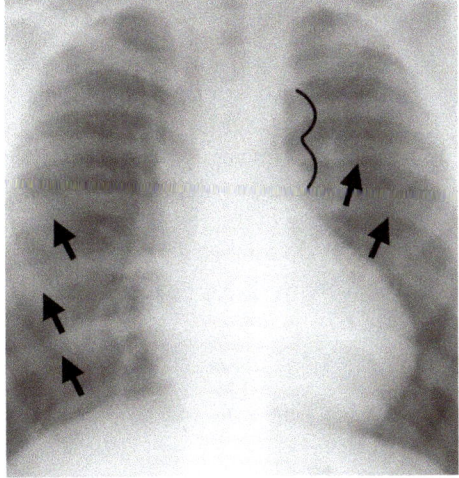

Fig. 8: Showing figure of 3 sign of descending aorta and notching over inferior border of ribs in Coarctation of aorta in an older child.

5. **Which Group of CHDs are Associated with Pulmonary Plethora on X-ray?**
   - *Acyanotic:* Left-to-right shunts like atrial septal defect (ASD), VSD, PDA (to have plethora left-to-right shunts should be at least 1.5:1)
   - *Cyanotic:* Admixture lesions like truncus arteriosus and transposition of the great arteries (d-TGA) without PS.
6. **Which Group of CHDs are Associated with Pulmonary Oligemia on X-ray?**
   - *Cyanotic:* TOF or TOF-like lesions and other complex cyanotic heart disease with severe PS; Eisenmenger syndrome.

7. **What Are the X-ray Features of CHD With Increased Pulmonary Blood Flow? (Figs. 9A and B)**

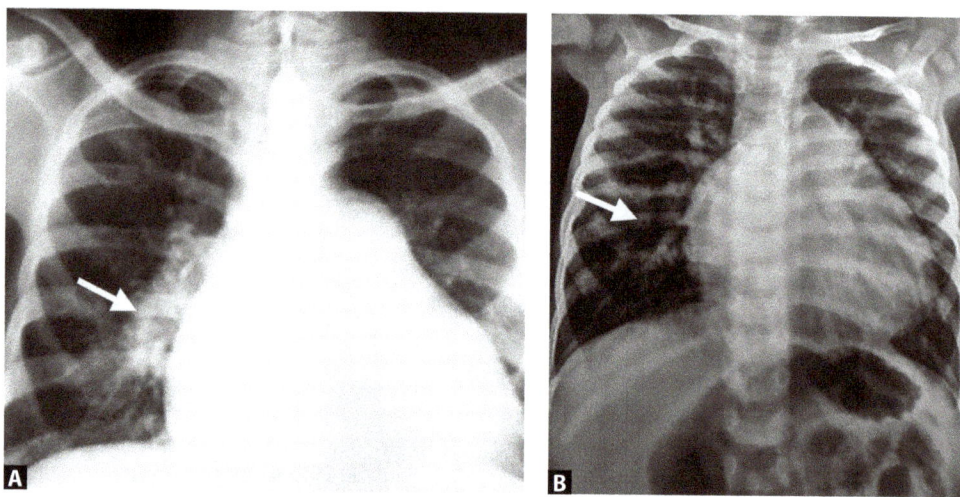

Figs. 9A and B: Showing pulmonary plethora with cardiomegaly. Arrows in these images showing dilated right pulmonary artery.

- Dilated main and branch pulmonary arteries
- Pulmonary arteries can be traced even in the lateral one third of the lung fields
- End on vessels are more in number (≥3 in one lung field or ≥5 in both lung fields)
- The end on vessel diameter is more than that of accompanying bronchus. Normally, it is 1.2:1 and in plethora it is ≥1.5:1
- The size of the right descending pulmonary artery (RDPA) is increased. If the ratio of RDPA to trachea is more than indicates significant left to right shunt.

8. **What are the X-ray Features of CHD with Decreased Pulmonary Blood Flow? (Figs. 10A and B)**

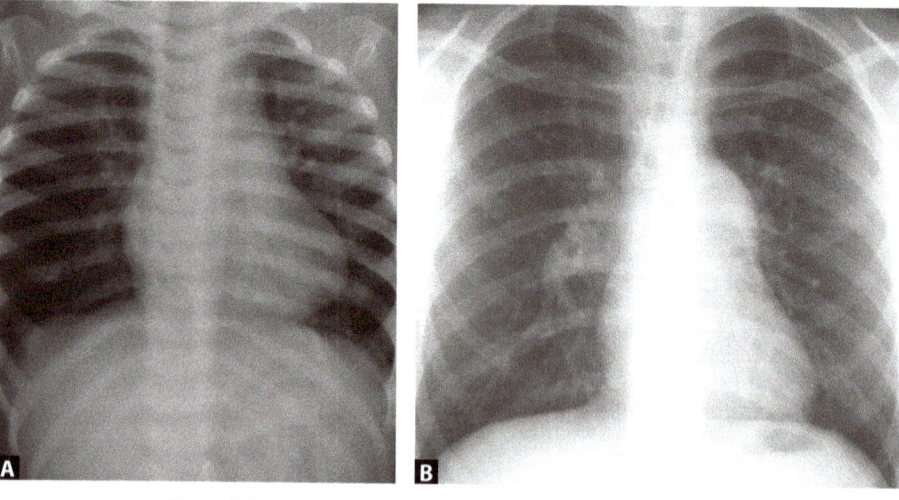

Figs. 10A and B: (A) Oligemic lungs; (B) Normal sized heart.

- In decreased pulmonary blood flow physiology, chest X-ray shows pulmonary oligemia (Fig. 10A) (i.e., vascular shadows are reduced). They are not seen even in the intermediate lung zones.
- Heart size will be normal (Fig. 10B).
- Main pulmonary artery (MPA), left pulmonary artery (LPA) and RDPA are of small size (normally RDPA is of the same size as the right lower lobe bronchus).
- Dilated MPA and RPA with oligemic lung fields are suggestive of Eisenmenger syndrome.

Congenital Hydrocephalus

Chapter 19

Darshan Vinodchandra Chauhan

CASE STUDY

A 24-hour-old neonate referred to the hospital with the complaint of large head since birth. The neonate had large head with open sutures and large bulging anterior fontanel. The child was having intrauterine growth restriction (IUGR), and birth weight was 1.9 kg. The child had no significant maternal and family history (Figs. 1A to D).

On examination, all the signs of hydrocephalus was there, which were not associated with myelomeningocele or any other malformations. Ophthalmic evaluation was suggestive of papilledema but no chorioretinitis. No other neurocutaneous markers were noted. The child was having setting sun sign, brisk deep tendon reflexes and extensor planters.

The brain imaging was suggestive of non-communicating hydrocephalus due to congenital stenosis of aqueduct of sylvius.

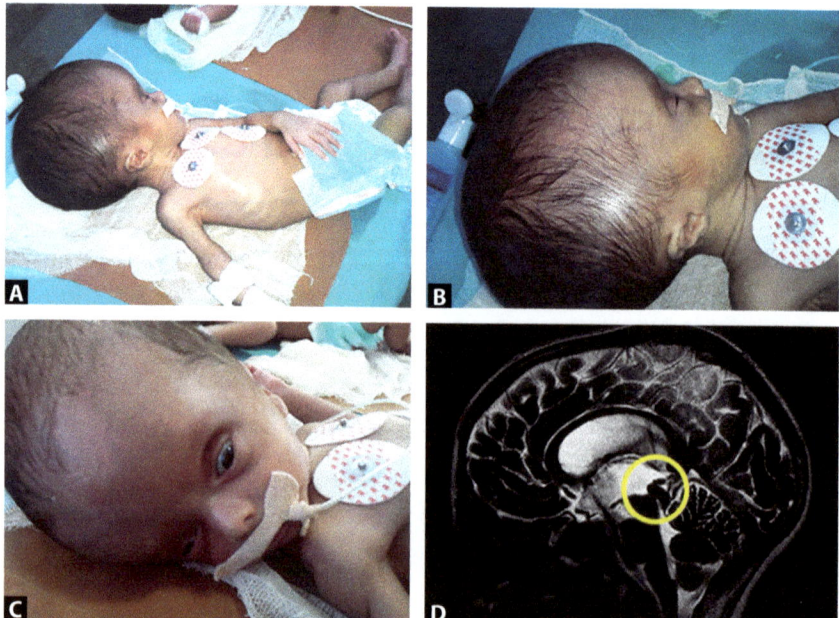

Figs. 1A to D: (A to C) Case of congenital hydrocephalus. (D) MRI brain of the same child.

1. **What is hydrocephalus?**
   Abnormal excess cerebrospinal fluid (CSF) accumulation in ventricular system mainly due to obstruction in CSF flow or due to poor absorption of CSF and rarely due to overproduction by choroid plexus.

2. **What is the difference between communicating and non-communicating hydrocephalus?**
   Most of the CSF is produced by choroid plexus in lateral ventricle and lesser amount is by choroid plexus in third and fourth ventricles and little by capillary endothelium.
   CSF flows from lateral ventricle to third ventricle by foramen of monro, from third to fourth ventricle by narrow aqueduct of sylvius and from fourth ventricle by two lateral foramina of luschka, and one midline foramen of magendie to basal cisterns and arachnoid space over the convexity of brain hemisphere.
   When the obstruction of CSF flows within the ventricular system, it is called obstructive hydrocephalus, and outside the ventricular system, it is called non-obstructive hydrocephalus.

3. **What are the common causes of non-communicating hydrocephalus?**
   - *Aqueductal stenosis:* X-linked recessive; neurofibromatosis
   - *Aqueductal gliosis:* neonatal meningitis; subarachnoid hemorrhage; intrauterine viral infection
   - Vein of Galen malformation can directly obstruct the aqueduct
   - *Posterior fossa lesion:* Chiari malformation; Dandy-Walker syndrome; posterior fossa tumors

4. **What are the common causes of communicating hydrocephalus?**
   - Subarachnoid or intraventricular hemorrhage
   - *Meningitis:* pneumococcal or tuberculous
   - Intrauterine infections
   - Leukemic infiltrates in arachnoid space

   All these cause damage to arachnoid villi and interfere with absorption of CSF.

5. **Why there is setting sun sign in hydrocephalus?**
   It is because of impingement of the dilated suprapineal recess on the tectum.

6. **What is Chiari malformation?**
   Type 1:
   - Displacement of cerebellar tonsils into cervical canal due to obstruction of the caudal portion of the fourth ventricle during fetal development.
   - Produces symptoms in adolescence or adult life—headache, neck pain, urinary frequency and progressive spasticity of lower limb.
   - It never causes hydrocephalus (Fig. 2).

   Type 2:
   - Anomaly of the hindbrain due to failure of pontine flexure during embryogenesis resulting in elongation of the fourth ventricle and kinking of brainstem.

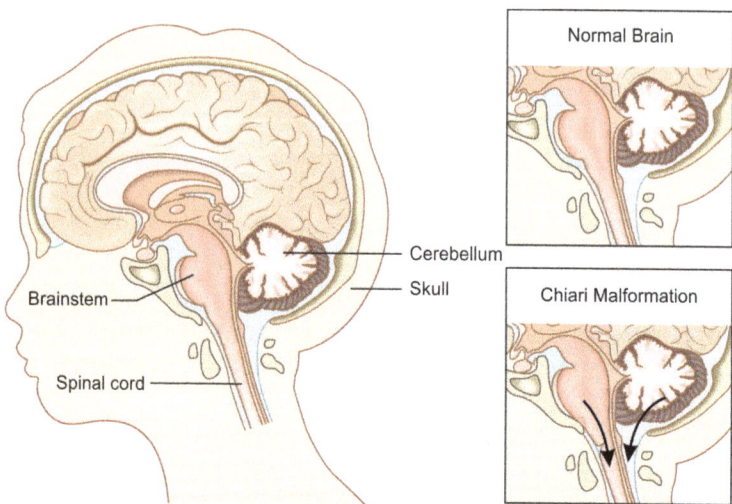

Fig. 2: Chiari malformation and normal brain.

- Produces symptoms in infancy—progressive hydrocephalus, frequently associated with myelomeningocele. It may case stridor, weak cry and apnea in infancy.
- Managed by operative procedure of posterior fossa decompression.

7. **What is Dandy-Walker malformation?**
   It is the cystic expansion of the fourth ventricle in the posterior fossa resulting in developmental failure of the roof of the fourth ventricle during embryogenesis, which is managed by shunting of cystic cavity (Fig. 3).

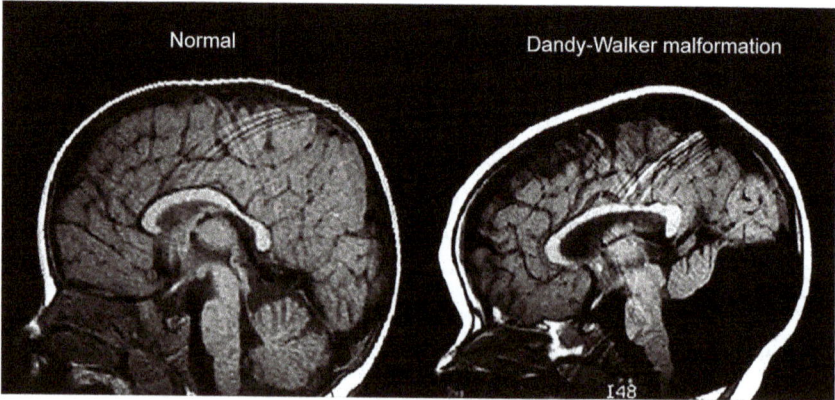

Fig. 3: Dandy-Walker malformation and normal brain.

8. **What is the difference between hydranencephaly and hydrocephalus?**
   In hydranencephaly, the cerebral hemispheres are absent or represented by membranous sacs with remnants of frontal, temporal and occipital dortex dispersed over their membrane. Midbrain and brainstem are relatively intact. This may be confused with massive hydrocephalus in brain imaging.

The cause of hydranencephaly is not much known but may be due to bilateral occlusion of internal carotid arteries during early fetal development.

9. **How the hydrocephalus can be managed?**

   Mostly, it depends of cause.

   Medical management: Acetazolamide and furosemide may reduce the CSF production and temporarily relives progression.

   Surgical management: Extracranial shunts.

Congenital Hypothyroidism

Chapter 20

Nigam Prakash Narain

CASE STUDY

A 1-month-old baby was brought with feeding problems, constipation and persistent jaundice and a hoarse cry. On examination, she looked pale and felt little cold with rough skin and odd looks with a large tongue. There was evident umbilical hernia also. Her hemoglobin (Hb) was 11 gm/dL and serum thyroid stimulating hormone (TSH) was raised at 18 mU/L.

Diagnosis: Congenital hypothyroidism (Fig. 1).

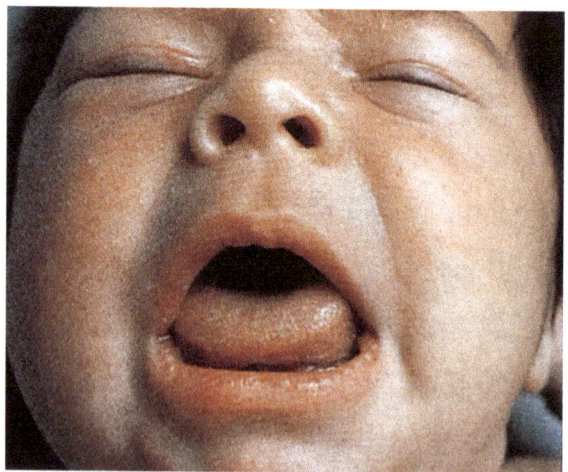

Fig. 1: Case of congenital hypothyroidism.

1. **How common is congenital hypothyroidism?**
   The incidence of congenital hypothyroidism is 1 in 2,000–4,000 live births, but in India, the incidence is on the higher side of this range, i.e., 1 in 2,000.
2. **What are the causes of congenital hypothyroidism?**
   Though there may be some rise in initial TSH due to maternal antibodies or antithyroid drugs, the permanent causes are maldescent or agenesis and dyshormonogenesis, in

which organification defect, iodide trapping defect, TSH unresponsiveness and defective thyroglobulin synthesis are included.

3. **How do we diagnose them at the earliest?**
   They can be suspected by newborn screening at birth but must be confirmed as early as 2 weeks of age, certainly by 4 weeks as the outcome of treatment started at that age is far more rewarding.

4. **In borderline cases or even in a single newborn screening if TSH is raised, how do we proceed?**
   In all preliminary suspected cases, a thyroid function test including both Free T4 and Total T4 along with serum TSH must be done to confirm the diagnosis. Serum T4 is usually low except in the cases of central pituitary induced hypothyroidism, a rare possibility.

5. **Why early treatment is of so much importance?**
   Early treatment is of immense importance as not only the physical growth but also the mental maturation may be permanently affected, and that is why this is the most important cause of preventable mental retardation.

6. **What other tests can be done to differentiate the causes?**
   Thyroid nuclear imaging can highlight the importance of lifelong treatment. ^{123}I with perchlorate discharge test will indicate defect of iodide organification.

7. **What is the treatment recommended?**
   Treatment for congenital hypothyroidism is replacement of deficient hormone as levothyroxine (10–15 µg/kg/day once daily), crushed and mixed with either breast milk or water preferably in empty stomach.

8. **What clinical or lab monitoring should be done, and how frequently?**
   Monitoring of the child both clinical and by TSH levels must be done at regular intervals; every 3–6 months.

9. **Will they require the treatment lifelong?**
   Yes. Definitely the treatment has to be pursued lifelong at all cost and the parents must realize it fully well.

10. **If thyroxine treatment has been instituted on suspicious grounds, what further actions can be taken?**
    If early treatment has been started on suspicious grounds without final confirmation, then thyroxine treatment has to be stopped for 4–6 weeks after 3 years followed by repeat thyroid function test to know that it was not transient hypothyroidism.

11. **What is the prognosis for such infants?**
    Prognosis is excellent with normal physical growth and intelligence if the treatment is instituted early and followed meticulously.

Chapter 21

Congenital Rubella Syndrome

Darshan Vinodchandra Chauhan

CASE STUDY

A 3-day-old neonate admitted in the neonatal intensive care unit (NICU) with complains of skin rashes, fast breathing, and refusal for feeding.

The mother was having significant history of fever with rash in the first trimester.

On examination: Neonatal purpura (Figs. 1B and C), bilateral congenital glaucoma (Fig. 1A), bilateral congenital cataract, hepatosplenomegaly and loud murmur [3 mm patent ductus arteriosus (PDA) was confirmed by two-dimensional (2D) echo].

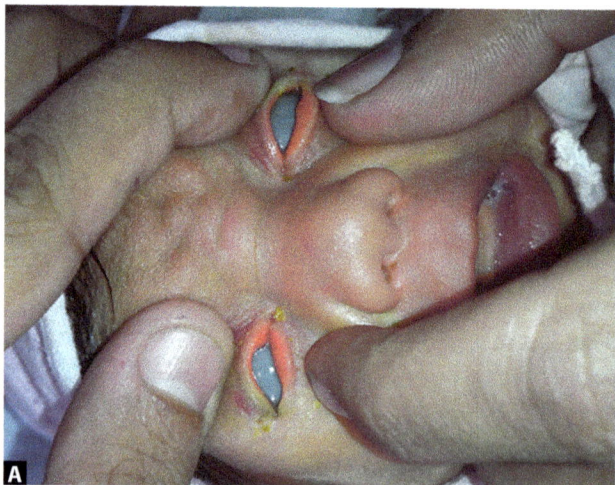

Fig. 1A: Bilateral congenital glaucoma in 3-day old neonate.

Congenital Rubella Syndrome

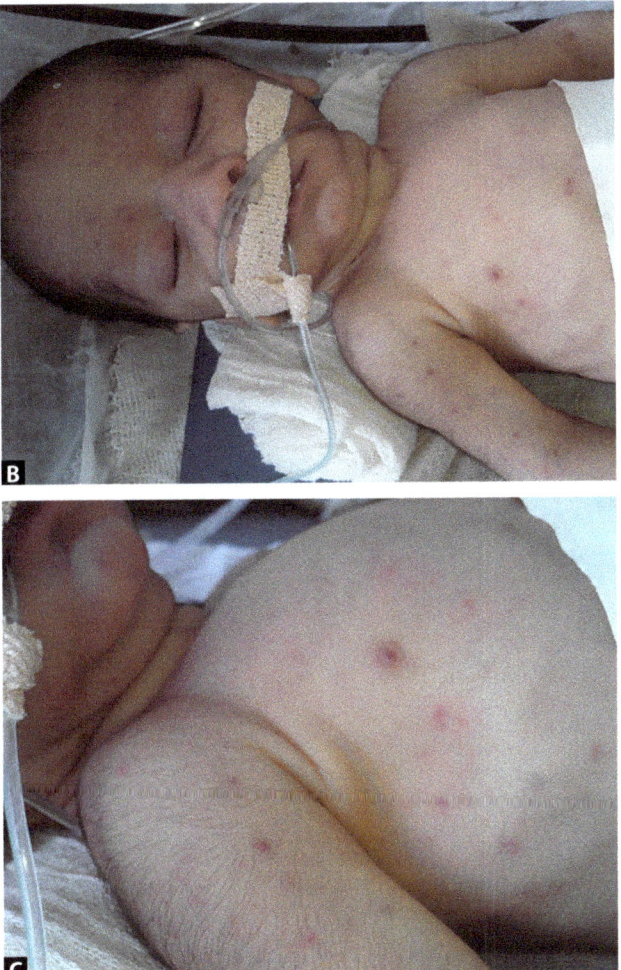

Figs. 1B and C: Neonatal purpura.

1. **What is congenital rubella syndrome?**
   It is a triad of congenital heart disease (PDA), congenital cataract, and sensory neural hearing deafness in neonate.
2. **What is the incidence and correlation with timing of maternal active rubella infection?**
   A neonate born with severe congenital defect when the mother suffers from active infection during the first 8 weeks of gestation.
   Afterwards, the chances of congenital defects in fetus gradually decrease from 90% for less than 11 weeks to 24% at 15–16 weeks of gestation.
   Defects occurring after 16 weeks of gestation are uncommon, even if fetal infection occurs.

3. What are the pathological findings associated with congenital rubella infection in fetus?

System	Pathologic findings
Cardiovascular	Patent ductus arteriosus
	Pulmonary artery stenosis
	Ventriculoseptal defect
	Myocarditis
Central nervous system	Chronic meningitis
	Parenchymal necrosis
	Vasculitis with calcification
Eye	Microphthalmia
	Cataract
	Iridocyclitis
	Ciliary body necrosis
	Glaucoma (Fig. 1A)
	Retinopathy
Ear	Cochlear hemorrhage
	Endothelial necrosis
Lung	Chronic mononuclear interstitial pneumonitis
Liver	Hepatic giant cell transformation
	Fibrosis
	Lobular disarray
	Bile stasis
Kidneys	Interstitial nephritis
Adrenal glands	Cortical cytomegaly
Bone	Malformed osteoid
	Poor mineralization of osteoid
	Thinning cartilage
Spleen, lymph nodes	Extramedullary hematopoiesis
Thymus	Histiocytic reaction
	Absence of germinal centers
Skin	Erythropoiesis in dermis

4. **How can it be prevented?**
Immunization against rubella by vaccine is the effective way to prevent the rubella infection during the pregnancy, and thus, prevent congenital rubella syndrome.

Congenital Varicella Syndrome

Chapter 22

Darshan Vinodchandra Chauhan

CASE STUDY

A neonate brought to the neonatal intensive care unit (NICU) for intrauterine growth restriction (IUGR) care with birth weight of 1.8 kg. The child was having typical skin lesions mostly over the bilateral lower limb and few in the upper limb. Regarding maternal history, the mother has suffered from Varicella during the fourth to fifth months of pregnancy with typical skin lesions and fever.

Skin lesions were typically cicatricial in character with hypopigmentation, and trunk was normal without any skin lesions. Brain imaging was done to rule out intracranial calcification, which was normal. Ophthalmologic examination was normal. The child was not having any other significant stigmata other than skin lesions due to intrauterine fetopathy (Figs. 1A and B).

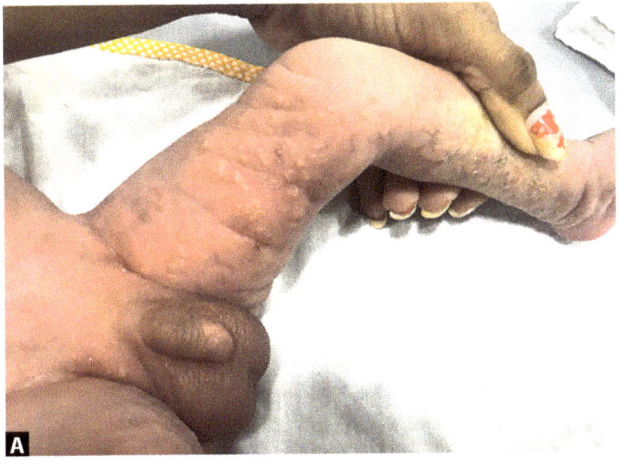

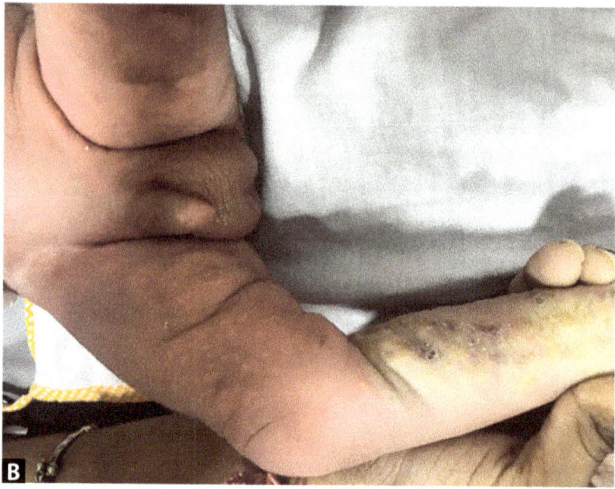

Figs. 1A and B: Case of congenital varicella syndrome.

1. **What is congenital Varicella and what is the incidence?**
   When a pregnant woman acquired chickenpox during the first trimester (up to 20 weeks of gestation), about 25% of the fetuses may get infection, and among them, 2% of the fetuses demonstrate congenital Varicella fetopathy.

2. **What is the effect to the fetus according to the timing of infection with Varicella in pregnant women?**
   - Greater than 6 weeks of gestation: Associated with abortion
   - Six to twelve weeks of gestation: Interruption with limb development
   - Twelve to twenty weeks of gestation: Damage to eye and brain, and sympathetic fibers in cervical and lumbosacral cord

3. **What are the stigmata of congenital Varicella syndrome?**
   Varicella zoster virus (VZV) is the neurotropic virus, and so most of the stigmata are due to infection of neural tissue of fetus. Viruses usually select the tissues that are rapidly developing, like limb buds and brain (Box 1).

BOX 1: Stigmata of congenital varicella syndrome.

Damage to sensory nerves
- Cicatricial skin lesions
- Hypopigmentation

Damage to optic stalk and lens vesicle
- Microphthalmia
- Cataracts
- Chorioretinitis
- Optic atrophy

Damage to brain/encephalitis
- Microcephaly
- Hydrocephaly
- Calcifications
- Aplasia of brain

Contd...

Contd...
> Damage to cervical or lumbosacral cord
- Hypoplasia of an extremity
- Motor and sensory deficits
- Absent deep tendon reflexes
- Anisocoria
- Horner syndrome
- Anal/urinary sphincter dysfunction

4. **What is the hallmark of congenital Varicella syndrome?**
   The hallmark of CVS is cutaneous lesion that has been called a cicatrix, a zigzag scarring, in a *dermatomal* distribution, often associated with atrophy of the affected limb.
   The characteristic cicatricial scarring may represent the cutaneous residua of VZV infection of the sensory nerves, analogous to herpes zoster.

5. **How to diagnose VZV fetopathy?**
   It is mostly based on the history of chickenpox to pregnant women with clinical presence of stigmata in newborn.
   The virus cannot be cultured from affected neonate but viral deoxyribonucleic acid (DNA) may be detected in affected tissue samples by polymerase chain reaction (PCR). Sometimes cord blood VZV specific immunoglobulin M (IgM) may be positive.

6. **Is the prenatal diagnosis possible? How much is it reliable?**
   VZV DNA PCR from chorionic villus sampling and fetal blood can be tested.
   Negative test is useful to rule out fetal infection but positive results do not differentiate fetal infection from embryopathy.
   Post-natal VZV immunoglobulin G:
   Persistent positive VZV immunoglobulin G (IgG) even 12–18 months after birth is the reliable indicator of intrauterine infection with VZV. Those children may develop zoster without clinically evident primary Varicella infection.

7. **Is there any role of acyclovir treatment or VZV immunoglobulin to susceptible mother exposed to chickenpox to prevent congenital Varicella syndrome?**
   No, it is not certain that administration of VZV immune globulin or acyclovir treatment to mother may modify the infection in the fetus and prevent congenital Varicella syndrome; therefore, both are not indicated.
   Rather administration of acyclovir in pregnancy is questionable because of its potential teratogenic effect.

Dental Caries

Chapter 23

Piyali Bhattacharya, Deval Arora

CASE STUDY 1

A 6-year-old female patient came with the chief complaint of decayed teeth in upper front tooth region since 2 months.

The patient gave the history of carious teeth which was asymptomatic and felt sensitivity on taking hot and cold foodstuff, and gets relieved after sometime. There is no history of continuous pain and no tenderness on percussion. The caries is reversible in nature showing mild involvement of enamel, dentin.

CASE STUDY 2

A 4-year-old female patient came with the chief complaint of decayed teeth in the lower right back tooth region and also complains of pain in the same since 1 week.

The patient was apparently asymptomatic when she felt pain while having food. The pain was sharp, continuous in nature and subsides on taking medication. There is no significant medical history. On clinical examination, deep carious lesion and tenderness to percussion were observed (Fig. 2A). Radiographic examination reveals carious lesion involving enamel, dentin and pulp as shown in Figure 2B. Tooth is diagnosed with irreversible pulpitis.

Both the cases showed dental caries; the first one is mild form of dental caries (Fig. 1) and the second one is severe form (Fig. 2) of dental caries.

1. **What is dental caries?**
   Dental caries is an irreversible microbial disease of the calcified tissues of the teeth, characterized by demineralization of the inorganic portion and destruction of the organic substance of the tooth which leads to cavitation.
2. **What are the etiological factors that cause dental caries?**
   There are four etiological factors that cause dental caries, which are as follows: host; microorganisms; substrate; time.
3. **Which bacteria are responsible for dental caries?**
   The oral cavity contains a wide variety of oral bacteria, but only a few specific species of bacteria are believed to cause dental caries; *Streptococcus mutans* and *Lactobacillus acidophillus* are the main responsible organisms along with a plethora of others.

Dental Caries

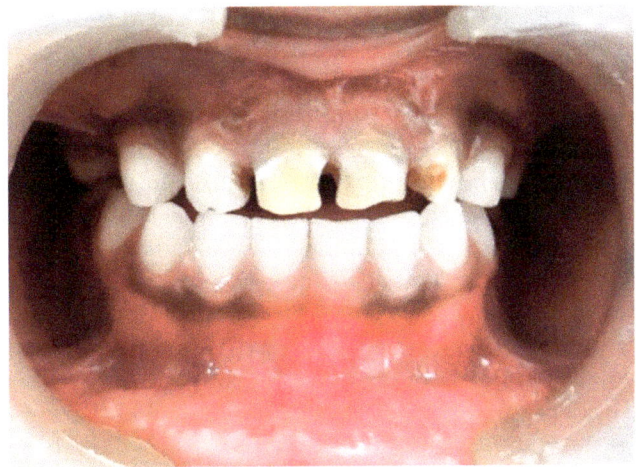

Fig. 1: Deep carious primary 1st molar.

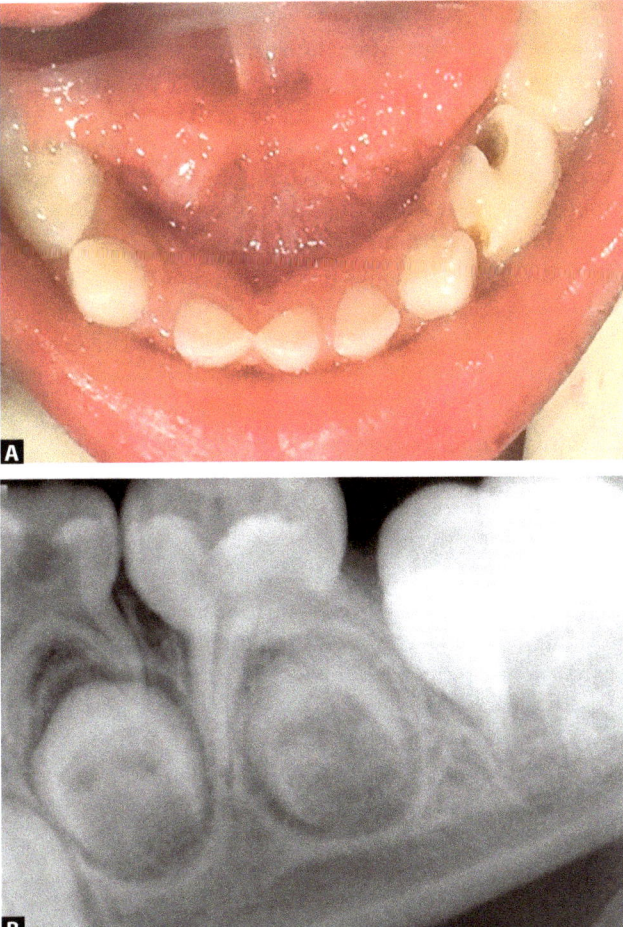

Figs. 2A and B: Clinical and radiograph showing carious involvement of enamel and dentin extending till the pulp of primary 1st molar.

4. **How caries causing bacteria cause demineralization of tooth, i.e. tooth decay?**
   Cariogenic bacteria in the plaque bio-film convert sugar to harmful acids that lower the pH of the oral cavity below the critical level (pH 5.5) and initiate demineralization or tooth decay.

5. **How are cavities diagnosed?**
   Cavities can be diagnosed by using an explorer (diagnostic instrument) to feel tooth structure that has been softened by tooth decay. If a cavity forms in between the teeth, it may only be visible in an X-ray (intra-oral-peri-apical radiograph). Other diagnostic tools that are used to detect cavities include fluorescence, fiber optic transillumination (FOTI), digital FOTI, ultrasound, electrical conductance (EC), etc.

6. **What do you understand by the reversible and irreversible pulpitis?**
   The term reversible pulpitis means mild inflammation of the tooth pulp, and is characterized by hypersensitivity to thermal (i.e., hot or cold) or sweet stimulus, which rapidly disappears when the stimulus is removed; however, in the case of irreversible pulpitis, pain is severe, continuous and can be radiating in nature, and after the removal of stimulus, it subsides by taking medication but needs immediate dental treatment.

7. **How is the nursing bottle caries different from rampant caries?**
   Nursing bottle caries is also known as nursing bottle syndrome or maternally derived streptococcus mutans disease; it is a specific form of caries which involves only primary dentition. The most striking feature is that even after generalized involvement, lower incisors are not affected due to the protective action of tongue and saliva, while in rampant caries, both primary and permanent dentitions are involved along with upper and lower incisors which are generally immune to ordinary decay.

8. **Does sucrose promote dental caries? If yes, then how?**
   Yes, sucrose promotes dental caries by increasing the mutans streptococci and lactobacillus count, and simultaneously decreases the buffering capacity of saliva to neutralize the acids produced as a product of cariogenic bacteria metabolism causing a fall of pH of oral cavity, which makes the tooth more susceptible to dental caries.

9. **When should a child have first dental visit?**
   According to the American Academy of Pediatric Dentistry (AAPD), the first dental visit should occur within 6 months after the baby's first tooth appears, but no later than the child's first birthday. This concept is also known as Dental Home.

10. **How can you prevent dental caries?**
    There are a variety of ways to help prevent caries, which includes: brushing and flossing daily, use of fluoridated toothpaste, which strengthens teeth, as well as fluoride treatments provided by the dentist and by using antibacterial mouth rinse along with regular check-up and visit to the dentist.

11. **What are the complications of dental caries if left untreated?**
    If left untreated, a cavity will cause the tooth to decay significantly. Eventually, uncontrolled decay may destroy the tooth completely. There is also the risk of developing an infection related to an abscess when the infection spreads to the root of the tooth and may go on to become a sinus opening perforating soft tissues.

12. **What are the drugs that cause increased risk of dental caries?**
    There are certain drugs which increase the risk of caries, namely: antihistamines, antidepressants, sedatives, decongestants, H_2 blockers and antacids.

13. **How does saliva help in the prevention of dental caries?**
    Saliva helps in cleaning the oral cavity and also contains certain immunoglobulins which act as a defense mechanism for oral cavity. Additionally, saliva contains bicarbonates which neutralize the acids produced by cariogenic bacteria and help in remineralization as it is supersaturated with calcium and phosphate ions.

14. **What are the dietary implications in dental caries?**
    Food has a definite role in the initiation and advancement of dental caries. Nutrition education and counseling for the purposes of reducing caries in children is aimed at teaching parents the importance of reducing high-frequency exposures to obvious and hidden sugars. Consumption of food high in sugar content or sticky food which has low level clearance from the oral cavity increases the risk of caries. Snacking in between meals with high sugar containing food also increases the risk of the same.

15. **How can we prevent dental caries from conception to 3 years of age?**
    It is important to educate the parents so that they can make appropriate decisions regarding the management of their infants and toddler's oral health. The parents should be counseled regarding cleaning of the infant's gum pads daily before the eruption of first primary tooth. A wet clean cloth is wrapped around the index finger and gum pads are massaged gently. Periodic recall to a qualified pedodontist minimizes the risk of dental infections.

FURTHER READING

1. Guideline on caries-risk assessment and management for infants, children, and adolescents. Chicago: American Academy of Pediatric Dentistry; 2013. pp. 123-30.
2. Marwah N, Bhatia R. Early childhood caries. In: Marwah N (Ed). Textbook of Pediatric Dentistry, 2nd edition. New Delhi: Jaypee Brothers Medical Publication; 2006. pp. 404-14.
3. Newbrun E. Substrate: diet and caries. In: Cariology, 3rd edition. New York: Quintessence Publishing; 1989. pp. 99-124.
4. Peter S. Epidemiology etiology and prevention of dental caries. In: Peter S (Ed). Essentials of Preventive and Community Dentistry, 3rd edition. New Delhi: Arya Publishing House; 2006. pp. 222-61.
5. Tandon S, Bhalla S. Dental caries in early childhood. In: Tandon S, (Ed). Textbook of Pedodontics, 2nd edition. New Delhi: Paras Medical Publication; 2001. pp. 192-205.

Dermatitis Herpetiformis

Chapter 24

Kosha Gajera

CASE STUDY

A 12-year-old boy has presented with itchy, burning, crusted papulovesicular lesions over knees, hands and elbows for 4–5 months. He is k/c/o celiac disease and insulin-dependent diabetes mellitus (IDDM). The patient is not following proper strict gluten-free diet. On clinical basis, the patient is diagnosed as having dermatitis herpetiformis (DH) (Figs. 1A and B) and treated with dapsone and strict gluten-free diet.

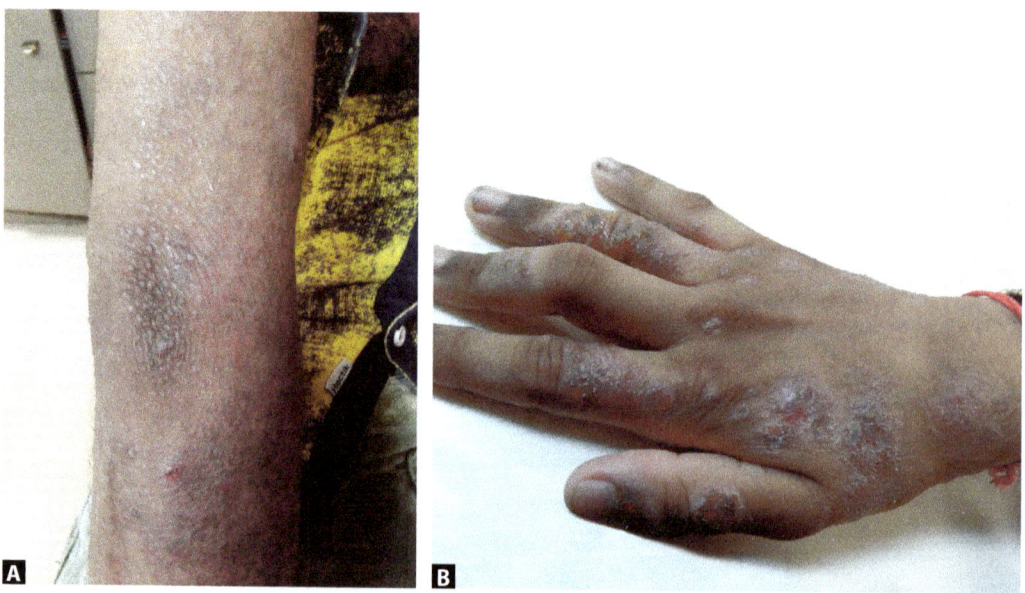

Figs. 1A and B: Case of dermatitis herpetiformis.

1. **What is dermatitis herpetiformis?**
   DH or Duhring-Brocq disease is an inflammatory cutaneous disease with a chronic relapsing course, pruritic polymorphic lesions, typical histopathological and immunopathological findings. It is considered as the specific cutaneous marker of celiac disease.

2. **How do the lesions look?**
   There are grouped vesicles and tense blisters with centrifugal growth, whose contents may be serous or hemorrhagic, with symmetrical distribution. Bullous elements rupture, culminating in denuded areas of exulcerated skin and crust. Itching of variable intensity and scratching and burning sensation immediately preceding the development of lesions are common. The affected extensor areas—lower limbs (anterior thigh and knee), elbows, buttocks and sacral region, although the shoulder, scapular region and scalp—may also be affected.

3. **What is the age of development of lesions?**
   It can affect individual of any age. Approximately 27% of the patients were below the age of 10, and 36% below the age of 20. Males are more affected, with a ratio of 2:1, but in patients under 20, the ratio is 12 females for every 8 males.

4. **In which other diseases it develops?**
   High association autoimmune diseases include thyroid (5–11%), pernicious anemia (1–3%), type 1 diabetes (1–2%) and collagen tissue disease. Screening for autoimmune diseases in patients with DH, as determination of antiperoxidase antibodies (present in 20% of cases), thyroid-stimulating hormone (TSH), T4 and T3, anti-gastric parietal cells (10–25% positive), atrial natriuretic factor (ANF), anti-Ro/SSA and glucose is suggested.

5. **What is the etiopathogenesis?**
   It is an IgA-mediated cutaneous disease, with immunoglobulin A deposits appearing in a granular pattern at the top of the dermal papilla in the sub-lamina dense area of the basement membrane, which is present both in affected skin and healthy skin. The same protein IgA1 with J chain is found in the small intestinal mucosa in patients with adult celiac disease, suggesting a strong association with DH. There is higher incidence of genotypes HLA DR3, HLA DQw2 in 80–90% of patients, HLA B8 and HLA DQ8 in 10–20% of cases.

6. **How is it diagnosed?**
   Skin biopsy showing IgA1 deposits in granular pattern, duodenal biopsy for celiac histopathology and serum anti-tTG antibodies. Direct immunofluorescence (DIF) of uninvolved skin collected in the perilesional site is the gold standard for the diagnosis of DH. DIF has a sensitivity and a specificity close to 100% for the diagnosis of DH. According to the European Society for Paediatric Gastroenterology Hepatology and Nutrition (ESPGHAN) guidelines for celiac disease, a positive DIF in a patient with suspected DH allows for the diagnosis of celiac disease without the need of duodenal biopsy.
   One hundred percent of patients with DH exhibit histopathological changes of celiac disease, i.e., villous atrophy.

7. **What are the differential diagnoses in children?**
   The main differential diagnoses in children are atopic dermatitis, scabies, papular urticaria and impetigo.

8. **How is it managed?**
   Dapsone and lifelong gluten-free diet. Gluten-free diet is able to resolve both the gastrointestinal and the cutaneous manifestations, as well as to prevent the development of lymphomas. Dapsone is considered a valid therapeutic option for patients with DH during the 6- to 24-month period until the gluten-free diet is effective. The starting dose should be 50 mg/day in order to minimize the potential side effects. Then the dosage can

be increased up to 200 mg/day until the disease is under control; in the maintenance phase, 0.5-1 mg/kg/day generally can control itching and the development of new skin lesions. Patients who cannot tolerate the use of dapsone may benefit from sulfapyridine (1-1.5 g/day, tetracycline 2 g/day, together with nicotinamide 1.5 g/day or cyclosporine for resistant cases).

9. **What is the prognosis?**
   It takes an average of 1-2 years of a gluten-free diet for the resolution of the cutaneous lesions, which invariably recur within 12 weeks after the reintroduction of gluten.
   Prognosis courses with periods of remission and exacerbation. An emotional event or infection may trigger a new worsening of the disease.

Desquamating Rash

Chapter 25

M Indra Shekhar Rao

CASE STUDY

A 6-year-old male child was admitted with the complaints of fever for about 2 weeks associated with redness of eyes. He had rashes all over the body on day 2 of fever and have subsided in 3–4 days. The child did not have lymphadenopathy, strawberry tongue or lip cracking. The child was treated elsewhere with antibiotics for 5 days. He had desquamation of skin all over the body from day 8 of fever. Two-dimensional (2D) echo was done after 10 days, and was normal (Figs. 1A and B).

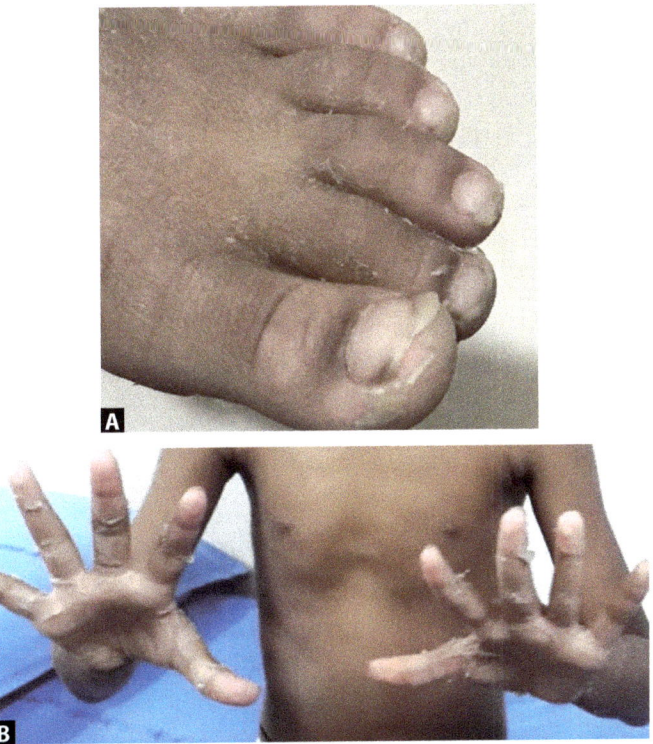

Figs. 1A and B: Desquamating rashes.

At admission, he had fever, tachycardia, conjunctival congestion and desquamation of skin all over the body. Blood investigations showed leucocytosis (18,000), platelet count was 3 lakhs/cu mm, high C-reactive protein (CRP) (102) and erythrocyte sedimentation rate (ESR) (60). Anti-streptolysin O (ASO) titer was normal and antinuclear antibody (ANA) was negative. Repeat 2D echo done after 2 weeks showed diffuse dilatation of coronaries LAD (4 mm) and right coronary artery (RCA) (4 mm), minimal pericardial effusion and dilated chambers.

The child was treated with intravenous immunoglobulin (IVIG) and aspirin. Fever subsided after 1 day and is on follow-up. Repeat 2D echo done after 2 weeks showed diffuse dilatation of coronaries LAD (3.3 mm) and RCA (2.6 mm), and minimal pericardial effusion.

1. **What are the possible differential diagnosis of desquamating rash?**
   Kawasaki disease (KD), scarlet fever, allergic or drug reaction and staphylococcal scalded skin syndrome.

2. **What are the diagnostic criteria for KD?**
   KD is diagnosed in the presence of fever for at least 5 days together with at least four of the five following principal clinical features:
   - Erythema and cracking of lips, strawberry tongue and/or erythema of oral and pharyngeal mucosa
   - Bilateral bulbar conjunctival injection without exudates
   - *Rash:* Maculopapular, diffuse erythroderma or erythema multiforme-like.
   - Erythema and edema of the hands and feet in acute phase and/or periungual desquamation in subacute phase
   - Cervical lymphadenopathy (≥1.5 cm diameter), usually unilateral.

   KD may be diagnosed with fewer than four of these features if coronary artery abnormalities are detected.

3. **What is incomplete or atypical KD?**
   Diagnosis of incomplete or atypical KD might be made in children with fever for ≥5 days and two or three compatible clinical criteria along with other compatible laboratory, clinical signs and echocardiographic findings on exclusion of other febrile illness.

4. **How is atypical or incomplete KD diagnosed?**
   A CRP ≥3.0 mg/dL and ESR ≥40 mm/hour are supportive of KD.
   Patients with these laboratory findings and (1) a positive echocardiogram, or (2) ≥3 supportive laboratory findings can be treated as KD.

5. **What are the supportive lab findings?**
   - Anemia for age
   - Platelet count of ≥450,000 after the seventh day of fever
   - Albumin ≤3.0 g/dL
   - Elevated alanine aminotransferase (ALT)
   - White blood cell count ≥15,000/mm^3, or
   - Urine with ≥10 white blood cell/hpf.

6. **What are the other clinical signs compatible with KD?**
   Important clinical signs compatible to KD are irritability, erythema and induration at site of Bacillus Calmette-Guérin (BCG) immunization. Other clinical signs are arthritis, aseptic meningitis, pneumonitis, uveitis, etc.

7. **What are the echocardiographic findings in KD?**
   Coronary artery aneurysms (CAA) occur in 15–25% of untreated cases. Other cardiac features are pericardial effusion, electrocardiographic abnormalities, pericarditis, myocarditis, valvular incompetence, cardiac failure and myocardial infarction.
8. **What are the other vessels involved in KD apart from coronaries?**
   Though rare, other vessels such as the axillary arteries, pulmonary artery, iliofemoral arteries can be involved.
9. **What is the treatment of KD?**
   IVIG 2 g/kg as a single infusion, usually given over 10–12 hours.
10. **What is the schedule for aspirin in KD?**
    Moderate (30–50 mg/kg/day) to high (80–100 mg/kg/day) dose of aspirin should be continued until the patient is afebrile for 2–3 days, followed by anti-platelet dose (3–5 mg/kg) until the patient has no evidence of coronary changes.
11. **How frequently should echocardiogram be done?**
    Echocardiography should be performed when the diagnosis of KD is considered, and repeated at 1–2 and 4–6 weeks after treatment.
    If aneurysms are developed, they require long-term follow-up till they recover.
12. **What is refractory or IVIG resistant KD?**
    Patients who have persistent or recurrent fever even after 48 hours of primary therapy with IVIG plus aspirin.
13. **What are the indications for corticosteroids in KD?**
    - IVIG-resistant patients
    - Patients with features of the most severe disease
      - Very young (<1 year old)
      - Those with markers of severe inflammation, including: persistently elevated CRP despite IVIG, liver dysfunction, hypoalbuminemia, and anemia
      - Patients with hemophagocytic lymphohistiocytosis (HLH) and/or shock.
    - Patients who already have evolving coronary and/or peripheral aneurysms with ongoing inflammation at presentation.
14. **How do you treat refractory KD?**
    A second dose of IVIG or high-dose pulse steroids, longer course of steroids, infliximab, cyclosporine and immunomodulatory monoclonal antibody therapy.
15. **What is Kobayashi risk score?**
    Kobayashi risk score is a scoring system for predicting IVIG resistance.
    A score greater than or equal to 5 is high risk.
    - Sodium < 133—2 points
    - ALT > 100—1 point
    - Platelet count < 3 lakhs/cu mm—1 point
    - <4 days of illness—2 points
    - CRP > 10 mg/dL—1 point
    - Age < 12 months—1 point
16. **What are the specific immunization recommendations after treating KD?**
    All vaccines should be deferred for at least 3 months following an episode of KD treated with IVIG.

Varicella zoster virus (VZV) vaccine and influenza vaccines should be considered in patients who require long-term aspirin.

17. **What are the complications of KD?**

    Coronary artery stenosis or thrombosis.

    In children with giant aneurysms, risk for myocardial infarction in young adulthood is high.

18. **What is the other name for KD?**

    The original name given is mucocutaneous lymph node syndrome by Tomisaku Kawasaki in 1967.

19. **What is the cause of KD?**

    KD most commonly develops in children, although its specific cause is still unclear. It is supposed to be caused by coxsackievirus A4.

Duchenne Muscular Dystrophy

Chapter 26

Piyali Bhattacharya

CASE STUDY

- 10 years old; male; sporadic case
- Progressive proximal muscle weakness: onset 5–6 years
- Gower sign + (Fig. 1A); calf pseudo hypertrophy + (Fig. 1B)
- Serum creatine phosphokinase (CPK) = 6,600 U/L; electromyography (EMG)—myopathic pattern.

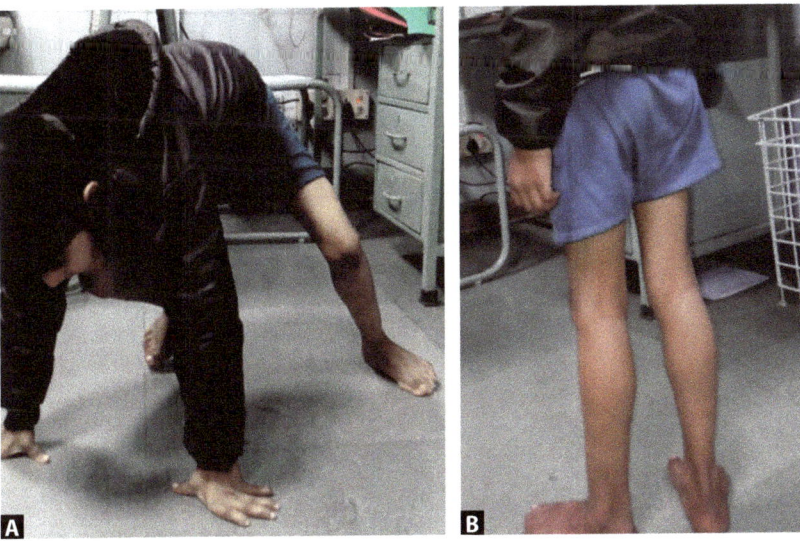

Figs. 1A and B: Case of Duchenne muscular dystrophy. (A) Gower's sign; (B) Prominent calf muscle.

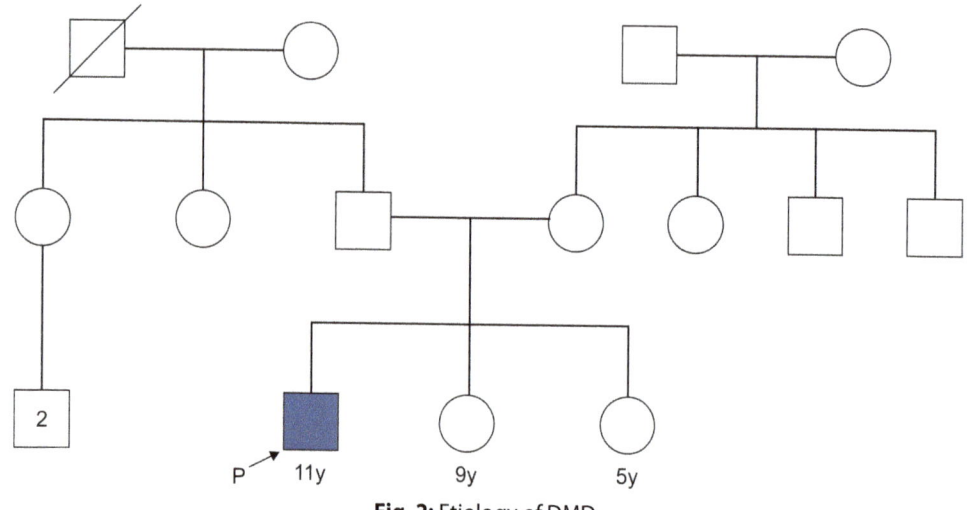

Fig. 2: Etiology of DMD.

Clinical diagnosis: Duchenne muscular dystrophy (DMD)

1. **What is muscular dystrophy (DMD)?**
   Muscular dystrophies are inherited progressive disorders of muscles usually caused by defects in cytoskeletal proteins or enzymes leading to degeneration and regeneration of muscle fibers. Muscular dystrophies lead to progressive muscular weakness and chronic disability as muscles are gradually replaced by adipose and fibrous tissue as disease advances.

2. **What is the incidence of DMD?**
   The incidence is about 1 in 3,500 live male births.

3. **Is DMD an inherited disease? Can DMD manifest in females?**
   It is an x-linked recessive trait and seen almost exclusively in males.
   Manifestation in females has also been documented.
   Females manifesting disease may have only one X chromosome as in Turner's syndrome (XO) which carries the Duchenne gene or there is inactivation of the unaffected paternal X chromosome allowing expression of mutated Duchenne gene from the maternal X chromosome.

4. **What is the etiology of DMD?**
   Mutation in the short arm of X chromosome at *Xp21* gene leads to DMD. The gene product is dystrophin, a protein, expressed in skeletal, cardiac and smooth muscles of the body and also in the brain (Fig. 2).
   Deletion/duplication of gene segments are seen in two- third of patients. Duplication is less common than deletions and a smaller number of patients may have point mutation as well. Absence of dystrophin leads to delocalization of dystrophin associated protein from membrane, disruption of cytoskeleton, and resultant instability and increased susceptibility to mechanical stress. In addition, altered membrane permeability and abnormal calcium homeostasis are thought to play a role.

5. **What are the clinical features of DMD?**
   Motor delay or an abnormal gait—boys present with difficulty in running or getting up from the ground and frequent falls.
   - At birth, there is no symptom. However, the motor milestones may be delayed in infancy. The problem becomes visible when children begin seeking support while getting up from the ground and rise with support of the hand: *Gower's maneuver*. At this stage, calf hypertrophy can be seen.
   - By 5-6 years, children have considerable difficulty in rising up or in climbing stairs.
   - By 6-7 years, lordosis develops and abdomen seems to be protuberant as paraspinal muscles weaken. A waddling gait appears due to weakness of gluteal muscles.

   The boy may experience episodes of buckling of knee and spontaneous falls due to weakened quadriceps. Gradually, extensors of knee and hip joints weaken, and the child takes to the wheel chair. Contracture is seen in many muscles, initially, in the tendo-Achilles. Spinal deformities increase and kyphoscoliosis adds to the problem of respiratory dysfunction.

6. **Which muscles are affected?**
   - Muscles of calves, deltoid, brachioradialis, infraspinatus, glutii, temporalis and tongue are affected.
   - Weakness initiates in the lower limbs with quadriceps and gluteal muscles. Foot drop occurs due to tendo-Achilles muscle weakness with resultant toe walking.
   - Weakness then ascends to the serratus anterior, lower trapezius and rhomboid causing winging of scapula.

7. **Which muscles are spared?**
   - Ocular
   - Facial
   - Bulbar
   - Hand muscles.

8. **Can reflexes be elicited?**
   Deep tendon reflexes are depressed in weak muscles, but ankle reflex can be elicited till late in the disease.

9. **What are the associated systemic findings?**
   Cardiac:
   - Dilated cardiomyopathy.
   - Hypocontractility starts early but overt symptoms appear by 10 years of age.

   Respiratory findings:
   - Restrictive lung disease is common.
   - Vital capacity decreases by 10 years of age and continues to decline.
   - Obstructive sleep apnea is seen in first decade with hypoventilation in the second decade.

10. **What is the milder variant of muscular dystrophy called?**
    Becker muscular dystrophy is a milder form of muscular dystrophy. The onset is much later, by about 12 years of age.
    Life span is almost normal and cardiac involvement is less frequent.

11. **How can we diagnose DMD?**
    Thorough examination of index case and a detailed family history are essential for diagnosing DMD.

The following investigations are diagnostic:
- Serum creatine kinase is increased since birth which progressively decreases as muscle mass is lost.
- Serum glutamic oxaloacetic transaminase/serum glutamic pyruvic transaminase (SGOT/SGPT) increased with increasing creatine kinase.
- Molecular genetic testing by polymerase chain reaction (PCR) techniques to study dystrophic gene.
- Multiplex ligation dependent pulse amplification (MLPA) is important for carrier detection.
- Prenatal chorionic villi sampling.
- Nerve conduction velocity is normal in early DMD, but in advanced disease, compound muscle action potentials may tend to decrease in amplitude.
- EMG shows short duration, low amplitude and polyphasic motor unit potentials particularly in proximal muscles.
- Muscle biopsy: Biopsy is done from muscles which have grade 3 or 4 power. It is indicated if clinical phenotype is atypical or genetic test is negative.

12. **What are the findings of muscle biopsy?**

    Muscle biopsy shows degenerating necrotic muscle fiber with basophilic cytoplasm and clusters of regenerating muscle fires which have basophilic cytoplasm.

    In advanced stages, there is replacement of muscle fiber by fat and endomysial connective tissue. Immunostaining shows absence of dystrophy.

13. **Outline the management in DMD.**
    - General supportive care
    - Physiotherapy
    - Surgical tendon release or surgical intervention for scoliosis (if degree is greater than 25%)
    - Early management of respiratory tract infections
    - Influenza and pneumococcal vaccination
    - Noninvasive positive pressure ventilation (NIPPV)
    - Annual ECG and ECHO
    - Prednisolone
    - 1.25 mg/kg and 2.5 mg/kg alternate day doses (10 days on and 10 days off, then 10 days on and 20 days off and thereafter 5 mg/kg/day twice weekly)
    - Care must be taken to rule out tuberculosis for fear of flare up
    - Deflazacort—0.9 mg/kg/day is an alternative medication.

Ectodermal Dysplasia

Piyali Bhattacharya

ECTODERMAL DYSPLASIA: X-LINKED

CASE STUDY

A 11-month-old child presented to the outpatient department (OPD) with the complaint of fever since birth. There was no history of sweating. On examination, the child was febrile, and had sparse hair and eyebrows, pointed conical incisors and a saddle nose with some frontal bossing.

1. **What is ectodermal dysplasia?**
   Ectodermal dysplasia is a heterogeneous group of disorders in which there is anatomical or functional impairment of one or more epidermal appendages such as hair (Fig. 1), nail, teeth (Fig. 2), and sweat glands.
   The most common ectodermal dysplasia is X-linked recessive hypohidrotic ectodermal dysplasia/anhidrotic ectodermal dysplasia or hidrotic ectodermal dysplasia.

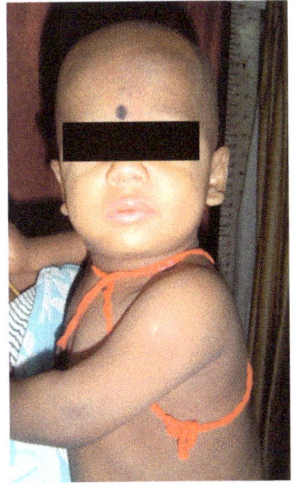

Fig. 1: Absent eyebrows.

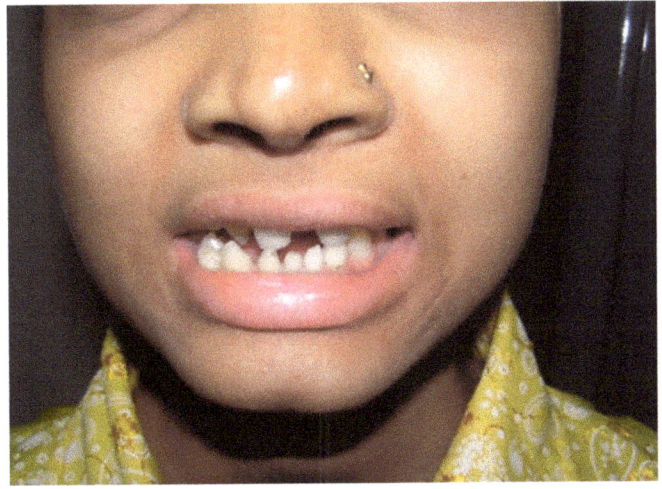

Fig. 2: Abnormal teeth with peg-shaped or conical incisors.

2. **What is hypohidrotic ectodermal dysplasia or Christ-Siemens-Touraine syndrome?**
   Hypohidrotic ectodermal dysplasia (Christ-Siemens-Touraine Syndrome) is a triad of the following:
   - Absent/reduced sweating leading to heat intolerance causing recurrent fever and febrile convulsions
   - Hypotrichosis
   - Defective dentition.
3. **What is the inheritance pattern in hypohidrotic ectodermal dysplasia?**
   Most patients are males and have X-linked recessive forms. However, autosomal dominant (AD) and autosomal recessive (AR) forms also exist.
4. **What are the signs and symptoms of hypohidrotic ectodermal dysplasia?**
   - Absence of sweating causes heat intolerance
   - Patient may present in childhood with a recurrent fever (PUO) and/or febrile convulsions
   - Alopecia, sparse eyebrows and normal hair lashes
   - Dentition is delayed and anomaly may vary from complete to partial absence of people with peg-shaped or conical incisors
   - *Facies:* Frontal bossing, saddle nose, sunken cheek, thick everted lips, large ears and sparse hairs
   - *Skin:* Small, dry, firmly wrinkled and may appear prematurely aged. Atopic eczema is often present
   - *Glands:* Hypoplastic lacrimal and salivary glands may lead to decreased tears, dry mouth and atrophic rhinitis
   - *Eye:* Corneal and lenticular opacities
   - Respiratory system complaints of asthma often coexist
   - Mental retardation is present in 30–50% cases
   - Life expectancy normal or slightly decreased.
5. **How can we diagnose hypohidrotic ectodermal dysplasia?**
   Clinical diagnosis can be done when the child develops teeth and hair abnormalities. The characteristic facies with lack of sweating make the diagnosis evident in hypohidrotic ectodermal dysplasia.
6. **What tests are diagnostic in hypohidrotic ectodermal dysplasia?**
   - *Sweat test:*

   X-linked hypohidrotic ectodermal dysplasia (XHED) affects many epithelial functions, including sweat gland formation. Female carriers who manifest XHED may have defective dentition or a patchy distribution of sweating or both, as determined by starch and iodine sweat testing.

   Sweat testing can be useful in assigning carrier status to at-risk females in XHED families. The advantages of diagnosing female carriers of XHED include the optimization of neonatal and pediatric care for affected male infants, who may be at substantial risk of death in infancy.

   - *Skin biopsy:*

   Sweat glands are absent/sparse, and hair follicles and sebaceous glands are reduced in number.

7. **How can we treat hypohidrotic ectodermal dysplasia?**
   - Temperature regulation is the mainstay of the treatment. Avoid heat by cool bathing multiple times every day, light clothing, air-conditioned home or school environment will prevent hyperthermia to some extent
   - Dry eyes may be treated with artificial tears
   - Liberal application of emollients
   - Dental prophylaxis for caries
   - Prosthodontic intervention with dentures.
8. **Are there any variants of ectodermal dysplasia?**
   Yes, hidrotic ectodermal dysplasia (Clouston syndrome) is a variant of hypohidrotic ectodermal dysplasia.
9. **What is the inheritance pattern of hidrotic ectodermal dysplasia?**
   It is a rare AD disease.
10. **Describe the characteristic features of hidrotic ectodermal dysplasia variant?**
    Characteristics:
    - Nail dystrophy—thickened, discolored and striated nails. Nails grow slowly with persistent paronychial infections.
    - Defects of hair—the scalp hair is sparse, fine, brittle and slow-growing. Total alopecia may occur, eyebrow lashes are thin or absent and body hair is sparse.
    - Palmoplantar keratoderma—skin tends to be dry and rough; skin may be thickened over knees, elbows and knuckles.
    - Teeth can be normal but dental caries is often present.
    - Sweating is normal.
    - Mental development is usually normal but may be retarded sometimes.
    - Additionally, oral leukoplakia, sensorineural hearing loss, poly/syndactyly may be associated.
11. **Enumerate the various management options for hidrotic ectodermal dysplasia?**
    Treatment/management:
    - Keratolytic agents and emollients
    - Dental prophylaxis for caries
    - Ocular lubrication
    - Control of onychomycosis.

Empyema Thoracis

Chapter 28

Aroon Narendra Trivedi

CASE STUDY 1

A 16 year man admitted with viral hepatitis , cough,cold and fever. On admission his X-ray chest was normal (Fig. 1)

He developed coagulopathy and pneumonia with synpneumonic effusion (Fig 2).

CT guided aspiration of 300 mL fluid was done (Fig. 3).

CT scan picture shows empyema with collapsed lung (Fig. 4).

A thoracoscopic decortication was done (Fig. 5).

On thoracoscopy pus in flakes and liquid form is seen (Fig. 6).

Suctioning of liquid pus and removal of pus flakes is done (Fig. 7).

Peeling of the parital pleura and attached pus is undertaken (Fig. 8).

To achieve complete decortication visceral pleura is peeled off (Fig. 9).

Complete clearance of empyema with decortication is done (Fig. 10).

Postoperative X-ray shows complete expansion of lung with clearance of empyema (Fig. 11).

ICD is removed on fourth postoperative day with normal X-ray (Fig. 12).

After two weeks post surgery on follow-up a normal chest X-ray is documented (Fig. 13).

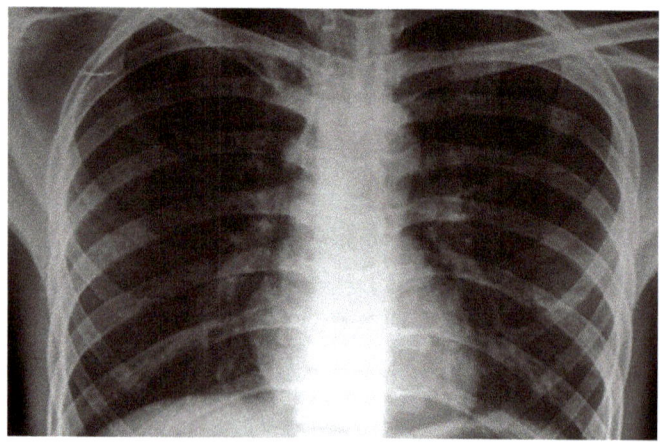

Fig. 1: Normal X-ray.

Empyema Thoracis

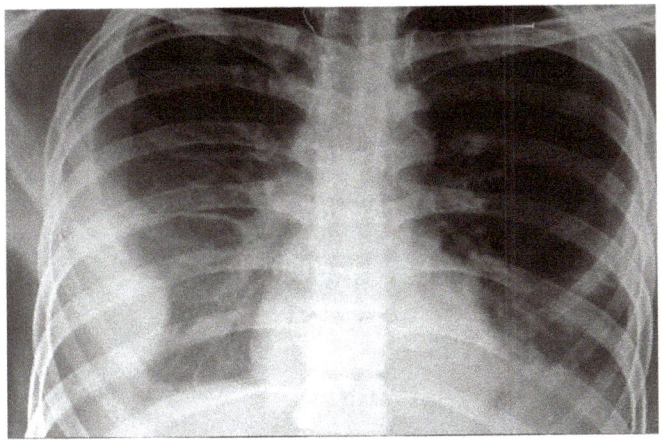

Fig. 2: Synpneumonic effusion.

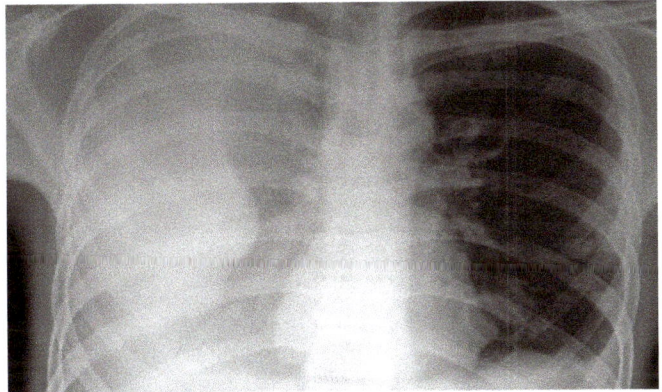

Fig. 3: A computed tomography (CT) guided ICD done. Removed 300 mL pus.

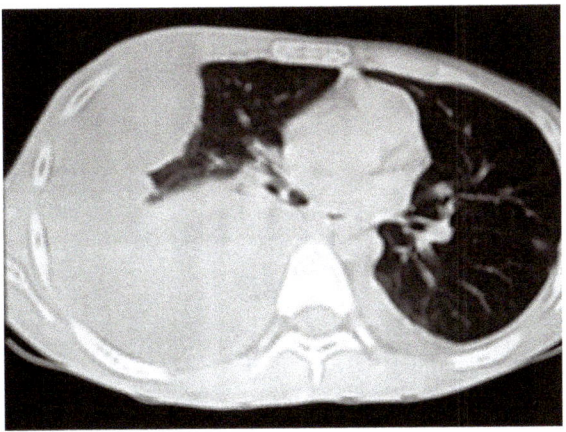

Fig. 4: CT Scan showing extensive empyma with collapsed lung.

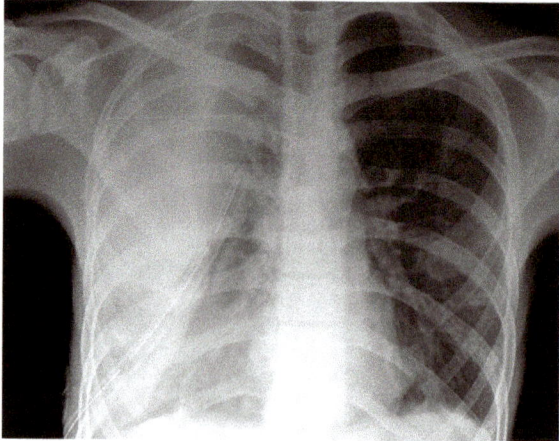
Fig. 5: Post-thoracoscopic decortication. First X-ray.

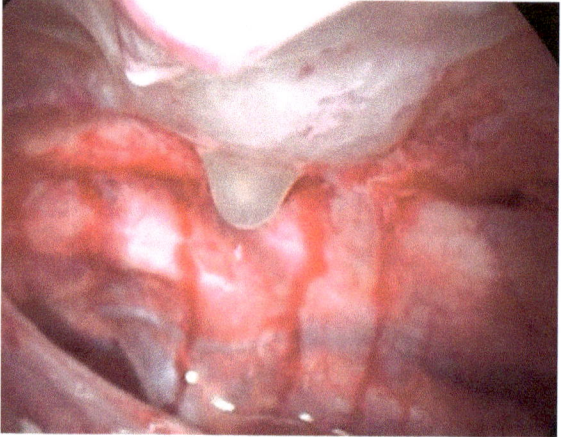
Fig. 6: First look on introduction of thoracoscope.

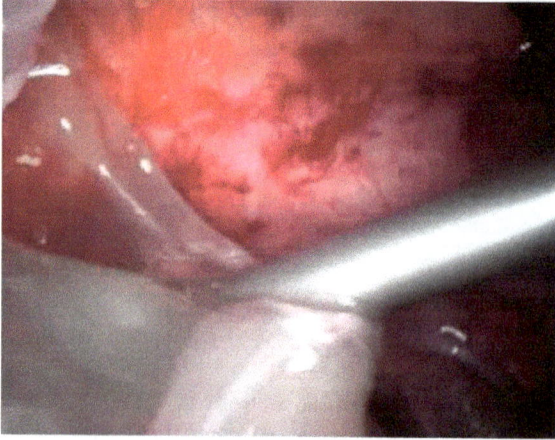
Fig. 7: Suctioning and removal of pus. The pus flakes are then removed.

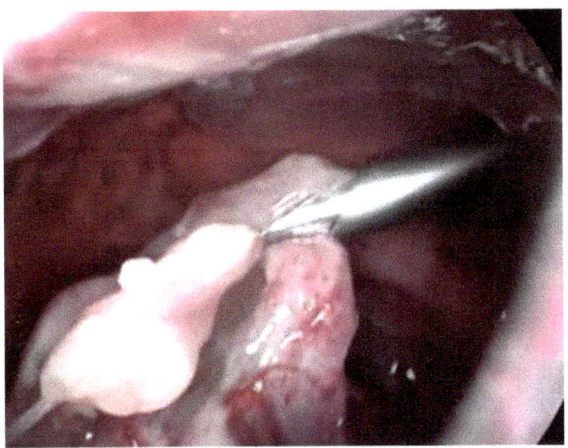

Fig. 8: Peeling of parietal pleura.

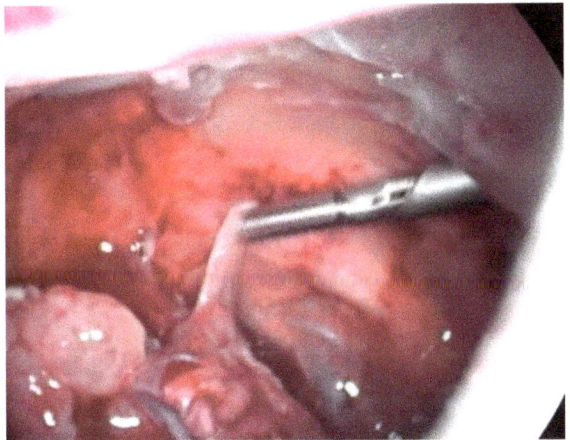

Fig. 9: Removal of visceral pleura.

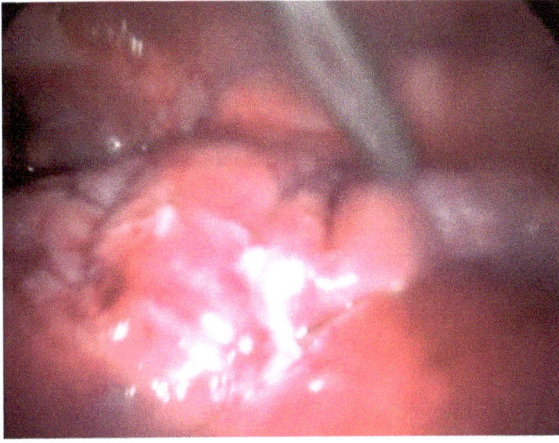

Fig. 10: Complete clearance is achieved. Normal saline wash is given. ICD is placed under vision.

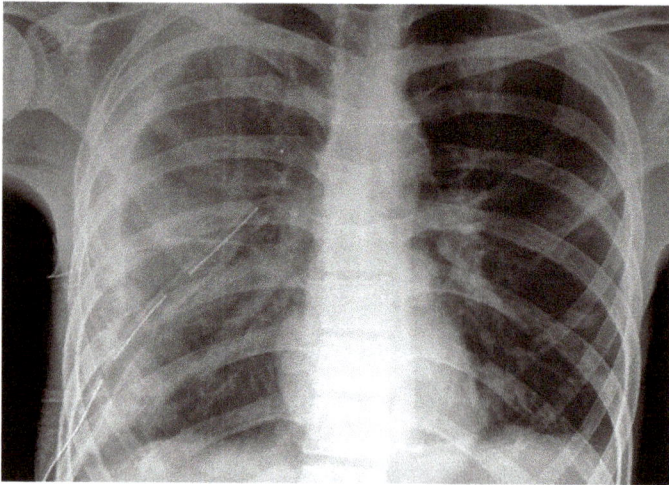

Fig. 11: Postoperative X-ray suggestive of complete expansion of lung with no residual collection.

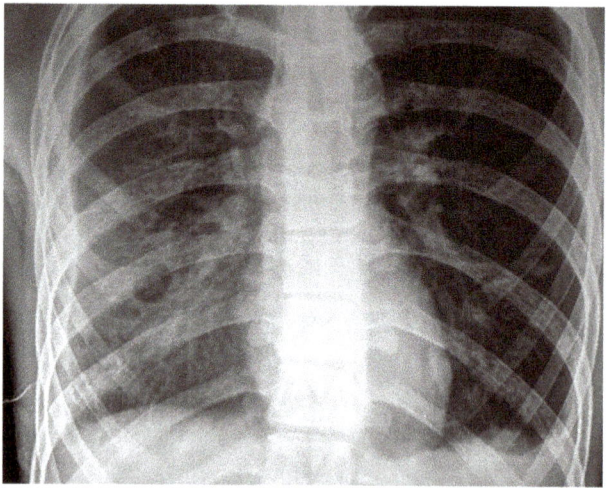

Fig. 12: ICD removed on 4th day. Post ICD removal X-ray.

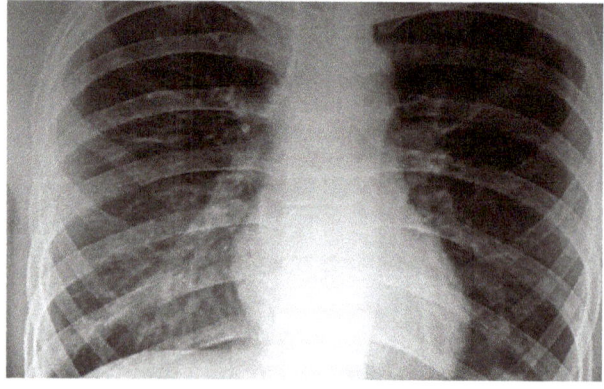

Fig. 13: X-ray after 2 weeks shows completely normal lung.

Empyema Thoracis

CASE STUDY 2

A 3-year-old child presented with cough and respiratory distress. X-ray was suggestive of pneumonia. (Fig. 14).

The child was started on antibiotics but had progressive increase in empyema (Fig. 15) and respiratory distress.

After computed tomography (CT) scan, a thoracoscopic decortication was done with perfect results as can be seen in post ICD removal X-ray (Fig. 16)

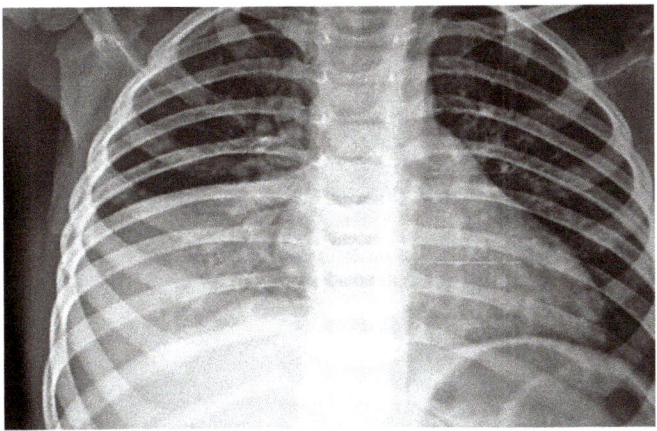

Fig. 14: X-ray showing pneumonia.

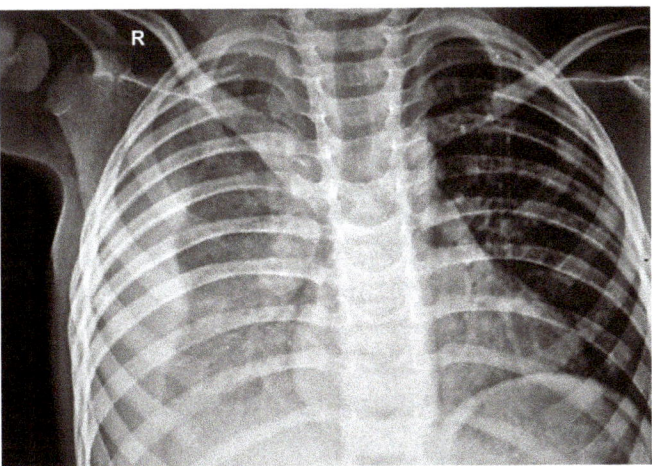

Fig. 15: Progressive increase in empyema.

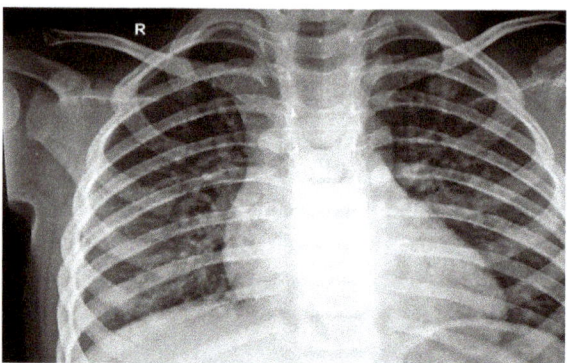

Fig. 16: Post decortication X-ray.

1. **What is Empyema Thoracis?**
   Empyema thoracis is the collection of pus in the thoracic cavity.
2. **What is the Presentation?**
   The child usually presents with cough and fever. As most empyemas are the consequence of pneumonia, the symptoms worsen. Respiratory distress may set in.
3. **What are the Investigations Required?**
   Complete hemogram, septic screen and X-ray care mandatory. Ultrasonography (USG) and CT scan are frequently needed.
4. **What is the Management?**
   Antibiotics form the mainstay of management. If the child does not respond, then aspiration, intercostal drainage (ICD) placement with or without thrombolytics are undertaken. Decortication (open or thoracoscopic) is done when the child does not respond.
5. **What is VATS?**
   Video-assisted thoracic surgery is the preferred treatment in fibropurulent stage of empyema. It is less painful, shortens hospital stay and hence is economical. Classical open decortication in this stage of empyema is rarely needed (Fig. 17).

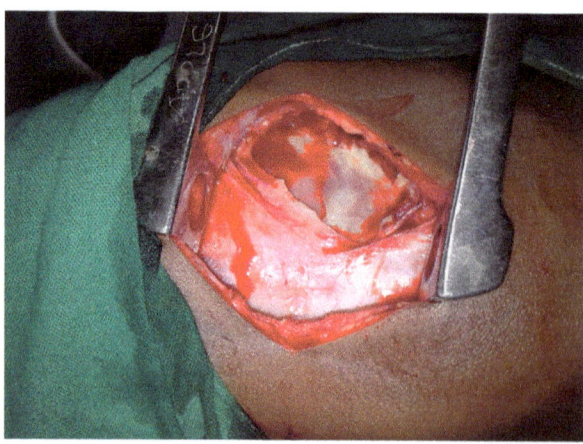

Fig. 17: On thoracotomy, the thickened pleura is seen. With VATS as the preferred modality of treatment, this surgery is getting to be of historical perspective.

Erb's Palsy

Chapter 29

Chetan Trivedi

CASE STUDY

A 3-day-old neonate brought with the complaint of decreased movement of right upper limb since birth, and with the history of difficult vaginal delivery with outlet forceps.

On examination, the neonate kept the right arm by the side of the body with little movement of fingers and hand (Fig. 1A). Deep tendon reflex (DTR) was absent in the right upper limb. The Moro's response was asymmetrical, with no active abduction of the right arm (Fig. 1B).

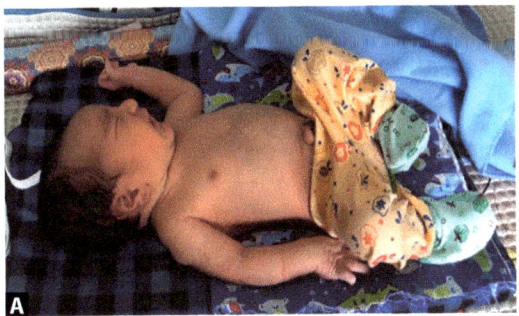 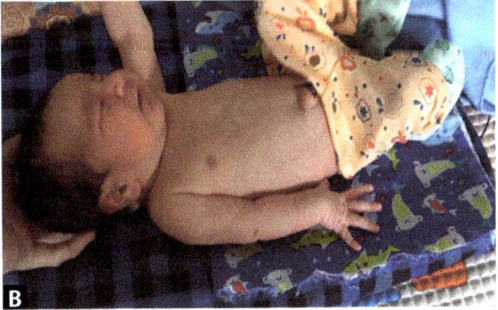

Figs. 1A and B: Erb's Palsy.

A CASE OF NEONATAL BRACHIAL PLEXUS PALSY OR BRACHIAL PLEXUS BIRTH PALSY

1. **What is Erb's palsy?**
   Erb's palsy Erb-Duchenne palsy is one of the types of brachial plexus birth palsy (BPBP), where there is a paralysis of the arm caused by injury to the upper group of the arm's main nerves, specifically the injury of the upper trunk C5–C6 nerves which is a part of the brachial plexus. These injuries arise most commonly, but not exclusively, from shoulder dystocia during a difficult birth.

2. **How to diagnose it?**
   The hallmark sign of BPBP is incomplete active range of motion but preserved passive range of motion. It is diagnosed by thorough physical examination and detailed gestational

and birth history. Imaging and electrodiagnostics can be used in special circumstances as add-on rather than replacement.

3. **What could be the clinical presentation?**
   - Characteristic position of the affected limb held close to the body rotated medially with elbow extended and pronated
   - Decreased movement of the affected limb can be elicited by asymmetric Moro's response
   - Associated features of Horner's syndrome (ptosis, miosis and anhidrosis)
   - Respiratory distress, feeding difficulties or asymmetric chest rise due to diaphragmatic weakness or paralysis with phrenic nerve damage
   - Orthopedic injuries like humerus fracture or clavicular fracture to be looked.

4. **What are the differential diagnoses?**
   Hemiparesis: A presence of DTRs, an absence of apparent abnormalities in electromyography (EMG) findings and an exaggerated (not a depressed) Moro's reflex.
   Hypotonia of central origin: Preserved DTRs and an absence of findings on EMG.
   Fracture, dislocation or epiphyseal separation of humerus and fracture clavicle: Pseudoparalysis due to pain.

5. **Can we predict which patient will improve without any residual damage?**
   Although there is no way to accurately predict, it depends on the number of nerve roots involved (C5–T1) and the type of nerve injury.
   Narakas grading (a system categorizing BPBP by root involvement) is given in Table 1.

TABLE 1: Narakas grading

Group	Roots	Clinical description
Group 1	C5, C6	Palsy of shoulder and biceps
Group 2	C5–C7	Palsy of shoulder, biceps and wrist/finger extension
Group 3	C5–T1	Total plexopathy with flail extremity
Group 4	C5–T1, Sympathetic chain	Flail extremity with Horner's syndrome

Grades 1 and 2 involving C5-C6 with better outcome; Grades 3 and 4 involving C5-T1 with poor outcome (except patients who have demonstrate antigravity biceps function (elbow flexion carries) before 2 months usually improve spontaneously).
Types of nerve injuries are given in Table 2.

TABLE 2: Types of nerve injuries.

	Neurapraxic injury	Axonotmetic injury	Neurotmetic injury
Damage	Disruption in myelin sheath around axons	Both disruption of myelin sheath with the axone but preservation of perineurium and epineurium	Complete rupture of nerve involving axon, myelin sheath and connective tissue
Severity	Least severe	Intermediate	Very severe
Functional loss	Reversible conduction loss	Variable sensory and motor loss	Complete motor and sensory loss
Spontaneous recovery	Within few weeks	Variable may be within few months	None

Fortunately 75% of the injuries are at root level C5-C6 involving neurapraxic and axonotmetic lesions which recover spontaneously.

In neurotmetic lesions and avulsions, muscle atrophy begins 3–6 months after injury, and by 1.5–2 years, it is irreversible.

Good prognosis:
- Presence of hand grasp at birth (outcome is good with surgery if hand function is preserved)
- Good antigravity function in biceps at 3 months
- Naraka's grade 1-2.

Poor prognosis:
Horner's syndrome, phrenic nerve palsy and winging of scapula suggest root avulsion.

6. **How to manage?**
   - Home/occupational/physical therapy
   - Serial examination and assessment of recovery
   - Implementation of surgical decision protocol with timely necessary surgical intervention.

7. **What is the new paradigm in the management of NBPP?**
   "All neonatal brachial plexus palsy recovers" and *"wait a year to see if recovery occurs"*—these statements do not hold true now. The improvement in surgical techniques and the need to intervene before permanent changes in the nerve, muscle and neuromuscular junction occur mean that early referral should be the new paradigm.

8. **How long the affected arm of NBPP injury should be immobilized after birth?**
   No need to immobilize unless associated with fractures. Early home-based passive physiotherapy by parents five times a day before feed as soon as the diagnosis is suspected. Goals of therapy include maintaining normal passive joint range of motion and promoting functional use of the affected extremity. No electrical stimulation till 2 months of age.

9. **What is the role of imaging in management algorithm?**
   - X-ray—fracture of clavicle or humerus or hemi paralysis of diaphragm
   - Magnetic resonance imaging (MRI) cervical spine to pick up a pseudomeningocele or a pseudomeningocele with absent rootlets. MRI can be done before surgical intervention but surgical decision is always based on clinical examination.
   - Electromyography (EMG) and nerve conduction velocity (NCV) in very selected situation as they over-optimize the outcome.
   - Ultrasonography (USG) only to confirm hemiparalysis of diaphragm.

10. **When to do surgery?**
    The decision to perform primary nerve surgery is a balancing act: on one end is the need to allow sufficient time for demonstration of spontaneous recovery, while on the other end, outcomes are improved with earlier intervention.
    - Panplexopathy with Horner's syndrome—surgery at 3 months
    - Flaccid wrist elbow persistent, i.e., no recovery at 6 months—surgery
    - Inability to complete cookie test at 9 months—surgery at 9 months

    Role of surgery decreases after 1 year of age. Surgery gives best result in a window period of 3–12 months.

11. **What is cookie test?**

    When the child is aged 9 months, a cookie is placed in his or her hand. The elbow is then held against the child's side. The test is successful if the child can get the cookie to his or her mouth without bending torso more than 45°. If the child cannot successfully complete the cookie test, primary nerve surgery is pursued.

12. **What are the surgical treatment options?**
    - Nerve grafting (resection of neuroma and sural nerve cable grafting)
    - Nerve transfer

    Finally, do not miss to screen the patient with NBPP for torticollis and speech delay which occurs with increased frequency in this population.

13. **What is the role of medicine in the management of NBPP?**

    No role.

Eruptive Xanthomatosis

Chapter 30

Ashok Kapse

CASE STUDY

A 7-year-old male child presented with waxy pea-sized bumps on extensor surface of knees, elbows and hips. He also had corneal arcus. His family history revealed that his father had similar swellings. His paternal uncle died of cardiac arrest few years back. Considering eruptive xanthomatosis, he was investigated for detailed biochemical profile. His triglycerides were 1,580 mg/dL and his father's levels were 2,750 mg/dL (Figs. 1 and 2).

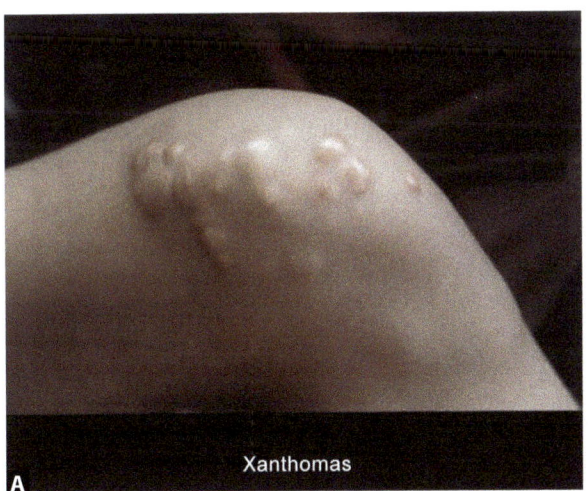
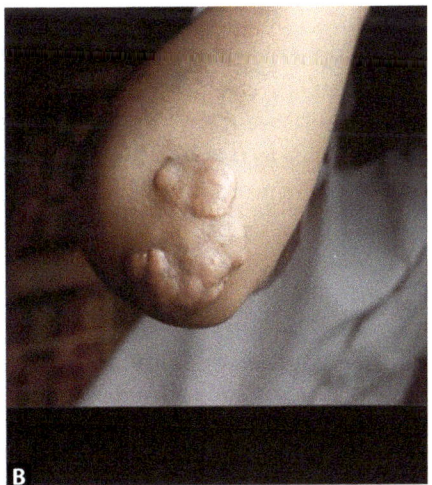

Figs. 1A and B: Xanthomas.

1. **What is eruptive xanthomatosis?**
   Eruptive xanthomatosis is a firm, yellow, waxy pea-like swellings on the skin which are surrounded by red halos and are itchy. Common sites for eruptions are eyes, elbows, face and buttocks. They can also appear on the back side of the arms and legs, particularly elbows and knees.

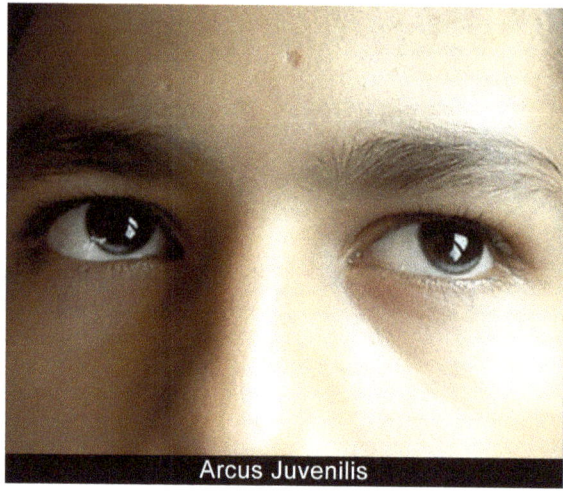

Fig. 2: Arcus juvenilis.

2. **What causes xanthomas?**
   A very high level of blood lipids causes xanthomas; they could be the manifestation of underlying systemic medical disorders like hypertriglyceridemia, hypercholesterolemia, uncontrolled diabetes, nephrotic syndrome, etc.

3. **What is corneal arcus?**
   Corneal arcus is a greyish or yellowish opaque colored ring or arc around the peripheral cornea of both eyes. The corneal arcus ring consists of lipid/cholesterol deposits in the periphery of the cornea stromal layer. It is known as arcus senilis.

4. **What is arcus juvenilis?**
   Corneal arcus developing in young age is called arcus juvenilis.

5. **What risks these patients may have?**
   They are prone for early onset coronary artery disease and pancreatitis.

6. **Is there any risk to other family members?**
   Many of the conditions that cause xanthomas are hereditary and familial; similar pathologies may exist in other members of the family, and it is very important to investigate and treat other family members.

7. **What is the most common differential diagnosis?**
   Molluscum contagiosum is the commonest confusing condition. Although both conditions have firm dome-shaped papules, molluscum contagiosum is invariably umbilicated. In histopathology, xanthomas have lipidized dermal.
   Macrophages, while molluscum has Henderson-Patterson inclusion bodies.

8. **What investigations should be done?**
   The patient needs to be investigated for lipid profile, blood sugar, thyroid profile and urinary proteins.

9. **How to treat such patients?**
   The treatment of eruptive xanthomas is focused on lowering triglycerides with medications such as fibrates, omega-3-fatty acids and nicotinic acid.

Erythema Infectiosum

Chapter 31

Atul Kulkarni

1. **What is erythema infectiosum?**
   It is the most common manifestation of human parvovirus B19, which is a benign self-limited exanthematous illness of childhood, sometimes in adults and pregnant women. It is called "fifth day disease."

2. **How is the disease transmitted?**
   Fifth disease is transmitted primarily by respiratory secretions (saliva, mucus, etc.), but can also be spread by contact with infected blood. The incubation period is usually between 4 and 21 days. Individuals with fifth disease are most infectious before the onset of symptoms. Typically, school children, day-care workers, teachers and parents are most likely to be exposed to the virus. When symptoms are evident, the risk of transmission is small; therefore, symptomatic individuals do not need to be isolated.

3. **What are the symptoms of fifth disease?**
   Fever, headache, sore throat itching, cough, diarrhea, nausea, vomiting, conjunctivitis, muscle aches, rash on the face also called as slapped cheek rash, rash over the chest, back, arms and legs, and joint pain (Figs. 1A to C).

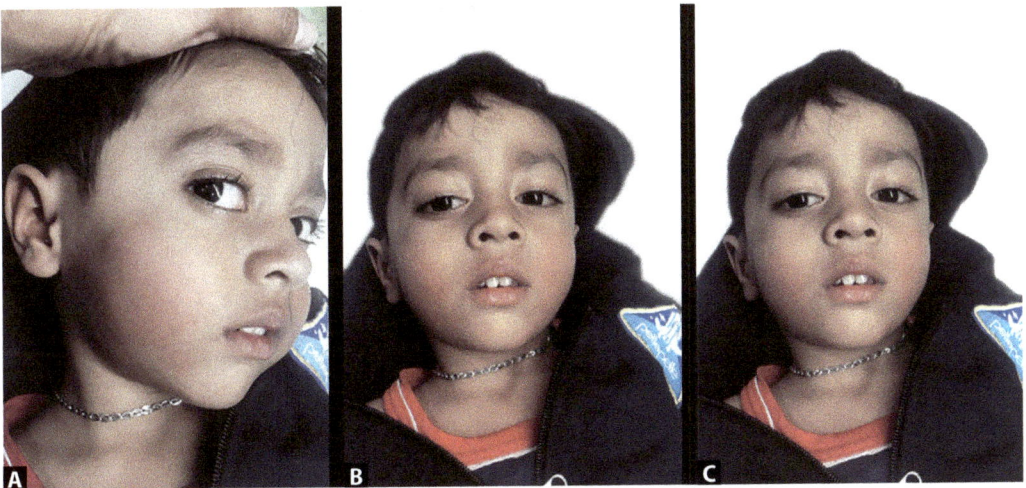

Figs. 1A to C: Case of erythema infectiosum.

4. **What is the course of illness?**
   Erythema infectiosum generally affects children between 4 and 10 years of age and manifests as a biphasic illness. Approximately 1 week after the infection occurs, a non-specific febrile illness with headache, malaise and myalgia develops; these symptoms last for 2–3 days and coincide with the onset of viremia. This is followed by an asymptomatic period of approximately 7 days and then the exanthematous phase of illness begins. The rash is immunologically mediated.
   Biphasic illness—occurrence of viremia—exanthematous illness—viremia resolves.
5. **What are the stages of exanthema?**
   - Erythematous flushing of face—slapped cheek appearance with relative circumoral pallor
   - Diffuse macular erythema—spreads to trunk and proximal extremities. Palms and soles are spared. It lasts for 1—3 weeks
   - Central clearing of lesion—reticulated lacy appearance. It lasts for 1—3 weeks.
6. **What are the causes for the recurrence of rash?**
   Rashes recur in response to a variety of non-specific environmental stimuli such as sunlight, heat, exercise or emotional stress (Fig. 2).

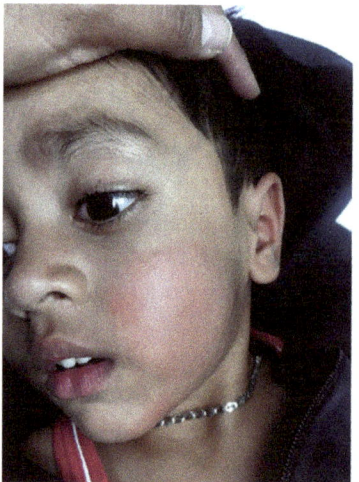

Fig. 2: Slapped cheek rash.

7. **What is the treatment of erythema infectiosum?**
   Treatment is supportive, as the infection is frequently self-limiting. Antipyretics are commonly used. The rash usually does not itch, but can be mildly painful. No specific therapy is recommended.
8. **How can the fifth day disease be prevented?**
   - Washing hands often with soaps and water, or using an alcohol hand rub.

Erythema Multiforme

Chapter 32

Ashok Kapse

CASE STUDY 1

A 3.5-year-old female child presented with mild fever, and annular non-itchy erythematous rash erupted 5 days back.

The child had history of mild upper respiratory tract infection 2 weeks back. Presently, the child has typical target lesions over thigh and buttocks, lesions started in legs and gradually ascended up. Physical examination was unremarkable except for typical rash. Lesions were limited only to skin, and mucosal involvement was absent. There was no history of drug exposure. Considering provisional diagnosis of erythema multiforme, blood samples for complete blood counts (CBC) and herpes simplex virus (HSV) and mycoplasma immunoglobulin M (IgM) were sent (Fig. 1).

The CBC was within normal limits; IgM for mycoplasma, and HSV-1 and HSV-2 were negative.

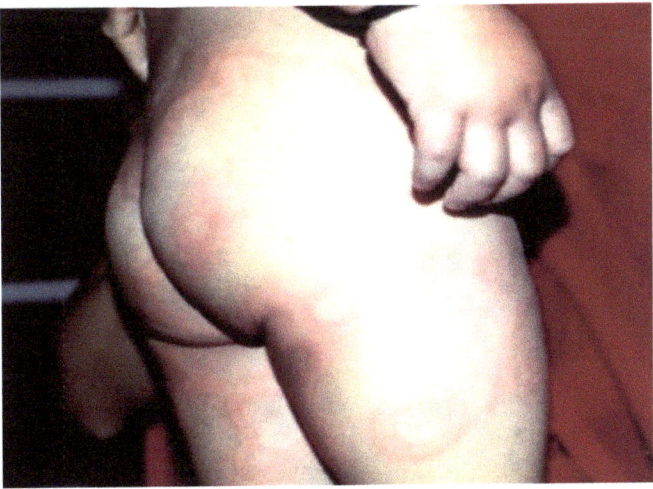

Fig. 1: Annular non-itchy erythematous rash.

CASE STUDY 2

A 2-year-old female child presented with polymorphous erythematous papular lesions; at places, lesions had incomplete targetoid character (Fig. 2).

The child had mild crusting of lips, and no other mucosa was involved. CBCs were within normal limits; HSV-1 IgM was positive.

Both cases have erythema multiforme, where first one is minor while second one is major.

1. **What is erythema multiforme (EM)?**
   Erythema multiforme is a dermal hypersensitivity reaction which presents as annular maculopapular skin eruption. There could be various triggers to erythema multiforme; however, HSV is the commonest culprit.

2. **What is the hallmark character of erythema multiforme (EM)?**
   Erythematous, maculopapules which tend to evolve into classic iris or targetoid skin lesions are the hallmark characteristics of erythema multiforme (Fig. 1).

3. **What differentiates erythema multiforme (EM) minor from erythema multiforme (EM) major?**
   Mucus membrane involvement (Fig. 2) differentiates erythema multiforme (EM) major from erythema multiforme (EM) minor.
   Major may have incomplete target lesions, two instead of three rings.

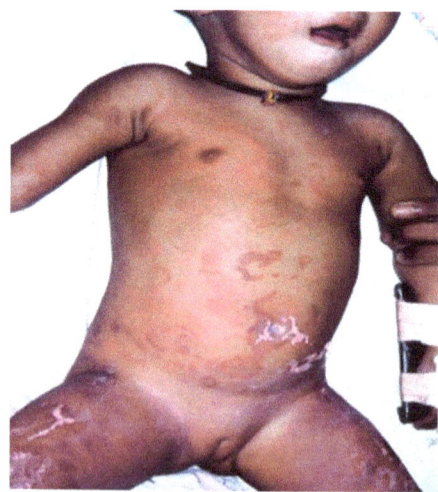

Fig. 2: Polymorphous erythematous papular lesions.

4. **What are the other features of erythema multiforme (EM) lesions?**
   Rashes are distributed symmetrically and acrally, concentrating on palms and soles, dorsum of the hands, and extensor surfaces of extremities and face. Lesions tend to have centripetal spread. Lesions are non-pruritic but may be associated with a burning sensation.
   Mucous membrane blistering occurs in about 25% of cases of EM; it is usually mild, and typically involves the oral cavity.
   Post-inflammatory hyperpigmentation or hypopigmentation may occur.

5. **Erythema multiforme (EM) and Stevens-Johnson syndrome, are they different diseases or spectrum of same disease?**
   EM and Stevens-Johnson syndrome (SJS) are different diseases; both have differing skin lesions, as against edematous maculopapular lesions of erythema multiforme. SJS is characterized by "acute disseminated epidermal necrosis" or "exanthematic necrolysis." Toxic epidermonecrolysis (TEN) is extreme extent epidermolysis where more than 30% of body surface area is necrolyzed.

6. **What are the important causative agents for erythema multiforme?**
   Common causes for erythema multiforme are infections: HSV, EBV, mycoplasma, Histoplasma are commonly implicated in EM.
   Herpes simplex is the commonest viral infection, while mycoplasma pneumonia is the most prevalent bacterial precipitant.

7. **How important is HSV in the pathogenesis of erythema multiforme (EM)?**
   Herpes simplex infection is the commonest cause in children and young adults, and is strongly associated with recurrent EM.

8. **What are the common drugs which can cause erythema multiforme (EM)?**
   EM is commonly linked to drugs; sulfonamides, nonsteroidal anti-inflammatory drugs (NSAIDs) and anticonvulsants are the commonly implicated drugs.

9. **Which are the predisposing conditions for erythema multiforme (EM)?**
   Inflammatory bowel disease (IBD), human immunodeficiency virus (HIV), systemic lupus erythematosus (SLE), bone transplant and steroid therapy increase the risk for erythema multiforme.

10. **What is the prognosis of erythema multiforme (EM)?**
    EM minor disease subsides completely in 2–3 weeks without any complications. EM major disease usually takes 3–6 weeks to resolve. One third of the cases may have recurrences.

11. **Which investigation is helpful in diagnosing erythema multiforme (EM)?**
    There are no definitive diagnostic laboratory studies for erythema multiforme.

12. **Which histologic findings are characteristic of erythema multiforme (EM)?**
    HSV antigens and HSV deoxyribonucleic acid (DNA) could be detected within keratinocytes by immunofluorescence study and polymerase chain reaction, respectively.

13. **What are the therapeutic considerations for erythema multiforme (EM)?**
    Most of the cases do not need any treatment; the rash subsides by itself over few weeks without causing any complications.
    Suspected offending drug should immediately be stopped.
    Antimicrobials like acyclovir and macrolides may be considered for proven herpes and mycoplasma infections, respectively.

14. **How should the erythema multiforme (EM) lesions be treated?**
    Antihistamine or mild steroids may be applied for itchy or burning lesions.

15. **How the recurrences could be prevented?**
    Recurrent erythema multiforme needs prolonged nearly 6 months course of acyclovir in doses of 10 mg/kg BW.

Erythema Nodosum

Chapter 33

Bakul Jayant Parekh

CASE STUDY

A 6-year-old male presented with fever for 5 days and throat pain. The patient was treated with paracetamol and antibiotics by the family physician but he develops erythematous nodular rash as in picture, so the diagnosis is erythema nodosum (Figs. 1A and B).

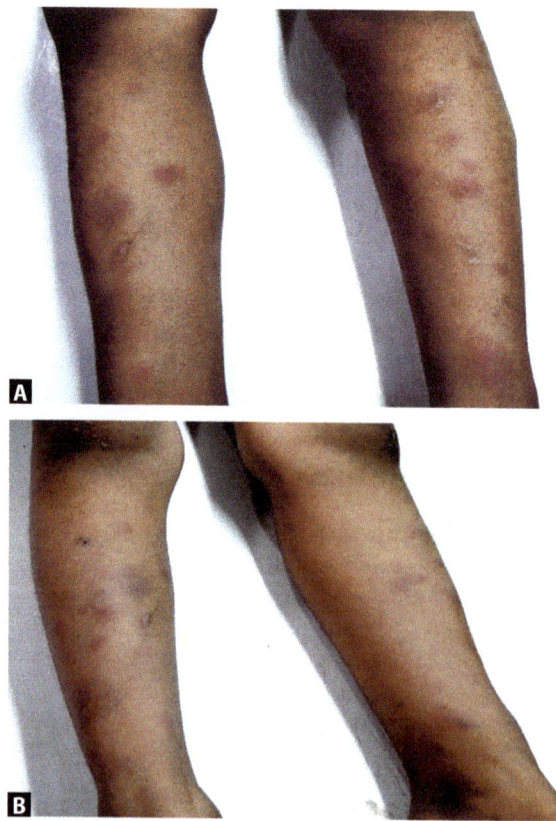

Figs. 1A and B: Cases of erythema nodosum.

1. **What is erythema nodosum?**
   Erythema nodosum is a nodular, erythematous, tender delayed type hypersensitivity reaction that typically appears with multiple lesions on the surfaces of the arms and legs, in the pretibial areas more common and less common in other cutaneous areas containing subcutaneous fat.

2. **What is the etiology of the erythema nodosum?**
   Infection is the most commonly identified etiology.
   - Bacterial—streptococcal (most common)
   - Others—tuberculosis, yersinia, cat scratch disease, leprosy, leptospirosis, tularemia, mycoplasma, whipple disease, lymphogranuloma venereum, psittacosis, brucellosis, etc.
   - Viruses—Epstein-Barr, mumps, hepatitis B, paravaccinia, etc.
   - Fungal—blastomycosis, sporotrichosis, histoplasmosis, coccidioidomycosis, etc.
   - Others drugs—oral contraceptives, penicillin, sulfonamide, bromides and iodides, tumor necrosis factor-alpha (TNF-alpha) inhibitors (rare)
   - Inflammatory bowel disease
   - Malignancy—lymphoma (Hodgkin's most common)
   - Leukemia [Acute myeloid leukemia (AML) most common]
   - Internal carcinomas
   - Miscellaneous—sarcoidosis, pregnancy, Whipple disease, Behcet's disease, sweet syndrome, etc.

3. **What is the epidemiology of erythema nodosum?**
   Erythema nodosum occurs in all age groups, sex and races; most common in women in second to fourth decades.

4. **What is the pathogenesis of erythema nodosum?**
   EN involves immune complex deposition in the septal venules of the subcutaneous fat, neutrophil recruitment with resulting reactive oxygen species formation, TNF-alpha production and granuloma formation. EN is predominantly septal panniculitis without primary vasculitis. Thrombophlebitis may be present in cases associated with Behcet's syndrome. Miescher's radial granulomas are a characteristic feature of early EN. With time, septal thickening occurs with mixed and granulomatous infiltrate leading to fibrosis and extension of inflammation into the adjacent fat lobules.

5. **What are the clinical manifestations of erythema nodosum?**
   Lesions appear initially bright or dull red but progress to brown or purple. They are tense and painful and usually do not ulcerate. The lesions vary in size from 1 to 6 cm, and are symmetric, oval with longer axis parallel to the extremity. Initial lesions may resolve in 1–2 weeks, but new lesions may continue to appear for 2–6 weeks; this secondary bruising is known as erythema contusiforms. Repeated episodes may occur weeks to months later. There may be systemic manifestations that include fever, malaise, arthralgias, upper respiratory infection symptoms, joint swelling and rheumatoid factor negative arthritis.

6. **How to diagnose erythema nodosum?**
   Clinical assessment: First, based on the history and the physical examination. They are present most commonly bilaterally on shins with absent ulcerations. Skin biopsy may be helpful for patients with atypical presentation. Evaluation of underlying disease is a must.
   Laboratory and radiological tests: Complete blood count (CBC), erythrocyte sedimentation rate (ESR), antistreptolysin O (ASO) titers, diagnostic test for streptococcal pharyngitis, chest X-ray, tuberculin test, etc.

7. **What is the differential diagnosis for erythema nodosum?**
   - Nodular vasculitis (erythema induratum/Bazin's disease)
   - Subcutaneous bacterial, fungal or mycobacterial infections
   - Cutaneous polyarteritis nodosa
   - Malignant subcutaneous infiltrates
   - Pancreatic panniculitis
   - Alpha 1 antitrypsin deficiency.

8. **What is the treatment of choice for erythema nodosum?**
   - Treatment of underlying disease, leg elevation, rest and compression.
   - First line is nonsteroidal anti-inflammatory drugs (NSAIDs) (ibuprofen, naproxen, indomethacin, etc.) and potassium iodide.
   - Others—salicylates, colchicines, intraintestinal injections of steroids, and in severe persistent cases, oral steroids.

Erythema Nodosum 2

Chapter 34

Aniruddha Ghosh, Ritabrata Kundu

CASE STUDY

A 6-year-old girl presented with fever and cough for last 10 days. She had associated myalgia and arthralgia for last 2 days. On examination, multiple nodular erythematous eruptions of 2–3 cm size were noted over bilateral shin bones. There was no history of any drug intake. Suspecting the lesions to be erythema nodosum and pulmonary tuberculosis to be the primary cause, tuberculin skin test (TST) was done which turned out to be positive, GeneXpert from induced sputum also became positive. As anti-TB therapy was started, gradually the lesions subsided.

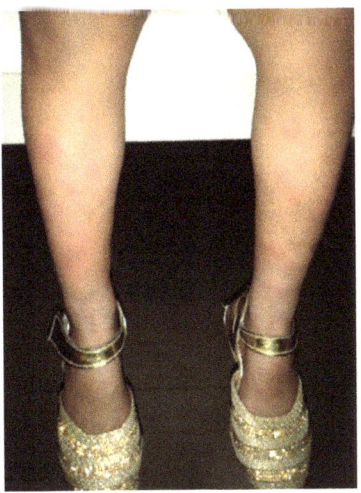

Fig.1: Case of erythema nodosum.

1. **How does erythema nodosum look like?**
   Erythema nodosum (Fig. 1) are tender nodules, bright to deep red in color (which may turn to purple and then brown with time), 1–5 cm in size, round to oval in shape, distributed most commonly over pretibial areas (pretibial areas > thighs/forearms > trunk > neck > face).
2. **What are the systemic symptoms most commonly associated with erythema nodosum?**
   Fever, arthritis, myalgia, etc., along with symptoms of any underlying disease.
3. **What is the pathophysiology of these lesions?**
   Erythema nodosum appears due to delayed type hypersensitivity to various stimuli.
4. **What are the stimuli that trigger erythema nodosum?**
   In 40% of the cases, erythema nodosum is *idiopathic* but there are other possible triggers, which are as follows:
   - *Infections:* Streptococcus, Salmonella, Yersinia, Campylobacter, tuberculosis, Chlamydia, cat-scratch fever, hepatitis B, Epstein-Barr virus, mycoses, mycoplasma, leishmaniasis, pertussis, syphilis, human immunodeficiency virus (HIV), etc.
   - *Drugs:* Sulfonamides, oral contraceptive pill (OCP), phenytoin, iodides, etc.
   - *Malignancy:* Leukemia, lymphoma, etc.
   - *Gastrointestinal disorders:* Ulcerative colitis, Crohn's disease, etc.
   - *Others:* Sarcoidosis, Bechet's disease, etc.
5. **What are the differential diagnoses of erythema nodosum?**
   Ecchymoses, cellulitis, erysipelas, deep mycoses, insect bites, thrombophlebitis, erythema induratum and other panniculitides.
6. **What are the histopathological findings of erythema nodosum?**
   Septal panniculitis in the dermis, subcutaneous fat, perivascularly in the septum and adjacent fat.
7. **What is the natural history of the lesions?**
   First warm tender nodules appear around pretibial area, and then gradually over 3–6 weeks, they subside with rest and leg elevation if the underlying disease is cured or the inciting drug is stopped.
8. **Can erythema nodosum recur?**
   Erythema nodosum may be recurrent if there is recurrent infection like in the cases of recurrent streptococcal infection.
9. **How do you manage erythema nodosum?**
   Skin lesions can be managed with rest, leg elevation, compression bandages, salicylates and other nonsteroidal anti-inflammatory drugs (NSAIDs) (NSAIDs are to be avoided in the case of inflammatory bowel diseases as they might cause disease flare). Identification and elimination of underlying cause is the most important treatment.
   Intralesional or systemic steroids can be used if infectious causes have been ruled out. Other treatment options include colchicines, potassium iodide, hydrochloroquine, cyclosporine A and thalidomide.

Fanconi Anemia

Chapter 35

Nirav Buch

CASE STUDY

A 7 year old boy referred for incidentally diagnosed pancytopenia for work up of fever. He was a known case of solitary kidney. He had short stature less than 3rd centile. He was born to a 3rd degree consanguineous wedlock. He had facial dysmorphism, extra digits (Figs. 1A and B). There was no organomegaly or lymph node enlargement. Complete blood count showed Hb 5.8 gm%, WBC 2600, polymorphs 25%, lymphocytes 65%, monocytes 7% and eosinophils 3%. RBC count 1.6 million/dL, mean corpuscular volume (MCV) 96 femtoliters (fL) and reticulocytes 0.5%. Bone Marrow examination revealed markedly hypocellular marrow with markedly reduced trilineage hematopoiesis. There was no increase in blasts. Cytogenetic evaluation showed normal 46; XY phenotype. Mitomycin C induced chromosomal break studies showed increased breakages. Diagnosis of Fanconi anemia was established.

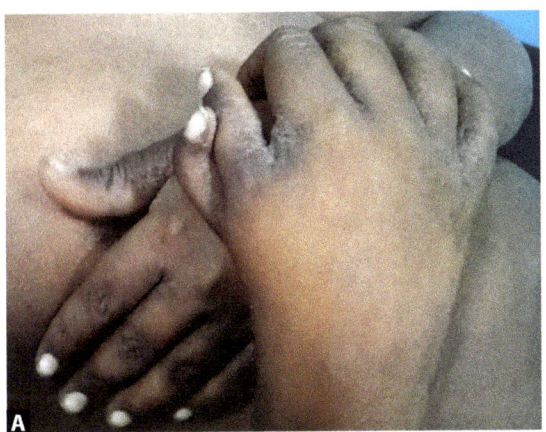 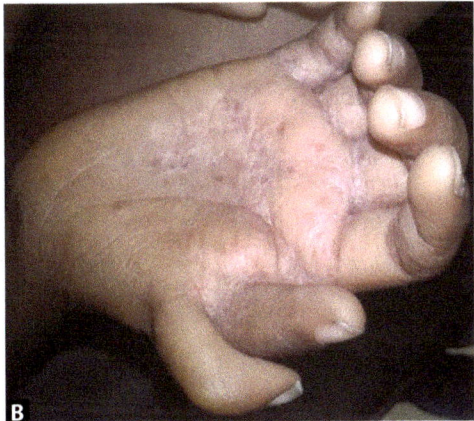

Fig. 1: Patient having extra digits.

1. **What is the function of Fanconi anemia genes in DNA repair pathway?**
   Fanconi anemia results from mutations in any of the sixteen FANC genes that produce an anchor complex that is involved in identification and repair of DNA. Interstrand crosslinks and maintaining genomic stability.

2. **Which patients should be evaluated for FA?**
   - Any patient with:

Height	Short stature microsomia
Skin	Café au lait spots skin pigmentation (hyper, hypo)
Upper limbs	Radius: absent, hypoplastic, absent or weak pulse Thumb: absent, hypoplastic, bifid, duplicated, rudimentary, attached by thread, triphalangeal, long, low set, digitized Thenar-eminence: flat, absent Hand: absent first metacarpal, clinodactyly, polydactyly Ulna: short, dysplastic
Skeletal	Head: microcephaly, hydrocephaly Face: triangular, birdlike, dysmorphic, mid-face hypoplasia Neck: Sprengel, Klippel-Feil, short, low hairline, web Spine: spina bifida, scoliosis, hemivertebrae, coccygeal aplasia small, strabismus, epicanthal folds, hypotelorism, hypertelorism
Eyes	Strabismus, cataracts, ptosis
Renal	Horseshoe, ectopic, pelvic, hypoplastic, dysplastic, absent, hydronephrosis, hydroureter
Gonads, male, urology	Hypogenitalia, undescended testis, hypospadias, micropenis, absent testis, infertility
Gonads, female, gynecology	Hypogenitalia, bicornuate uterus, malposition, small ovaries, late menarche, early menopause, infertility
Development	Mental retardation, developmental delay
Ears	Deafness: conductive, sensorineural, mixed Shape: abnormal pinna, dysplastic, atretic, narrow canal, abnormal middle ear bones Speech: delayed, unclear
Cardiopulmonary	Congenital heart disease: patent ductus arteriosus, atrial septal defect, ventricular septal defect, coarcta
Low birth weight	
Lower limbs	Hips: congenital hip dislocation Feet: toe syndactyly, abnormal toes, club feet
Gastrointestinal	Tracheoesophageal fistula atresia: esophagus, duodenum, jejunum, imperforate anus, annular pancreas Malrotation Poor feeding
Central nervous system	Pituitary: small, stalk interruption Structure: absent corpus callosum, cerebellar hypoplasia, hydrocephalus, dilated ventricles

   - Any patient with family history of:

Any suspicion or patient

   - Family history of Vacterl-H:

Any patient	Especially if both radial ray and renal anomalies are preset

   - Family history of hematology:

Aplastic anemia Acute myeloid leukemia Myelodysplastic syndrome	Any patient

- Family history of tumors:

Head and neck SCC	"Young"- less than 50 years old
Vulvar/vaginal SCC	
Cervical SCC	
Esophageal SCC	
Brain tumor midline	
Medulloblastoma	
Wilms tumor	
Neuroblastoma	
Retinoblastoma	

- Sibling or child of Fanconi anemia patient:

Sibling or child of FA patient cytogenetics	Abnormal chromosome tests (e.g., breaks) without DNA crosslinker in study done for non-FA purpose

3. **What are other disorders that are associated with chromosomal instability.?**
   Disorders that may share clinical features with FA and manifest with chromosome instability: Disorder Putative Genes Involved Ataxia-telangiectasia ATM, Ataxia-telangiectasia-like disorder MRE11, Bloom syndrome, BLM DNA ligase 4 syndrome, LIG4 Dubowitz syndrome, Dyskeratosis congenita DKC1, TERT, TERC, WRAP53, NOP10, NHP2, TINF2, RTEL1, CTC1, Nijmegen breakage syndrome, NBN Nijmegen breakage syndrome-like disorder, RAD50 Roberts syndrome, ESCO2 Rothmund-Thomson syndrome, RECQL4 Seckel syndrome 1 ATR Severe combined immunodeficiency NHEJ1 Warsaw breakage syndrome DDX11.

4. **What are the other inherited bone marrow failure syndromes?**
   Fanconi anemia, dyskeratosis congenita, diamond blackfan anemia, swachman diamond syndrome, severe congenital neutropenia, Kostmann syndrome, megakaryocytic thrombocytopenia, thrombocytopenia absent radii.

5. **How do we treat Fanconi anemia?**
   - Anabolic steroids
   - Stem cell transplantation
   - Supportive care depending on organs involved example skin oral hematopoietic endocrine locomotor nutritional and gastrointestinal and renal problems.
   - Prenatal diagnosis and family screening for careers status.

6. **How is Fanconi anemia inherited?**
   Most commonly Fanconi anemia is inherited as an autosomal recessive disorder however about 2% are inherited as X linked recessive condition (one of the 16 genotypes).

Foreign Body in Bronchus

Chapter 36

Aroon Narendra Trivedi

CASE STUDY 1

A 1-month-old child was brought with severe respiratory distress and with a history of foreign body insertion in the mouth by elder sibling (Figs. 1A and B). The child was resuscitated and a metallic foreign body was removed (Fig. 2).

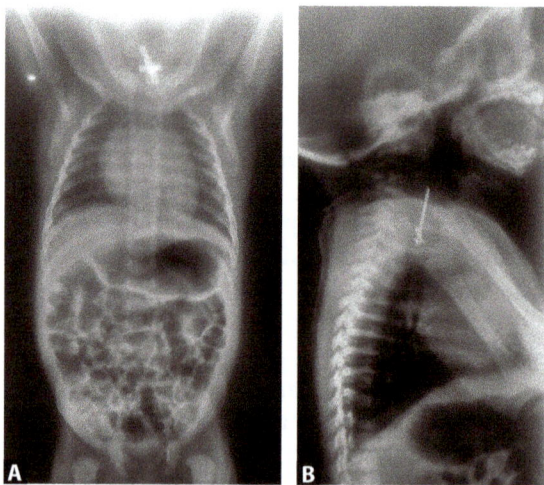

Fig. 1A and B: X-ray showing foreign body.

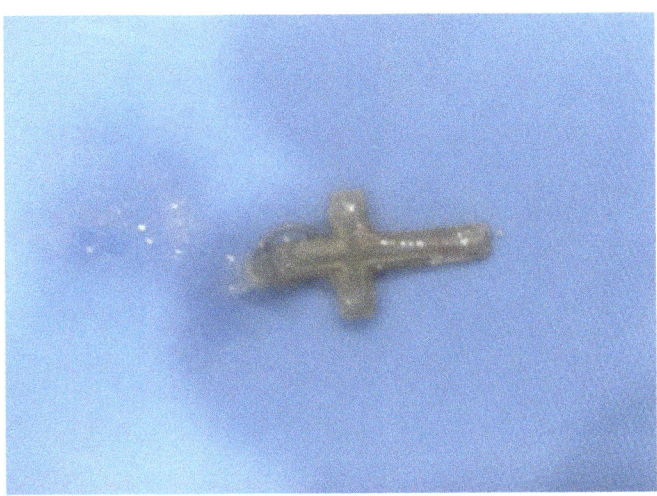

Fig. 2: Child was resuscitated and a metallic foreign body was removed.

CASE STUDY 2

A 13-month-old child presented with chronic cough, and no significant history. X-ray chest showed symptoms of hyperinflated right lung (Fig. 3). There was absence of air entry on right side. The child underwent a bronchoscopy and groundnut pieces were removed (Fig. 4).

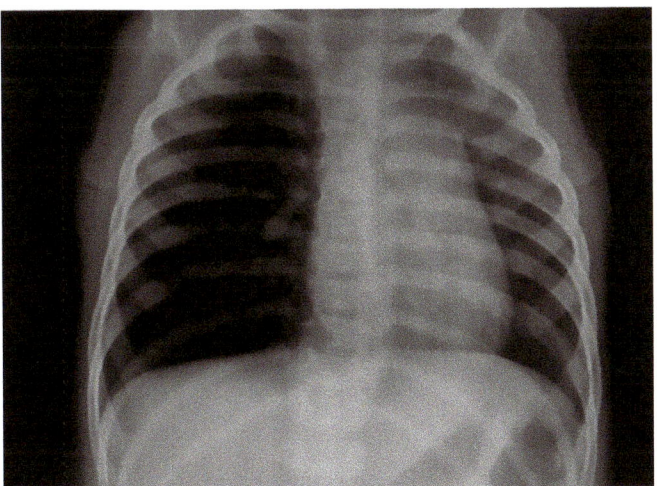

Fig. 3: Hyperinflated right lung.

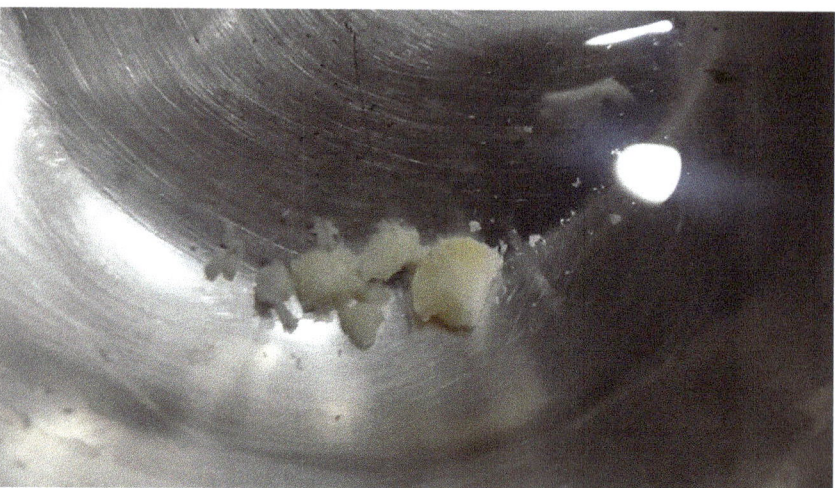

Fig. 4: Child underwent a bronchoscopy and groundnut pieces were removed.

CASE STUDY 3

A 2-year-old child came with cough, and no significant history. X-ray was not indicative of any anomaly. The child underwent computed tomography (CT) virtual bronchoscopy which confirmed the presence of a foreign body. It was removed by bronchoscopy (Figs. 5 and 6).

Foreign body bronchus is a life-threatening condition in which prompt diagnosis and urgent bronchoscopy is a must.

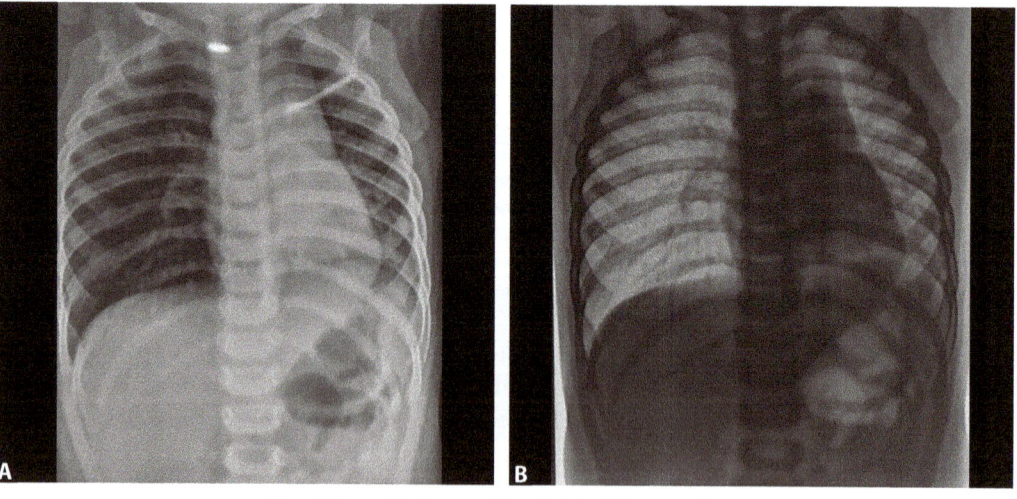

Figs. 5A and B: X-ray of the child of Case study 3.

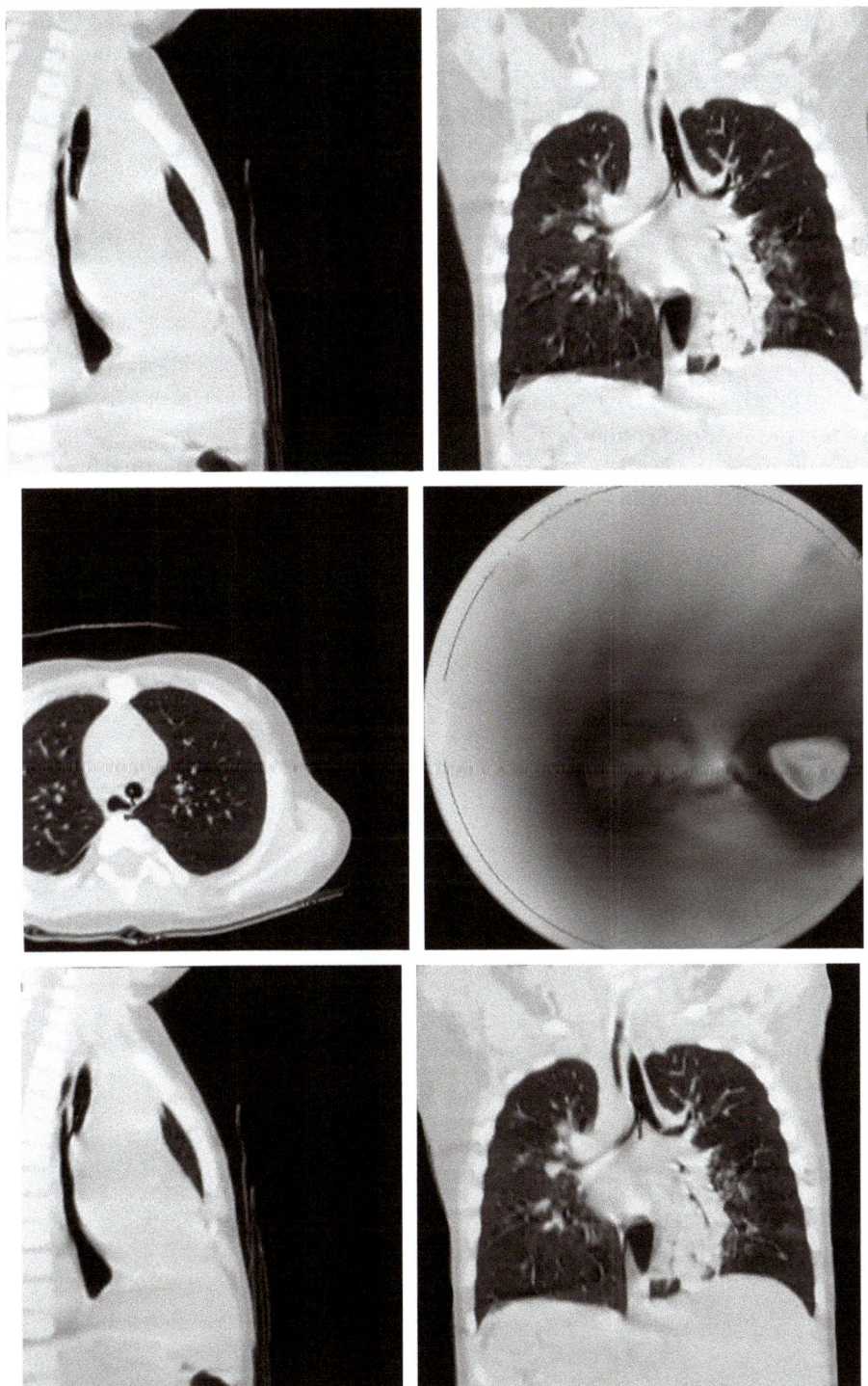

Fig. 6: Child underwent computed tomography (CT) virtual bronchoscopy which confirmed the presence of a foreign body (Case Study 3).

1. **What are the Diagnostic Features of Foreign Body Bronchus?**
   A confirmative history along with absent or grossly reduced air entry on the affected side will confirm the diagnosis.
   In the case of uncertain history and clinical findings, an X-ray chest may show hyperinflated lung on the affected side.
   A CT virtual bronchoscopy will confirm the diagnosis in all cases.
2. **Are Routine Blood Investigation of Any Help?**
   Routine blood investigations may show non-specific leucocytosis. They are helpful primarily for anesthesia purposes.
3. **What are the Distinctive X-ray Findings in FB Inhalation?**
   Chest X-ray will be normal in approximately 40% of the cases. In an expiration X-ray, there may be overinflated and hyper lucent lung with rib flaring and a depressed ipsilateral hemidiaphragm.
4. **What is the Role of Bronchoscopy in FB in Airway Foreign Bodies?**
   While flexible bronchoscopy remains the gold standard for diagnosis, rigid bronchoscopy is the preferred method for retrieval of foreign body.

Febrile Urticaria

Chapter 37

Vasant Khalatkar

CASE STUDY

A 13-year-old female admitted with acute onset of high-grade fever with urticarial patch all over body (Figs.1A and B). There was no other associated symptom related to fever. On examination child was febrile,103°F with multiple itchy wheals on the body. Wheals were erythematous with irregular border. Systemic examination was normal. Investigation: Total leucocyte count (TLC) 21,630/cu. mm with neutrophil 86%, C-reactive protein (CRP) was 54.2, serum IgE 162 IU/mL, urine showed pus cell with E. Coli, X-ray nasopharynx showed adenoid hypertrophy. Rest investigations like stool routine, dengue antibody and blood culture were negative.

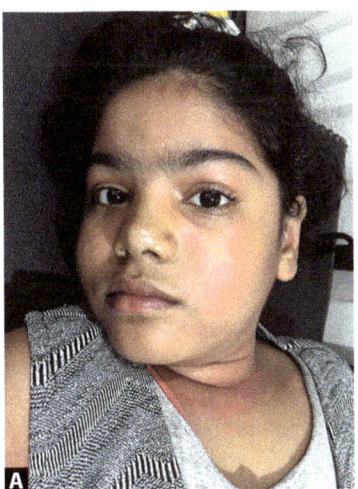 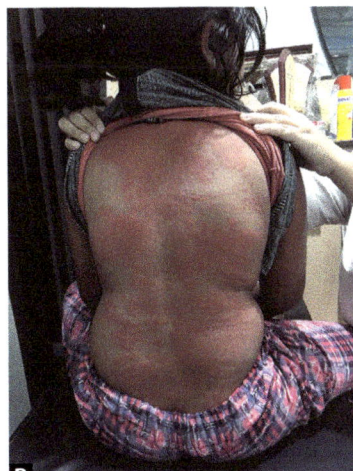

Figs.1A and B: Urticarial patch all over the body.

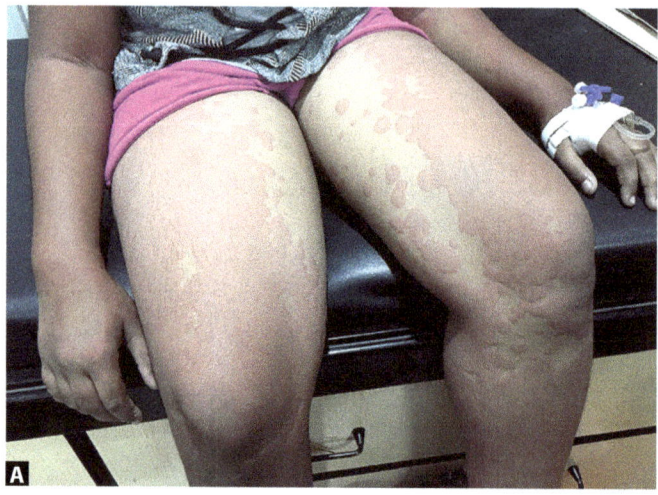
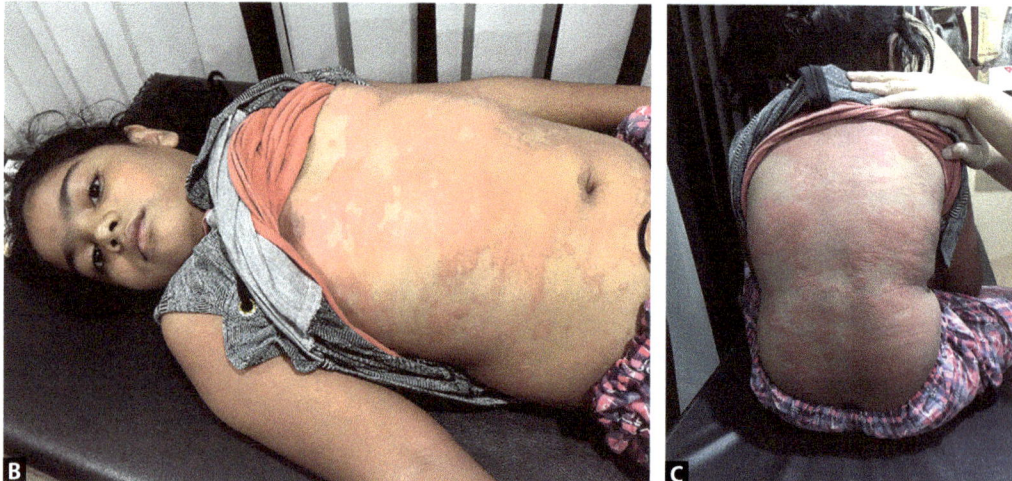

Figs. 2A to C: Itchy wheal seen on the thigh, stomach and on the back.

Diagnosis: Febrile Urticaria.

1. **What is febrile urticaria?**
   Febrile Urticaria is distinct skin reaction with occurrence of itchy wheals anywhere on the skin along with fever (Figs. 2A to C). Wheals are short lived elevated erythematous lesion, with irregular border ranging from a few millimeters to several centimeters in diameter and can become confluent. It is always associated with high grade fever. The itching can be pricking or burning but there is no excoriation of skin.

2. **What is pathophysiology of Urticaria?**
   It is the result of agranulation of mast cells and basophils with release of mediators like histamine. Degranulation is induced by immune mediated functional autoantibody against the high affinity IgE receptors.

3. **What is etiology of febrile Urticaria?**

   It can be infectious or noninfectious. It can be bacterial- Mycoplasma or viral like Entero virus, Adeno virus, Parvovirus B 19, EBV, Hepatitis, HIV, and Lyme disease. It can be noninfectious like allergy, vasculitis, malignancy, Influenza vaccination, or idiopathic. Dental sepsis, sinusitis upper respiratory tract infection, Urinary tract infection and cutaneous fungal infection can also lead to febrile urticaria.

4. **How will you investigate a patient with febrile urticaria?**

   Febrile urticaria is a self-limiting condition, but it may present with decreased ability to work or generalized malaise. It can present with dreaded angioedema at times so it is important to investigate. One need to do complete blood count (CBC), C-reactive protein (CRP), liver function test (LFT), Stool®, Urine® and X ray.

   Complete count shows leukocytosis, raise eosinophil counts. C. reactive protein and hepatic enzymes may be increase. Stool examination should be done to detect cva/cyst if there is eosinophilia as it helps to detect parasite. ESR may be raised in chronic infection, raised serum IgE level help to detect chronic urticaria. Blood culture and urine culture are important to rule out cystitis and septicemia. Sinus and Dental radiography should be done. Screening for *H. pylori* infection, and allergy testing is recommended for recurrent urticaria. Allergy skin testing for food can be helpful in acute urticaria.

   Besides a careful history for infections routine diagnostic work-up (i) differential blood count and C-reactive protein, (ii) *Helicobacter pylori* monoclonal stool antigen test, and (iii) serology for streptococci (antistreptolysin, anti-DNase B), staphylococci (antistaphylolysin), yersinia (IgA, IgG, immunoblot) has to be done. If an infection is identified, it should be appropriately treated, and it should be checked whether eradication has been achieved or not.

5. **What is differential diagnosis for Febrile Urticaria?**

   Cholinergic urticaria caused by increased body temperature after physical exercise and emotional stress is common in young adults Dermatographic urticaria (Urticaria facilitia) which occur after infection or drug intake (Penicillin). Cutaneous or systemic mastocytosis, complement mediated disorders, malignancies, mixed connective tissue diseases can present like febrile urticaria.

6. **How do you manage such patients?**

   Good history and examination along with investigation will help to diagnosis the disease. As it is self limiting condition nothing much has to be done. Antihistaminics-hydroxyzine and diphenhydromine can be given. Treat the infections, avoid provoking element. Immunomodulatory agents have to be used in refractory cases.

Forehead Hematoma: Unveiling as "Child Abuse"

Uma Siddhartha Nayak

PREAMBLE

We, pediatricians, are primarily caretakers of childhood illnesses as well as of the health of children. We all provide preventive and curative services. Should we be concerned with other issues of children like right to education, protection, safety, security and child rights in general? Probably yes. IAP themes in the past have been "child rights and protection," "Save the girl child" and "every child in school." Therefore, while treating our patients, our child patient's overall well-being and rights and protection are aspects that we need to attend to in certain situations. Here is one such patient.

CLINICAL PRESENTATION

Ria Nimeshbhai Patel (name changed), A 16-month-old girl was seen in our outpatient department (OPD) in February/March 2012. The father complained of a swelling on the forehead (Fig. 1) for the last 3 days.

The resident on duty in the OPD went into details of history and found out that the swelling was due to a fall. On examination, she also had ecchymosis around both eyes and no other significant findings (Fig. 2). She was admitted primarily for workup and observation. Her weight

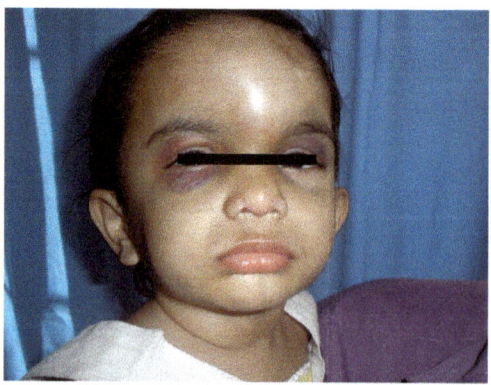

Fig. 1: Forehead swelling.

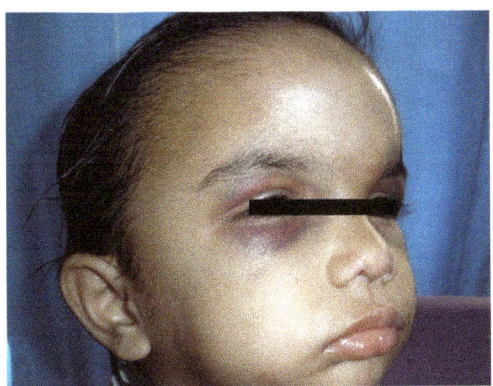

Fig. 2: Peri-orbital ecchymosis.

was 7.3 Kg, hemoglobin (Hb) was 9.3 g/dL. Routine complete blood count (CBC) and bleeding profile was normal. The family was a middle-class family, the father had a decent job and the delay in seeking medical help for this alarming looking condition could not be explained. *Neglect on the part of the family was clearly visible.* When I saw this child in rounds, I probed into further history and over the next few days after spending hours in talking to the family, the following relevant past and family history could be extracted.

Additional Past and Family History

- Significant past history of recurrent ecchymosis on different parts of the body was obtained. Paternal uncle (kaka) showed a photograph of the same. He seemed to be the only person concerned.
- On day 3, they brought two files of hematologists who had been consulted for previous episodes. However, all investigations done on two earlier occasions were all within normal limits.
- The father was 37 and the mother around 35, a little too old for a 16-month-old child—their only child.
- The parents did not seem to share a normal relationship but were overall subdued.
- Child abuse was a very likely possibility, and hence on day 4, on further probing the other family members (the kaka and kaki) came to meet and further alarming past history came out.
- Neither we nor the relatives had uttered the child abuse possibility yet. However, a past history, which is 6 months ago, of a fractured left humerus came up (Fig. 3). An old X-ray showed a spiral fracture, common in a case of injury in the form of a twisting force.
- *Differential diagnosis originally considered for the hematoma:* (1) Vitamin C deficiency; however, signs of scurvy were not seen on X-ray of the knee. (2) Idiopathic thrombocytopenic purpura (ITP) was not strongly considered as there were no petechiae (but ecchymosis) and platelet count was normal. (3) Platelet function disorders were kept as a remote possibility.
- *Child abuse and neglect was strongly suspected:* Physical and emotional abuse.
- Growth faltering in a family which was not resource restricted.

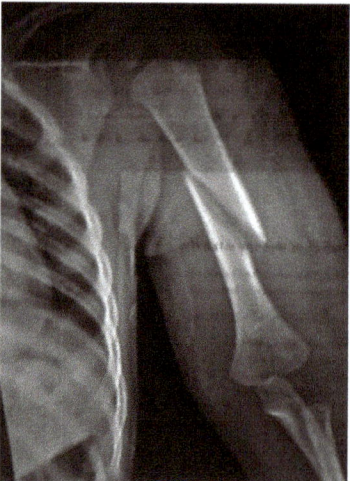

Fig. 3: Fracture humerus: spiral type.

- Recurrent ecchymosis with no hematological abnormality. But why and who was causing it still eluded us
- Fracture humerus and that too due to a twist injury
- Suspicious history of head trauma
- Mild developmental delay
- Some form of family disharmony.

Opening of the Pandora's Box

As the possibility of a police complaint for suspected child abuse strongly came up, the family finally opened up. The extended family thought that the mother was the culprit as she was a step mother. The mother then opened up for the first time after many episodes of health problems. She had two children from a previous marriage and was abusing this child in fits of rage as she was not allowed to meet her real children by the court. The husband, however, wanted to still save the marriage.

THE FINAL DIAGNOSIS: CHILD ABUSE BY STEP MOTHER: PHYSICAL AND EMOTIONAL

1. **What is child abuse and what are the different forms of child abuse?**
   The term child abuse refers to any act or failure to act that violates the rights of the child that endangers his or her optimum health, survival or development. A recent world health organization (WHO) estimate shows that 40 million children aged 0–14 around the world suffer from abuse and neglect, and require health and social care. The forms of abuse are: physical abuse, sexual abuse, neglect and emotional (psychological) abuse (Fig. 4).

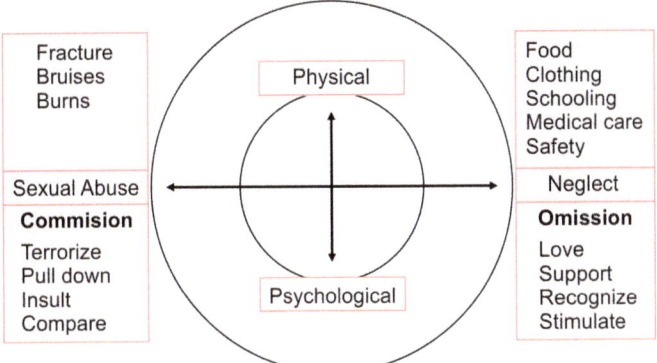

Fig. 4: Forms and types of child abuse.

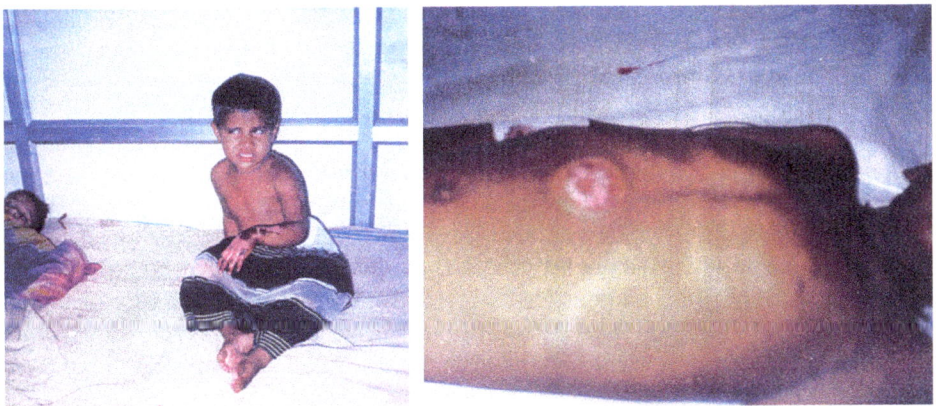

Fig. 5: Other forms of physical abuse: burns; branding.

2. **What is the magnitude of child abuse?**
A study of child abuse was conducted by Ministry of Women and Child Development (WCD) in 2007 in 13 states in India. Sound methodology was used, and child and young adult respondents were chosen from five environments, namely children from families, schools, institutional care, street children and working children. Out of 12,447 respondents, a whopping 69% suffered physical abuse, (50% by mothers, 32% by fathers and the rest by others), 50% reported sexual abuse and 50% reported some form of emotional abuse. *Two out of every three children were physically abused, one out of three girls and one out of six boys were sexually abused, and every second child was emotionally abused.*
In a study carried out at MS university, Baroda, India by Uma Nayak et al. from January 2003 to March 2005, 63 cases of child abuse were reported of which the distribution was: physical abuse 17% (Fig. 5), neglect 19%, emotional abuse 2% and sexual abuse 62%. Sexual abuse cases were picked up only from records of medicolegal OPD and surprisingly had not even been referred to Obstetric Department or Pediatric Department unless very sick.

3. **How is child sexual abuse (CSA) defined?**
   CSA is the involvement of a child in sexual activity that she/he does not fully comprehend, is unable to give informed consent to, or for which the child is not developmentally prepared, or that violate the laws or social taboos of society.

4. **What constitutes CSA?**
   CSA is evidenced by an activity between a child and an adult or another child who by age or development is in a relationship of responsibility, trust or power; the activity being intended to gratify or satisfy the needs of other person.

5. **What are the types of CSA?**
   Three types of CSA are often distinguished: (1) non-contact sexual abuse (e.g., threats of sexual abuse, verbal sexual harassment, sexual solicitation, indecent exposure and exposing the child to pornography); (2) contact sexual abuse involving sexual intercourse (i.e., sexual assault or rape); (3) contact sexual abuse excluding sexual intercourse but involving other acts such as inappropriate touching, fondling and kissing.

6. **What are characteristics of CSA?**
   Not only girls but boys too could be *victims* of CSA.
   Institutionalized children, differently abled children, those staying in hostels are at a *greater risk*.
   CSA is often carried out *without* physical force, but rather with manipulation and "grooming" (e.g., psychological, emotional or material).
   It may occur on a *frequent* basis over weeks or even years, as repeated episodes that become more invasive over time, and it can also occur on a single occasion.
   According to a study carried out by *RAHI, a Delhi-based organization* in 1997, focusing on English speaking upper- and middle-class ladies from five metro cities in the country, it was found that 68% of those who had been abused were living in nuclear families, 60% said their mothers were housewives and 54% of the survivors had told someone about the abuse.
   Child protection is needed at *all places* where CSA can occur: own home, home of a friend or relative, school, parks, school transport and public transport.
   The main reasons given *for not telling anyone* about the abuse were: wanting to forget it happened (23%), fear of what people would think of them (14%), self-blame for the abuse (11%) and not having anyone to trust (11%). Only 3% did not tell because the abuser had threatened them. Only 1% did not tell because they were bribed by the abuser.

7. **How can CSA be prevented?**
   By teaching and training parents, teachers and medical and paramedical professionals to recognize *warning signs* like a suddenly subdued child, school absenteeism, academic faltering, inappropriate sexual play and inappropriately close to "uncles," "neighbors," etc.
   It is also extremely important to orient children to CSA in an age-appropriate manner and teach them good touch and bad touch (swim suit area) as well as to learn to say NO in situations of discomfort and to YELL and RUN.

8. **What is POCSO?**
   Prevention of children from Sexual Offences (POCSO Act 2012), The Protection of Children from Sexual Offences Act, 2012, specifically addresses the issue of sexual offences committed against children, which until now had been tried under laws that did not differentiate between adult and child victims. In order to effectively address the heinous crimes of sexual abuse and sexual exploitation of children through less ambiguous and more

stringent legal provisions, the Ministry of Women and Child Development championed the introduction of the POCSO Act, 2012.

The *punishments* provided in the law are also stringent and are commensurate with the gravity of the offence. It deems a sexual assault to be "aggravated" when abuse is committed by a person in a position of trust or authority vis-a-vis the child, such as a family member, police officer, teacher or doctor. Different levels of punishment are included, which are more stringent in cases of aggravated assault.

Under this Act, various child friendly procedures are put in place at various stages of the judicial process. Also, the Special Court is to complete the trial within a period of *one year*, as far as possible.

Disclosing the name of the child in the media is a punishable offence, punishable by up to 1 year.

It clearly describes various forms of *sexual misconducts* including actual or attempted sexual intercourse, oral sex, fondling sexual parts, pornography and inappropriately photographing. POCSO is a comprehensive law, which besides expanding the scope and range of forms of CSA, makes its *reporting mandatory* and gives guidelines for various actions by the police and at courts. Physicians are made responsible for ensuring prompt and adequate response to child victims.

The law provides for *relief and rehabilitation* of the child, as soon as the complaint is made to the Special Juvenile Police Unit (SJPU) or to the local police. Immediate and adequate care and protection (such as admitting the child into a shelter home or to the nearest hospital within 24 hours of the report) are provided. The Child Welfare Committee (CWC) is also required to be notified within 24 hours of recording the complaint. Moreover, it is a mandate of the National Commission for the Protection of Child Rights (NCPCR) and State Commissions for the Protection of Child Rights (SCPCR) to monitor the implementation of the Act.

9. **What is a doctor's role in response to CSA?**

    Every case of sexual assault is a medical emergency for which free treatment is mandatory at government or private medical facilities, and no document or precondition is necessary for providing emergency medical care.

    A medical history is to be sought and examination carried out in utmost child friendly atmosphere without being judgmental and after informed consent by parents if <12 years old and also from the child if >12 years old.

    Forensic examination and sample collection for infections, sexually transmitted disease (STD) and human immunodeficiency virus (HIV) are to be done for evidence of sexual assault.

    Emergency management is to be offered and mandatory reporting is to be done by the doctor.

    Responding to CSA and the details of examination and treatment are described in detail in a recent WHO publication 2017 titled "Responding to children and adolescents who have been sexually abused: WHO clinical guidelines 2017."

10. **What is the "multidisciplinary approach" to CSA?**

    The POCSO envisages a multidisciplinary approach wherein there is a convergence of all stake holders like different departments within the medical facility like gynecologist, pediatrician, forensic expert, pediatric surgeon, psychiatrist and others like the police personnel, social worker, psychologist, counsellor and legal personnel. These comprehensive services are offered/will be offered through the development of "One stop crisis centers" (OSC) developed under the aegis of the Ministry of Women and Child Development, Govt. of India

11. **What are the long-term consequences of CSA?**
    Long-lasting effects of the sexual abuse are: lack of self-confidence, inability to express feelings, inability to trust people and feeling angry at the world most of the time. Other effects include: avoiding sex or compulsively seeking it out, experiencing chronic aches and pains, and use of drugs and alcohol.

KEY MESSAGES

When we come across a case of suspected child abuse, we should not under-report but act in the best interest of the child. We may need to take another colleague into confidence, work and record everything professionally, and get appropriate bodies to take over. The family needs to be taken into confidence. Appropriate communication will be necessary to prevent a backlash by the family. However, the child's interest is prime and we owe it to them.

Gastroesophageal Reflux Disease

Chapter 39

Bankim Parekh

1. **What is Gastroesophageal Reflux Disease?**
   When the stomach contents travel retrograde into the esophagus, it is called gastroesophageal reflux (GER) (Fig. 1). When the reflux leads to complications or problems, it is called gastroesophageal reflux disease (GERD). The common problems are:
   - Vomiting out so much of the feeds that the growth gets affected
   - The acid in stomach contents causing problems to esophagus, oropharynx, teeth, respiratory tract and lungs
   - Aspiration of stomach contents into airways leading to choking or breathlessness.

   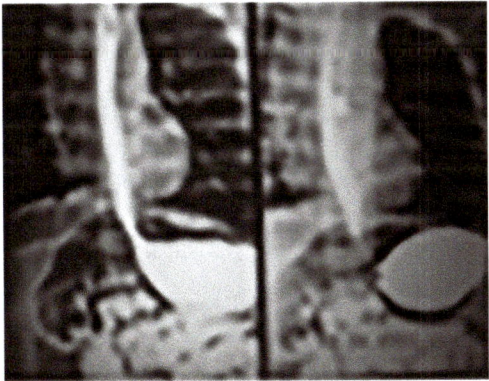

   Fig. 1: Dye study showing GER.

2. **What Causes GER?**
   - Lax lower esophageal sphincter (LES) tone
   - Transient LES relaxations
   - Hiatus hernia
   - Respiratory distress induces reflux
   - Chronic esophagitis due to acid reflux sets up a vicious cycle by inhibiting esophageal peristalsis.

3. **Are There Any Predisposing Factors That Cause GERD?**
   - Majority of premature babies have GERD
   - Prevalence of GERD is observed to be the maximum at 4 months. Vomiting and GERD reduces over the next few months and disappears in majority by 12–24 months
   - A gene named *GERD 1* is found to be correlated with the condition
   - Obese children, and those having asthma have higher incidences of GERD.
4. **What Are the Common Clinical Presentations?**
   - An infant having frequent effortless vomits is a common clinical scenario
   - Excessive irritability in an infant associated with arching, and paroxysmal dystonic movements due to GER is called Sandifer syndrome
   - GER can lead to choking, aspiration, esophagitis and associated complications; heartburn, manifested by crying after meals, or after certain foods, or on lying down. This can cause food aversion and failure to thrive
   - Older children can present with symptoms of chest pain, upper abdominal pain and heartburn, besides frequent vomiting
   - Sandifer syndrome—the baby arches backwards.
5. **How Is GERD Diagnosed?**
   - Clinical suspicion is diagnosis for most practical purposes. An effective trial of treatment confirms the diagnosis. Confirmation by investigations is needed when there is no response to trial of treatment or a doubt persists.
   - Investigations like upper gastrointestinal (GI) dye study, milk scan scintigraphy, endoscopy to look for ulcers, and multichannel intraluminal impedance and pH monitoring are available. Each of them has limitations. The results are best interpreted along with clinical correlation.
6. **How Is GERD Treated?**
   - Some general principles are: avoid sleeping/supine position soon after meals. Sitting position is not good—it increases reflux. Head raised position/upright position/prone when awake under observation reduces reflux
   - Reduce pressure over abdomen—avoid tight clothing/tight elastics
   - Weight control/loss if overweight
   - Treat asthma or other respiratory diseases (Figs. 2 and 3).

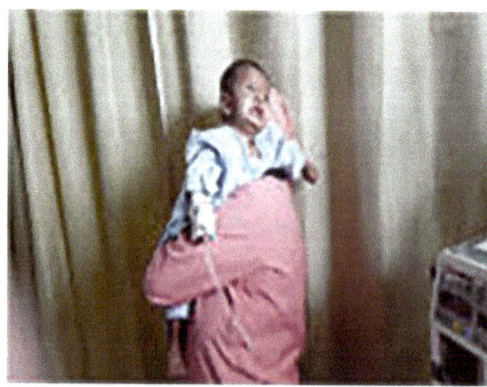

Fig. 2: Sandifer syndrome.

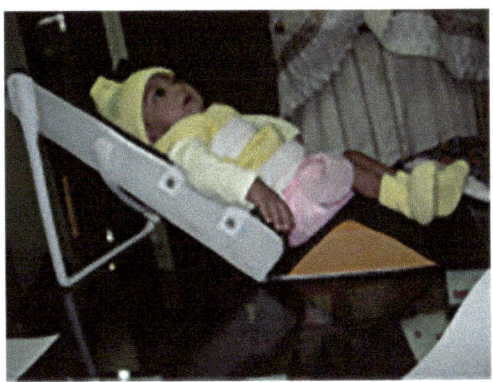

Fig. 3: Esophageal chair.

7. **What Changes in Diet Can Help?**
   - Small frequent feeds
   - Thickened feeds
   - Hypoallergic formula
   - Avoid cow's milk in mother's diet
   - Avoid acidic or reflux-inducing foods (tomatoes, chocolate, mint, etc.) and beverages (juices, carbonated and caffeinated drinks, alcohol, etc.)
   - Weight reduction and elimination of smoke exposure.

8. **What Medicines Can Help These Patients?**
   - Prokinetics like metoclopramide, cisapride and domperidone, erythromycin (motilin receptor agonist) increase LES tone, increase gastric emptying, but trials in GERD patients do not show much efficacy. Some are known to have side effects, e.g., increased QTc interval
   - Antacids like aluminum hydroxide, magnesium hydroxide, etc.
   - Barrier agents like sucralfate and alginate can help reduce the effect of acid reflux partially
   - H2 receptor blockers like cimetidine, ranitidine and famotidine and proton-pump inhibitors (PPI) like lansoprazole and omeprazole reduce the production of acid
   - Baclofen is a GABA receptor agonist that reduces transient LES relaxation
   - Surgical management like Nissan fundoplication can help in severe cases not responding to medical treatment or for child at risk of life-threatening events.

Griscelli Syndrome

Chapter 40

Ankit Kumar Parmar

CASE STUDY

An 11-month-old male child, third by birth order, born of non-consanguineous marriage presented with fever since 1 month, and not gaining weight since 1 month. On examination, the patient had failure to thrive, hypopigmentation of hairs of scalp and eyebrows noted (Figs. 1 and 2). Systemic examination shows sign of hepatosplenomegaly. On investigation, complete blood count (CBC) shows pancytopenia with deranged liver function test (LFT). Hair mount microscopy showed large clumped melanosomes mostly in the medulla of the hair shaft. Skin biopsy showed hyperpigmented basal melanocytes. We re-examined the peripheral blood smear thoroughly, but no inclusions were seen within leucocytes. Bone marrow examination suggested hemophagocytic cells and conformation of diagnosis of Griscelli syndrome was done by mutation RAB 27A by next generation sequencing.

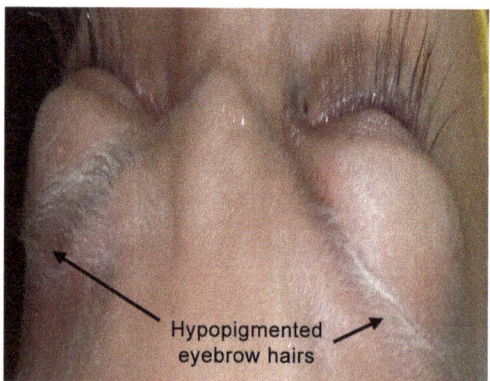

Fig. 1: Hypopigmented eyebrows.

Griscelli Syndrome

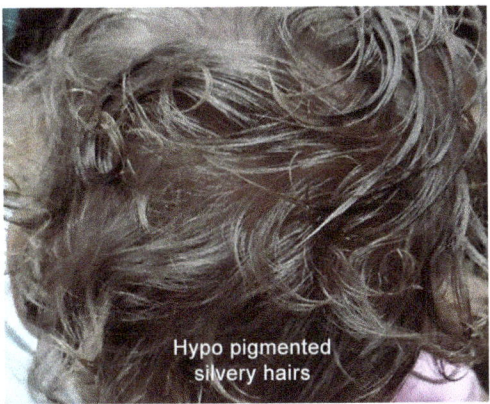

Fig. 2: Hypopigmented silvery hairs.

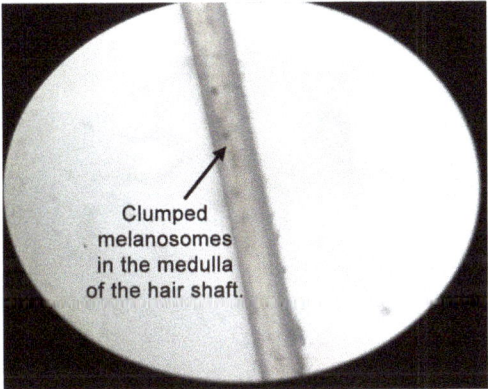

Fig. 3: Irregular clumped melanosomes in the hair shaft medulla.

1. **What is Griscelli syndrome?**
   Griscelli syndrome is an inherited condition characterized by unusually light (hypopigmented) skin and light silvery-gray hair starting in infancy.
2. **What are the other names of Griscelli syndrome?**
   - Hypopigmentation immunodeficiency disease
   - Partial albinism with immunodeficiency.
3. **What is the frequency and inheritance pattern?**
   Griscelli syndrome is a rare condition; its prevalence is unknown. Type 2 appears to be the most common. This condition is inherited in an autosomal recessive pattern.
4. **What are the signs and symptoms of this syndrome?**
   Griscelli syndrome is defined by the characteristic hypopigmentation, with frequent pyogenic infection, enlargement of the liver and spleen, a low blood neutrophils level, low blood platelet level and immunodeficiency.

5. **How to differentiate with other hypopigmentary immunodeficiency syndrome like Chediak-Higashi syndrome (CHS)?**
   - CHS is a rare genetic disorder, inherited as an autosomal recessive disorder. It is characterized by mild pigment dilution (partial oculocutaneous albinism), silvery blond hair, severe phagocytic immunodeficiency, bleeding tendencies, recurrent pyogenic infections and progressive sensory or motor neurological defects.
   - CHS and Griscelli syndrome share many common signs and symptoms like hypopigmented hairs, eyebrows, HLH, etc.
   - Hence, it is very important to differentiate both for sending confirmatory investigation.
   - Peripheral smear of CHS patient shows large clumps in leukocytes which is absent in Griscelli syndrome.
   - Hair microscopy also helps as in CHS melanin clumps regularly arranged in hair shaft, while in Griscelli syndrome, it is irregularly arranged in small clumps (Fig. 3).
   - Excess pigmentation of melanocytes at the basal layer of the skin (Fig. 4) is seen in Griscelli syndrome, whereas CHS shows large melanosomes in both melanocytes and keratinocytes.
   - Electron microscopy of the skin reveals mature melanosomes in Griscelli and large melanosomes in melanocytes and keratinocytes in CHS.

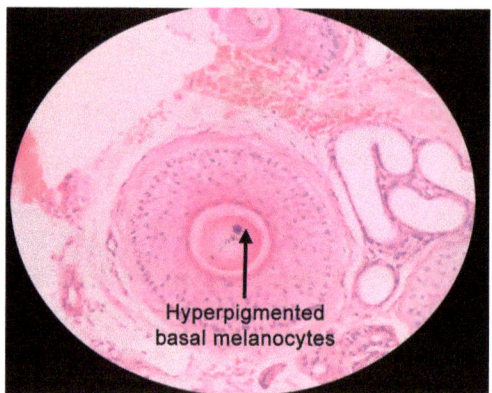

Fig. 4: Hyperpigmented basal melanocytes.

6. **How to diagnose a patient with suspected Griscelli syndrome?**
   - Peripheral smear, hair biopsy and microscopy
   - Bone marrow examination as patient can present with hemophagocytic syndrome
   - Specific mutation like Type 1 results from mutations in the *MYO5A* gene, Type 2 is caused by mutations in the *RAB27A* gene and Type 3 results from mutations in the *MLPH* gene
   - What is the treatment for the patient?
   - Treatment for Griscelli syndrome Type 1 is only symptomatic. In Griscelli syndrome Type 2, the hemophagocytic syndrome is often fatal, and the only cure is bone marrow transplantation.

Hair on End Appearance

Chapter 41

Ashok Kapse

> **CASE STUDY**
>
> A 14-year-old female child presented for enlarging head size; she was a known case of thalassemia intermedia. The child has been maintaining hemoglobin (Hb) between 9 g% and 11g%, and was not transfusion dependent. She had undergone splenectomy at the age of 8 years. She was subjected to X-ray skull which revealed classical "hair on end" appearance (Fig. 1).

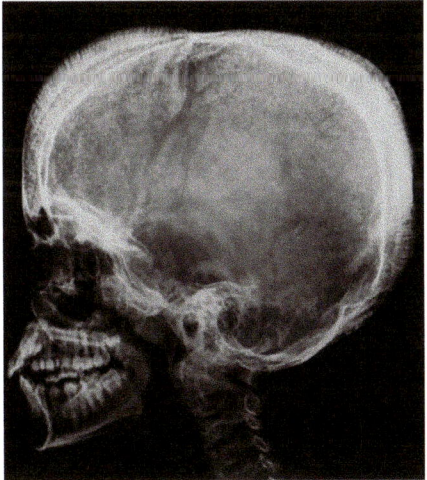

Fig. 1: Hair on end appearence.

1. **What is hair on end appearance?**
   A radiological finding the hair on end sign is seen in the diploic space on skull radiographs giving an appearance as if the hair is standing on the end.
2. **How is this appearance produced?**
   The changes are due to compensatory marrow hyperplasia, periosteal neo-osteogenesis of the outer cranial table transpire which results in marked calvarial thickening, external displacement and thinning of the inner table. Thin vertical striations of calcified spicules perpendicular to bone surface gives classical hair on end appearance.

3. **What are the conditions where this appearance could occur?**
   Hair on end appearance is mostly seen in hemolytic conditions; however, it could also occur in non-hemolytic conditions like congenital syphilis—syphilitic periostitis of tibia, metastatic neuroblastoma, iron-deficiency anemia, cyanotic—right-to-left shunt—congenital heart disease, osteomyelitis, polycythemia vera, thyroid acropachy and hemangiomas. Mnemonic HI NEST aptly represents clinical conditions causing hair on end appearance.
   H—Hereditary Spherocytosis
   I—Iron deficiency anemia
   N—Neuroblastoma
   E—Enzyme deficiency, e.g. G-6-PD deficiency
   S—Sickle cell disease
   T—Thalassemia major

4. **Would anemia correction reverse hair on end appearance?**
   It is less likely that appearance would be rectified by anemia correction; however, regular transfusion and chelation definitely prevent excessive bone marrow hyperplasia, and thereby occurrence of hair on end appearance.

5. **What are the common bony pathologies in thalassemia?**
   Osteopenia and osteoporosis leading to fractures are common bony complications of thalassemia.

Henoch-Schonlein Purpura

Chapter 42

Nigam Prakash Narain

CASE STUDY

A male child aged 7 years presented with purpuric rashes on gluteal region and lower limbs as shown in Figures 1A and B. These rashes were preceded by minor cough and cold for 3–4 days but there was no fever or itching in the rash. On examination of the child, there was no marked pallor or evident lymphadenopathy. After a few days, he started having pain in abdomen and had some pain in his knees with swelling. His blood counts were nearly normal (Hb%—11 g/dL; WBC—8,500/cmm; platelet—460,000/cmm).

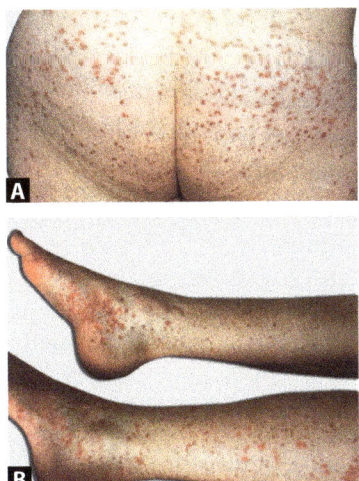

Figs. 1A and B: Purpuric rashes.

Diagnosis: Henoch-Schonlein Purpura

1. **Which type of disease is Henoch-Schonlein Purpura?**
   This is a leukocytoclastic type of vasculitis affecting small vessels.
2. **What is the epidemiology of this disease?**
   It is prevalent worldwide, incidence being 14–20/100,000 children per year with slight more preponderance amongst males. Ninety percent of the cases are found in children aged

3–10 years. Many cases follow upper respiratory infection, and hence, more common in winters and spring seasons.

3. **What are the causative agents?**
   Relation with upper respiratory infection suggests the causative agent as Group A β-hemolytic *Streptococcus* or common respiratory viruses.

4. **What are the salient features of this disease?**
   Non-thrombocytopenic purpura, arthritis or arthralgia of one or two bigger joints, abdominal pain and renal involvement are characteristic features of this disease.

5. **What is the pathophysiology behind these symptoms?**
   There is vasculitis of dermal capillaries with infiltrates of neutrophils and monocytes. In kidney, there is endocapillary proliferative glomerulonephritis. Immunofluorescence indicates immunoglobulin A (IgA) deposition in walls of small vessels; sometimes with C3, fibrin and immunoglobulin M (IgM).

6. **How do we diagnose this condition?**
   Diagnosis is always clinical and whatever pathophysiology may be there, no lab investigations except complete blood count (CBC) may be needed, which is mainly to exclude thrombocytopenia in these cases.

7. **What is the usual course of this condition and prognosis?**
   Palpable purpura or petechiae are the first signs usually lasting 3–10 days, but sometimes recur off and on for four months. Arthritis is usually oligo articular involving knees and ankles, and resolves within 2 weeks, even before disappearance of rash without any residual damage.

8. **What are the dreaded complications of this problem?**
   Gastrointestinal manifestations include colicky abdominal pain usually, but vomiting, diarrhea, ileus, intussusception or even perforation may be a complication of this disease. Renal involvement is seen in half of the cases in the form of microscopic hematuria. Rarely it may progress to proeinuria, hypertension, frank nephritis or nephrotic syndrome, or even renal failure. Very rarely neurological complications like seizures, headaches and behavior changes may appear.

9. **What are the treatment options?**
   Treatment is largely supportive with rest, analgesia for pains, adequate hydration and proper nutrition. Corticosteroids are only needed for severe abdominal complications, orchitis or renal involvement in the form of predinoslone 1–2 mg/kg/day, tapered in 2–3 weeks.

10. **What is the role of immunosuppressant?**
    Rarely in chronic situations of nephritis and proteinuria, azathioprine, cyclophosphamide or mycophenolate mofetil may have to be tried.

11. **Is there any follow up needed for these cases?**
    Ideally all cases but certainly those cases with renal involvement must be monitored for blood pressure and urinary abnormalities for at least 6 months.

Chapter 43

Hepatic Abscess

Dhanya Dharmapalan

> **CASE STUDY**
>
> A 4-year-old presented with pain in abdomen, fever with chills and vomiting on and off since 5 days. On examination, there was mild hepatomegaly with hypochondriac tenderness. Complete blood count (CBC) showed hemoglobin (Hb) 9.8 g/dL, TLC 22,400 with N74%, L25% and E1%. Serum glutamic oxaloacetic transaminase (SGOT) was 64, and serum glutamic pyruvic transaminase (SGPT) 58. Ultrasonography (USG) abdomen was suggestive of liver abscess 9.3 × 7.2 × 7.6cm in the right lobe.

1. **What are the clinical signs and symptoms of liver abscess?**
   The signs and symptoms can be nonspecific and include fever, abdominal pain, vomiting, loose motions, weight loss, loss of appetite and occasionally jaundice. On examination, there may be right hepatic tenderness. Ruptured hepatic abscess into the pleura may present like empyema with respiratory symptoms. On examination, icterus may be present, and there is usually hepatic tenderness.

2. **What are the etiologic organisms for liver abscess?**
   Liver abscess can be caused by bacteria, parasites or fungal organisms. The incidence of pyogenic liver abscess has been reported to be more than 79 per 100,000 pediatric admissions in India. Pyogenic abscesses tend to be polymicrobial; *Staphylococcus aureus* is the most frequently isolated organism in children. Other causative organisms are anerobes including microaerophilic streptococcus and Gram negative organisms like *E. coli, Klebsiella, Salmonella, Pseudomonas*, etc.
   Amoebic abscess is caused by invasion by the trophozoites of *E. histolytica* and accounts for 3–9% of all amoebiasis. In a small proportion, one can have mixed pyogenic and amoebic infections. Fungal abscesses are usually encountered in immunocompromised children. Tubercular hepatic abscesses have been reported in immunocompetent children.

3. **What are the predisposing factors for liver abscess?**
   In neonates, umbilical catheterization, abscesses are predisposing factors. In older children, malnutrition, genetic conditions like Papillon-Leferve syndrome, chronic granulomatous diseases, C1 complement deficiencies and hyper immunoglobulin E. Other factors are trauma causing direct or indirect hepatic injury, portal vein catheterization and recurrent cholangitis.

4. **What is the pathogenesis of liver abscess?**
   Most cases of liver abscesses result from direct extension of infection from either the biliary or intestinal tract or from hematogenous spread. Bacterial liver seeding by direct inoculation, from either penetrating trauma or an invasive procedure is another less common cause of hepatic abscess.
   Amoebic abscess results from invasion of *E. histolytica* trophozoites through the gut mucosal barrier which travel through the portal circulation to the liver.

5. **What are the diagnostic tests?**
   There is usually leukocytosis. Acute inflammatory markers are usually raised. There is usually mild elevation of liver enzymes, especially alkaline phosphatase. Blood cultures can be positive in bacteremic children and help to find out causative organism. Pus can be aspirated under USG guidance and subjected to gram staining and culture.
   Presence of anchovy sauce is classically described in amebic abscess. *E. histolytica* cysts or trophozoites in the stool are neither sensitive nor specific and can be confused with asymptomatic carriage. Similarly, antibody testing for *E. histolytica* though has reported high specificity and sensitivity in the developed countries, have limited role in endemic countries like India as they cannot reliably distinguish from past infections and confirm extraintestinal amebiasis.
   X-ray chest may reveal raised right dome of diaphragm (Fig. 1).

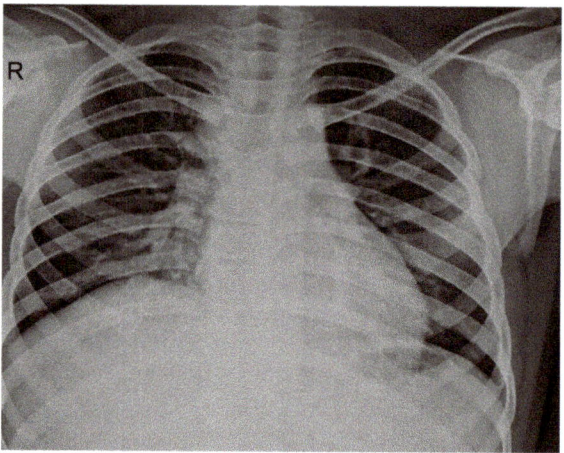

Fig. 1: X-ray chest in a child with hepatic abscess. Note the raised right hemidiaphragm due to abscess in right lobe of liver.

Ultrasonography is a very good modality to detect the size, location, number and the characteristic features of the abscess (Fig. 2). It can also guide aspiration. Computed tomography (CT) abdomen is more sensitive than USG to detect very small abscesses. Pyogenic abscesses are usually multiple and have thick abscess wall compared to amoebic abscess which are usually solitary, and oval with thin abscess wall. Though presence of multiple abscesses does not rule out amoebic liver abscesses, most of the abscess are located in the right lobe of liver probably due to direct continuation of portal vein into the right lobe.

Hepatic Abscess

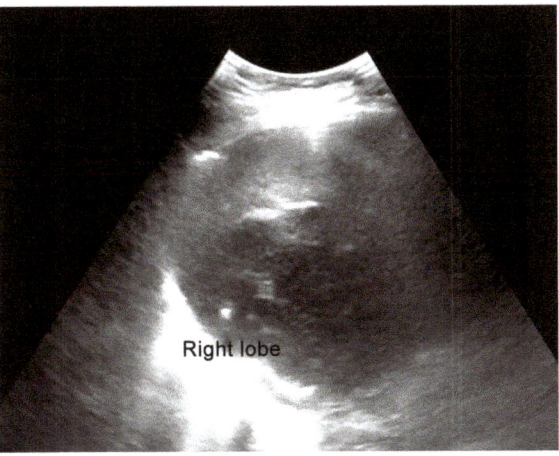

Fig. 2: Hepatic abscess in right lobe of liver on ultrasonography.

6. **What is the empirical choice of antibiotics?**
   Antibiotics must be empirically started to cover Gram positive (especially *Staphylococcus*), Gram negative and anerobes. Cloxacillin (if available) or co-amoxiclav/ceftriaxone with metronidazole with amikacin broadly covers most of the susceptible organisms. In the case of suspected methicillin-resistant *Staphylococcus aureus* (MRSA), vancomycin is the first-line antibiotic.
   The treatment should be modified as per the culture reports. The total duration of treatment is 4–6 weeks. Intravenous (IV) antibiotics should be given at least for 2 weeks before shifting to oral medications. C-reactive protein (CRP) trend can be used for monitoring purpose. The radiological resolution on sonography can take longer time from 3 months to 2 years. In case of amoebic abscess, metronidazole should be given for 14 days and should be followed by a lumen active agent against intracolonic cysts like diloxanide furuoate or paromomycin for 10 days.

7. **What are the indications of surgical drainage?**
   Surgical drainage is indicated in any abscess which has a chance for rupture, large volume abscess, left lobe abscess, or if, no improvement with medical management with clinical signs of persistent sepsis or enlarging abscess. Percutaneous catheter drainage is the mainstay of management in these cases. Percutaneous catheter drainage is not indicated when there is presence of ascites or if abscess is close to the pleura.
   Open laparotomy is rarely required and is reserved for only those that display a poor response to percutaneous drainage and antibiotic therapy; when the pus is thick, there is rupture into peritoneal cavity.

8. **What are the complications of hepatic abscess?**
   Hepatic abscess can rupture into the pleura or peritoneum or pericardium and cause death if left untreated. Large hepatic abscesses can cause inferior vena caval obstruction leading to ascites.

Herpes Simplex Infection

Chapter 44

Aniruddha Ghosh, Ritabrata Kundu

CASE STUDY

A term appropriate for gestational age (AGA) baby boy delivered by normal vaginal delivery presented with shock on day 6 of life. Multiple vesicles and pustules over abdomen and thighs (Fig. 1) were noted along with hepatomegaly, splenomegaly and purpuric rash. On investigation, prothrombin time (PT) and activated partial thromboplastin time (APTT) were prolonged, conjugated hyperbilirubinemia was present and deoxyribonucleic acid (DNA) polymerase chain reaction (PCR) of serum for herpes simplex virus (HSV) was found to be positive. Lumbar puncture and magnetic resonance imaging (MRI) brain were within normal limits. Patient was admitted in the neonatal intensive care unit (NICU) and was treated with intravenous (IV) acyclovir, fresh frozen plasma (FFP) along with other supportive measures. A diagnosis of neonatal HSV infection was made. The baby survived and was discharged from NICU on day 27 of life.

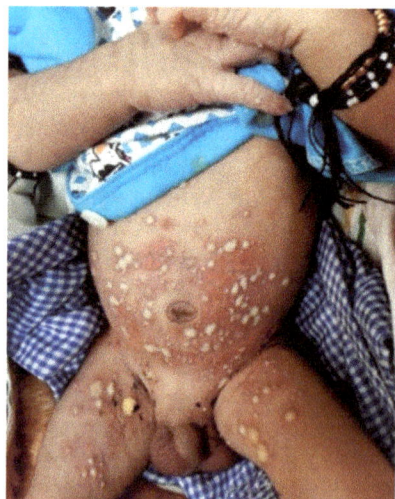

Fig. 1: Multiple vesicles and pustules over abdomen and thighs.

Herpes Simplex Infection

1. **What are the types of HSV?**
   The two types of HSV are HSV-1 and HSV-2. Both are equally capable of causing initial infection. HSV-1 causes recurrent oral infections more commonly, whereas HSV-2 has greater propensity to cause recurrent genital infections. HSV-1 spreads by contact with oral secretions and HSV-2 by anogenital contact.

2. **What are the types of infections caused by HSV?**
   - *Primary infection:* It occurs in previously uninfected seronegative persons, either by HSV-1 or HSV-2. It is often severe as the host immunity is very low to HSV.
   - *Non-primary first infection:* When a person has already been infected by one type of HSV (HSV-1), the person acquires the other type of HSV infection (HSV-2). Due to cross immunity between the two types, the host has certain amount of protection against the new infection and it tends to be less severe than true primary infection.
   - *Recurrent infection:* During primary or non-primary first infections, the virus establishes dormancy inside regional sensory ganglions. These viruses reactivate and can cause recurrent symptomatic or asymptomatic infections. Symptomatic recurrent infections become less severe with each recurrence and asymptomatic recurrent infections seldom cause any distress to the host, but these second groups may transmit the virus to other susceptible hosts.

3. **What are the hallmarks of HSV skin or mucosal lesions?**
   Shallow ulcers and skin vesicles. Vesicles are classically 2–4 mm in size and are surrounded by erythematous base. Lesions on moist mucous membranes may have fleeting lesions.

4. **Which factors determine clinical manifestations of HSV?**
   - Portal of entry
   - Primary or non-primary infection
   - Host immunity
   - Type of virus
   - In the case of newborns, gestational age of neonate and maternal immunity.

5. **How does oropharyngeal HSV infection present?**
   - Presents as herpetic gingivostomatitis in 6 months to 5 years age group commonly
   - Extremely painful lesions appear in gums, lips, tongue, palate, tonsils, pharynx and perioral skin along with high grade fever, drooling, refusal to feed and odynophagia
   - Vesicles evolve into shallow ulcers with yellowish gray membrane
   - Regional lymph nodes are enlarged
   - Dehydration is the most common indication of hospitalization in these patients
   - In older children and adolescent, this infection may present as pharyngitis and tonsillitis rather than gingivostomatitis.

6. **What is herpes labialis?**
   Herpes labialis or fever blisters or cold sores are the most common reactivation lesions of HSV-1 (Fig. 2).

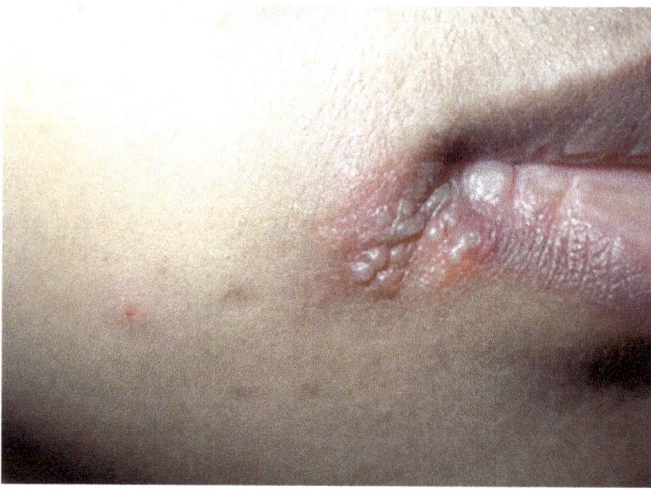

Fig. 2: Herpes labialis.

- Usually asymptomatic, sometimes paraesthesia before skin eruptions
- Small groups of erythematous papules develop first involving most commonly the outer edge of the vermillion border of lips and ophthalmic division of trigeminal nerve
- Papules or blisters heal by crusting.

7. **What is herpetic whitlow?**
   - It is the herpetic paronychia of fingers and toes (Fig. 3)
   - It is seen most commonly in infants and toddlers who have habit of thumb sucking and clinical or subclinical oral HSV-1 infection

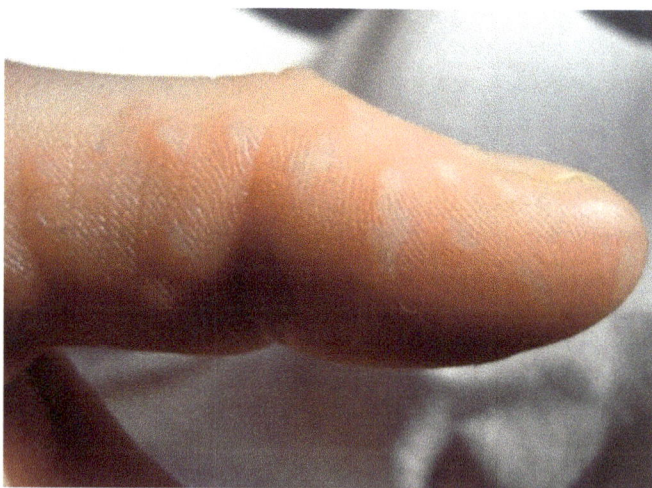

Fig. 3: Herpetic whitlow.

- HSV-2 whitlows may be seen in adolescents who have genital lesions
- Incising the lesions are not recommended as it delays natural healing.

8. **In which group of patients cutaneous herpes can be life threatening?**
   It can be life threatening in patients with skin diseases like:
   - Eczema (eczema herpeticum)
   - Pemphigus
   - Darier disease
   - Burns
   - Following laser procedures of skin.

9. **How Does Genital Herpes Present?**
   - Usually caused by HSV-2, sometimes HSV-1
   - Adolescents are the common sufferer; genital herpes in a small child should raise the suspicion of sexual abuse
   - Males have lesions over shaft of penis, females have lesions on cervix, vaginal mucosa, mons pubis and labia. Sometimes dysuria due to genital herpes may be severe to cause urinary retention
   - Inguinal lymph nodes get enlarged during second or third week
   - Non-primary and recurrent infections often remain unnoticed and these cases shed the virus for a long time.

10. **What Are the Central Nervous System Involvements Seen in Herpes?**
    - HSV encephalitis is an acute to subacute necrotising infection of frontal and/or temporal lobe and limbic system
    - Beyond neonatal age group almost exclusively caused by HSV-1
    - Apart from non-specific clinical features of acute encephalitis syndrome, some features may be suggestive of HSV encephalitis: anosmia, peculiar behavior, memory loss, speech problems, hallucinations, etc.
    - If left untreated, in 75% of the cases, coma or death occurs
    - CSF picture shows moderate number of mononuclear and polymorphonuclear cells, mildly elevated protein, slightly decreased glucose and often moderate number of red blood cells
    - MRI brain often shows classical frontotemporal involvement by HSV
    - HSV can also cause recurrent aseptic meningitis known as Mollaret meningitis.

11. **What Are the Severe Manifestations of HSV in Immunocompromised Patients?**
    Immunocompromised patients may have fulminant HSV infection with multiple organ involvement.
    - Rash and ulcers are extensive and reach deeper tissues
    - Tracheobronchitis
    - Pneumonitis
    - Sepsis like picture with septic shock
    - Hepatitis
    - Adrenal gland involvement
    - Disseminated intravascular coagulation.

12. **What Is the Prevalence of Neonatal Herpes Infection?**
    1 in 3,000–5,000.

13. **How Does Neonatal Infection Occur?**
    Infection may transmit in utero, peripartum or postpartum, often during passage through infected maternal birth passage. Neonates are more commonly affected where mother had

recent infection rather than in cases of recurrent maternal genital herpes. Risk is higher with intrapartum interventions like forceps, and babies with low gestational age.

14. **What Are the Patterns of Neonatal Herpes?**

    There are three patterns often with overlap between them:
    - Skin, eye and mouth disease: Presents during 5–11 days of life. Presents with few blisters over presenting part or parts where electrodes are placed. Leaving untreated may spread causing encephalitis or disseminated disease. Despite treatment, neonates may have keratoconjunctivitis, chorioretinitis, cataracts, retinal detachment, etc.
    - CNS infection with or without skin lesions: Neonates present during 14–21 days of life with focal and intractable seizures, lethargy and irritability. CNS involvement is global rather than frontotemporal in the case of neonatal encephalitis.
    - Disseminated HSV infections: Newborns present during 5–11 days of life with shock, organomegaly, bleeding, icterus, respiratory distress, etc.

15. **How to Diagnose HSV Infections?**

    Viral culture is the gold standard for diagnosis. Use of DNA PCR methods is highly sensitive and specific. It is the test of choice in examining CSF samples derived from cases of suspected HSV encephalitis. As most of the diagnostic tests take time to yield result, treatment should not be delayed if clinical suspicion is high.

16. **How to Treat HSV Infections?**

    Acyclovir is the drug of choice. Depending upon severity of infection, it may be used through IV or oral routes. Hydration status of patient is crucial during therapy as renal function may deteriorate.
    - Acute mucocutaneous herpes:
        - Gingivostomatitis: Oral acyclovir (15 mg/kg/dose five times a day PO for 7 days). If the patient cannot take orally then only IV therapy is indicated
        - Herpes Labialis: Topical acyclovir is used. In case of recurrent disease, oral therapy is indicated
    - Herpetic whitlow: High dose oral acyclovir is to be used
    - *Extensive eczema herpeticum and other skin diseases with herpes* infection should be treated with parenteral acyclovir
    - Herpetic genital lesions: Oral acyclovir (400 mg TDS for 7–10 days)
    - CNS infection: IV acyclovir 500 mg/m^2 or 10 mg/kg/dose TDS for 14–21 days
    - Immunocompromised patients with severe or disseminated infection: IV acyclovir 250 mg/m^2 every 8 hourly
    - Perinatal infections: High dose IV acyclovir (20 mg/kg/dose TDS). Infants with HSV infections of skin, eyes and mouth should receive 14 days of therapy, whereas those with disseminated disease or encephalitis would receive 21 days of therapy. These patients should be monitored for neutropenia. Suppressive oral acyclovir therapy 300 mg/m^2 per dose for 3 times daily for 6 months with regular monitoring of neutrophil at weeks 2 and 4 is warranted in all cases of neonatal herpes infection.

Chapter 45

Herpes Zoster Infection

Aniruddha Ghosh, Ritabrata Kundu

CASE STUDY

A 6-year-old boy, a case of frequent relapsing nephrotic syndrome (at present in remission with alternate day tapering dose of oral prednisolone) presented with painful vesicular rash with erythematous surrounding on the right half of forehead (Fig. 1) along with low-grade fever for last 2 days. Right eyelid was involved, but there was no ocular involvement. He had history of chickenpox at the age of 9 months. Suspecting it to be a case of herpes zoster infection involving right ophthalmic division of trigeminal nerve, antipyretics were prescribed along with oral acyclovir. Gradually, the lesions subsided by crusting and there was no pain or burning sensation afterwards.

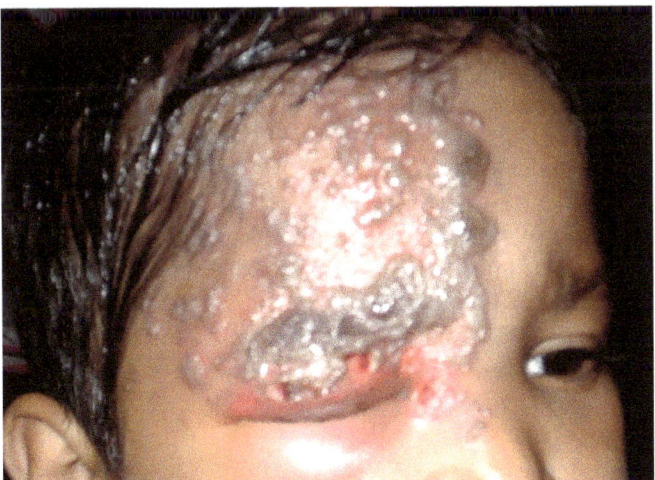

Fig. 1: Vesicular rash with erythematous surrounding on the right half of forehead.

1. **What is Herpes Zoster?**
   Herpes zoster (synonym: shingles) is a reactivation of varicella zoster virus (VZV) and is characterized by localized unilateral pain with vesico-bullous eruption limited to a dermatome innervated by a corresponding sensory ganglion.

2. **How common is it in Children?**
   It is not common in healthy children younger than 10 years of age, only exception being those infected with VZV in utero or in the first year of life. Immunocompromised children [human immunodeficiency virus (HIV), immunodeficiency disorders, immunosuppressive therapy, etc.] have much higher chances of developing herpes zoster, sometimes multiple times.

3. **What is the pathophysiology of the condition?**
   VZV ascends via the sensory nerves to corresponding ganglia during primary infection (chicken pox) and remains dormant there. If humoral and cellular immunity ebbs, viruses start replicating within the ganglia and travel to the dermatome via the sensory nerve trunk resulting in pain followed by rash.

4. **What are the clinical features of Herpes Zoster?**
   Symptoms:
   Pain, paraesthesia and tenderness may precede eruption by 3–5 days. Rarely, "zoster sine herpete" can occur with just pain in the involved dermatome. Fever, malaise, headache, etc. might be there as associated systemic features.
   Signs:
   - Skin lesions evolve from papules (24 hours) to vesicles and bullae (48 hours) to pustules (96 hours) and finally form crusts (7–10 days).
   - Vesicles are of 2–5 mm size, and have red base along with clear fluid inside them.
   - Lesions affect specific dermatomes: thorax (50%), trigeminal (20%), lumbosacral/cervical (20%). Very few stray outside of dermatome.
   - Oral, genital and rarely bladder mucosa may get involved.
   - Ophthalmic involvement: Keratitis, scleritis, iritis, conjunctivitis may occur. Vesicles on the tip of the nose (Hutchinson's sign) are very much indicative of nasociliary branch of trigeminal nerve involvement where ocular involvement is most common. Ophthalmic zoster may lead to blindness; that is why aggressive treatment is needed.
   - Sensory or motor nerve changes may occur although postherpetic neuralgia is less common in case of children compared to affected adults.
   - Regional lymph nodes are enlarged.

5. **What is disseminated Herpes Zoster?**
   Disseminated zoster, defined as 20 or more lesions outside the affected or adjacent dermatome, may occur in immunocompromised children having cutaneous as well as systemic involvement like pneumonia, encephalitis, hepatitis, disseminated intravascular coagulation, etc.

6. **Can it infect other children?**
   Fluid contained in zoster vesicles is contagious and contacts can develop primary varicella (chickenpox) but not zoster.

7. **How to diagnose Herpes Zoster?**
   Clinical features along with past history of chickenpox are suggestive of the condition. Viral isolation and culture, and VZV titers more than four times in convalescent versus acute condition can confirm the diagnosis. Tzanck preparation of scraping of lesion shows giant cells but cannot differentiate VZV from HSV.

8. **How to Treat Herpes Zoster?**
   Some experts do not recommend antiviral therapy in uncomplicated cases due to lesser chance of postherpetic neuralgia in children compared to adults. If treatment is decided, then it may be done with oral acyclovir (20 mg/kg/dose TID-QID) to shorten duration of illness. But zoster in immunocompromised children should be always treated with intravenous (IV) acyclovir (500 mg/m^2 or 10 mg/kg/dose every 8 hours) to prevent dissemination of infection which can be life-threatening. Neuritis with zoster should be managed with analgesics. Corticosteroids are not recommended for treatment of herpes zoster in children.
9. **Can Varicella Vaccine Cause Herpes Zoster in Later Life?**
   The chance of having herpes zoster is much less with vaccine virus than wild virus.

Hereditary Angioedema

Chapter 46

Ashok Banga, Usha Banga

CASE STUDY

A 14-year-old girl presented with swelling of lips and eyelids. She was apparently well 7 years back when she started developing multiple episodes of swelling of upper and lower limbs which were spontaneous in onset, gradually progressive, involving hands and feet first, and extending proximally. Swelling resolved spontaneously over a course of 2–3 days. Swelling was not associated with pain or itching. Antihistamine LCZ gave little relief.

In the last 2 years, she had two episodes of swelling of face and lips with mild respiratory difficulty for which hospitalization was required. Nebulization and hydrocortisone provided some relief and the child improved in 2–3 days.

- Complete blood count (CBC) tested was within normal limits
- Liver function test (LFT), electrolytes, urea, creatinine and lipid profile were normal
- Ultrasonography (USG) abdomen and pelvis, electrocardiography (ECG) and X-ray chest were normal
- Prothrombin time/international normalized ratio (PT/INR)—13.6/1.224
- Urine and stool normal

The patient was referred to AIIMS and investigated at Derma outpatient department (OPD), and was diagnosed hereditary angioedema (HAE).

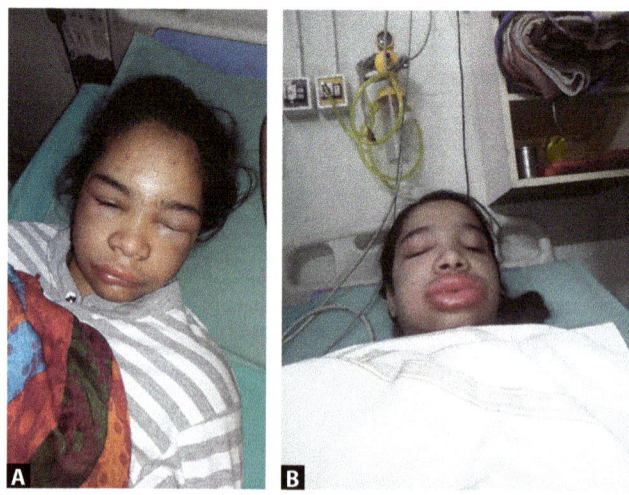

Figs. 1A and B: Swelling of lips and eyelids—case of hereditary angioedema.

Hereditary Angioedema

1. **What is HAE?**
   HAE (type-1 and type-2) is an inherited autosomal dominant disease caused by low functional levels of plasma protein C1 inhibitor (C1-INH).

2. **What are the signs and symptoms of HAE?**
   Typical presentation is in the form of episodic attacks of deep localized swelling, most commonly on hands or feet. *This is non-pitting edema and has no itching* or urticaria. Swelling usually progresses over 36 hours and then gradually resolves over the same period of time. In some patients, this is preceded by erythematous rash that is not raised and not pruritic.
   The second major symptom complex for presentation is in the form of severe abdominal pain because of edema of mucosa at any point of gut. It is like acute abdomen but resolves in 2–3 days.
   The most feared complication of HAE is laryngeal edema that can be life-threatening. More than half of such patients may experience it once in their lifetime. It can be spontaneous but dental work with procaine injection is the common precipitant.
   Symptoms begin typically during childhood and become more severe during adolescence.

3. **What causes attacks?**
   The cause is mostly unknown but in some patients trauma and emotional stress clearly precipitate the attack. Drugs like angiotensin converting enzyme inhibitors and estrogen make the disease worse. In some, menstruation also induces attack. Frequency of attacks varies from weekly to once in many years.

4. **What is the management?**
   - Avoidance of precipitating factors—angiotensin-converting-enzyme (ACE) inhibitors, estrogens, mental and physical stress, trauma, dental infections, etc.
   - Steroids, anti-histamines and epinephrine do not work in this condition.
   - Infusion of C1-INH concentrate
   - Patients and close household contacts should be immunized against *H. influenzea*, *S. pneumonie* and *N. meningitides*. Repeat immunization is advised as complement deficiency may blunt the vaccine response.

   In the case of acute airway compromise:
   - C1 inhibitor concentrate is the first line therapy (Ciniryze; Berinert)
   - Twenty units/kg (each vial is 500 units) cost 500 euros (Rs. 35,000). Shelf life 30 months before reconstitution
   - Given intravenous (IV) over 10 min even at home. In 95% of the patients, one dose is sufficient
   - Bradykinin B2 receptor antagonist Icatibant (Firazyr): 30 mg slow SC injection in abdominal wall (Cost Rs. 63,569).

   Or

   FFP 2 units initially and then repeated 2–4 hourly till relief. Cost Rs. 400/unit
   In the case of Bowel wall angioedema: Symptomatic therapy, rehydration, diclofenac or tramadol, butylscopolamine, metoclopramide, etc.

5. **How can one be alert and prepared before?**
   - Dental procedures
   - Abdominal surgeries
   - Any surgical intervention

6. **What is the maintenance treatment?**
   - Stanazolol 2 mg OD
   - Benazol 100 mg OD
   - Tenexamic acid 1 g BID
   - To maintain a log book with description of attacks and treatment response
   - Monitor blood pressure (BP), weight, LFT, renal function test (RFT), fasting lipid profile (FLP) and urinalysis every 6 months
   - Serum alpha-fetoprotein (AFP) and USG abdomen yearly
   - Inform the doctor if planning pregnancy
   - Regular follow up with treating physician every 4 months.

Hereditary Methemoglobinemia

Chapter 47

Sanjay Bafna

CASE STUDY

- An 18-month-old girl was brought to us with severe respiratory distress, stridor and cyanosis requiring intubation and ventilation. The child was undernourished, hemodynamically stable, irritable and had spasticity, microcephaly without focal deficit. Rest of the examination was unremarkable.
- Till now, the child was managed by her primary pediatrician and was referred to us for pediatric intensive care unit (PICU) management. Birth and neonatal periods were uneventful.
- At 3 months, she was detected with cyanosis for which X-ray chest, two-dimensional (2D) echo and computed tomography (CT) pulmonary angiography were done, which were normal. At 6 months, the child was referred to neurologist for neurodevelopmental delay. Magnetic resonance imaging (MRI) brain showed inferior cerebellar vermis hypoplasia and large posterior fossa cerebrospinal fluid (CSF) space which was reported as Dandy Walker variant. Since then she was on anticonvulsant, gabapentin, and physiotherapy.
- On present admission, it was noticed that blood was chocolate brown, persistent SpO_2 of 85% and ABG by co-oximetry showed methemoglobin of 47% (Figs. 1A and B). Hence, diagnosis of hereditary methemoglobinemia type 2 was entertained and vitamin C was started. Methemoglobin gradually declined and was 5% on discharge. The child was sent home on day 7 with no cyanosis. She was advised to continue levetiracetam, vitamin C and syndopa.
- Diagnosis of type 2 methemoglobinemia was confirmed by genetic analysis.

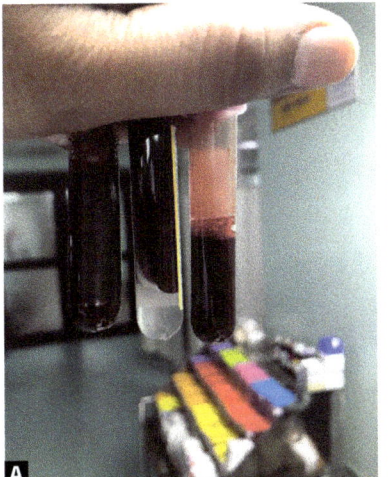

Figs. 1A and B: (A) Blood samples; (B) Report of the same sample.

1. **What is methemoglobinemia?**
   Methemoglobinemia is a clinical syndrome caused by increase in the serum concentration of methemoglobin.

2. **What is the pathophysiology of methemoglobinemia?**
   The iron molecule in hemoglobin is normally in the ferrous state (Fe^{2+}) which is essential for oxygen transport. In normal individuals, oxidation of hemoglobin to methemoglobin occurs at a slow rate which is countered by methemoglobin reduction to maintain a steady state of 1% methemoglobin. The newly formed metHb has a reduced ability to bind oxygen. The predominant intracellular mechanism for the reduction of methemoglobinemia is NADH-dependent reaction catalyzed by cytochrome 5b reductase.

3. **What is the etiopathogenesis of methemoglobinemia?**
   - Hereditary methemoglobinemia:
     - Due to deficiency of reductive pathways, such as NADH-cytochrome b5 reductase deficiency
     - Due to abnormal hemoglobin—called structural methemoglobinemia—they are referred to as M-hemoglobins
   - Acquired or toxic methemoglobinemia:
     - Results from excess production of methemoglobin due to exposure to toxic substances/drugs.
     - Drugs—nitrates, dapsone, sulfonamides, nitric oxide
     - Severe AGE and acidosis, sepsis
     - Aniline dyes, industrial chemicals, pesticides.

4. **What are the manifestations of methemoglobinemia?**
   Cardinal feature is central cyanosis. When methemoglobinemia levels are greater than 1.5 g/24 hour, cyanosis is visible (15% methemoglobin); a level of 70% methemoglobinemia is lethal. The level is usually reported as a percent of normal hemoglobin, and the toxic level is lower at a lower hemoglobin level.

Level of methemoglobin	Signs and symptoms
15–20%	Clinical cyanosis and chocolate brown blood
>20–45%	Headache, dizziness, weakness
>45%	Anemia, cardiac arrhythmia, seizure, dyspnea, acidosis
55–70%	Coma, seizures, arrhythmias, shock
>70%	Death if untreated

5. **What Are the manifestations of hereditary methemoglobin due to deficiency of NADH CYTOCHROME b5 reductase?**
   There are two types—Type I and II

Type 1	Type 2
• Most common type	• 10% of all congenital cases
• Enzyme deficient only in RBC	• Enzyme deficient in all tissues
• Mostly asymptomatic, headache, fatigue and exertional dyspnea	• Unremitting, progressive neurologic deterioration, mental retardation, microcephaly, opisthotonos, athetoid movements and generalized hypertonia
• May present in late age	• Significant symptoms begin in infancy, death by 10 years in most of the cases

6. **What are the manifestations of methemoglobin due to abnormal hemoglobin?**
   They are abnormal hemoglobin variants causing cyanosis resulting from point mutations in one of the globin chains—α, β or ɤ in the heme pocket. These unstable hemoglobins lead to hemolytic anemia, especially if β chains are involved. Clinically these children are cyanotic since birth, but otherwise they are asymptomatic.
7. **How is methemoglobin diagnosed?**
   These children have central cyanosis since birth with normal cardiorespiratory status. Due to peculiarity of methemoglobin, SpO_2 constantly stays around 85% on pulse-oximetry. Blood gas analysis by co-oximetry will show raised level of methemoglobin which can be confirmed by blood level of methemoglobin.
   Confirmatory diagnosis of enzymatic deficiency is by genetic analysis.
   Unstable Hb are diagnosed by high performance liquid chromatography (HPLC) which may not be reliable. Diagnostic confirmation may require DNA sequencing or mass spectrometry.
8. **What is the treatment of methemoglobin?**
   Daily oral *treatment* with ascorbic acid (200–500 mg/day in divided doses) is used in enzymatic deficiency.
   Ascorbic acid should not be used for treatment of toxic methemoglobinemia. Methylene blue given intravenously (1-2 mg/kg initially) is used to treat toxic methemoglobinemia. An oral dose can be administered (3-5 mg/kg/24 hour) as maintenance therapy.
   Methylene blue should not be used in patients with glucose-6-dehydrogenase deficiency.

Hand–Foot–Mouth Disease

Chapter 48

Ketan Shah

CASE STUDY 1

A 2-year-old child came with history of high fever, difficulty in swallowing and pain in mouth. The child goes to day-care center. The mother also noticed eruption on leg and hand. The child had multiple ulcers in oral cavity (Fig. 1) with surrounding edema. Child had vesicular eruptions on hands legs and buttocks (Fig. 2).

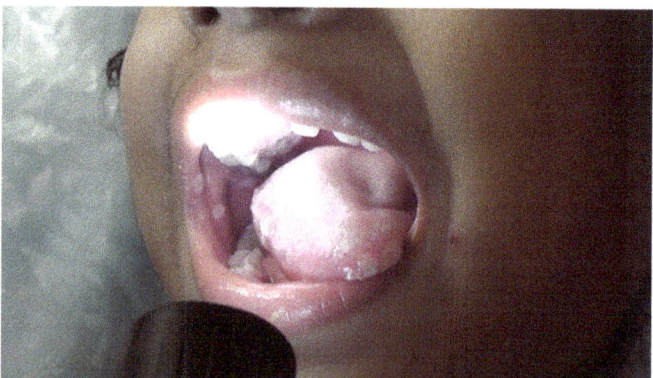

Fig. 1: Ulcers on tongue.

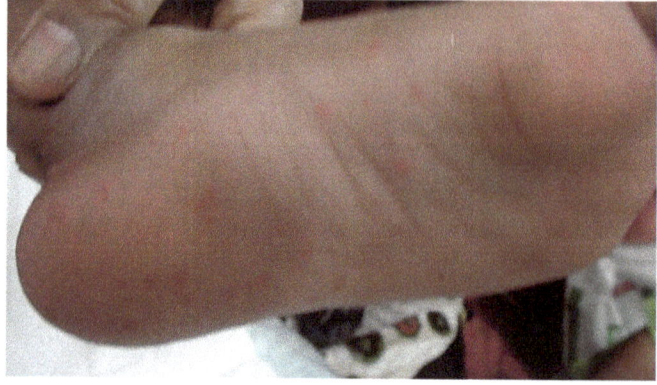

Fig. 2: Eruptions on soles.

Hand–Foot–Mouth Disease

CASE STUDY 2

A 12-month-old female came with history of high fever and irritability. Her mother noticed multiple vesicular eruptions on buttocks (Fig. 3) and hand (Fig. 4). She had mild itching on eruption. Oral cavity shows palatal redness and ulcerative lesions.

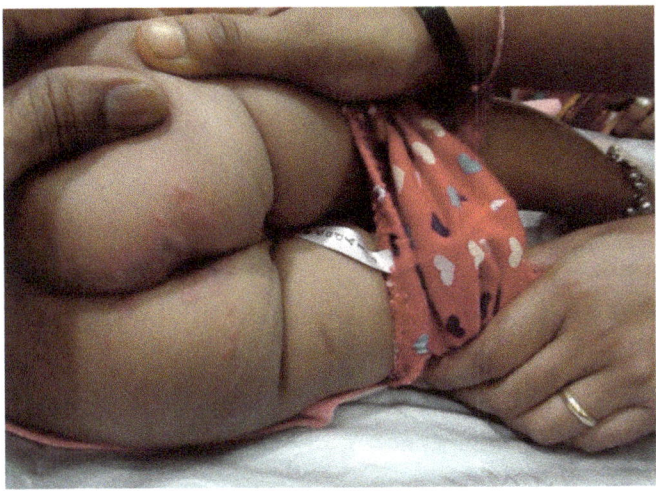

Fig. 3: Eruptions on buttocks.

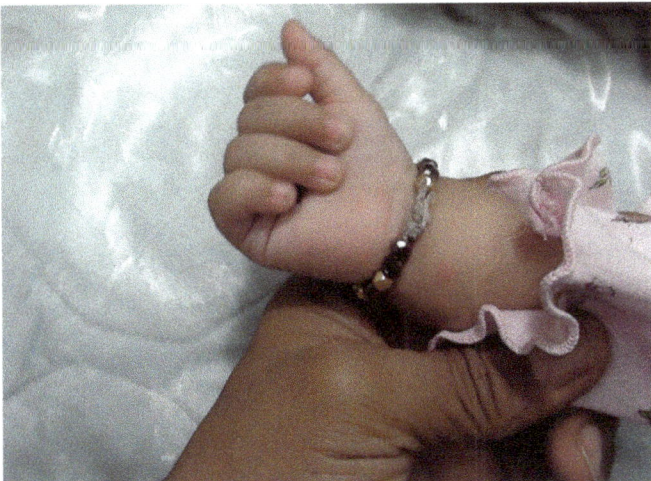

Fig. 4: Eruptions on hand.

1. **What is the characteristic of the disease?**
   It is the most distinctive rash syndrome. It is characterized by vesicles or ulcers in oral cavity, palate, buccal mucosa, posterior pharynx, gingiva and/or lips. Ulcerative lesions are 4–8 mm in size and surrounding inflammation may be seen. Maculopapular, vesicular lesions may occur on palm, sole, buttocks and groin.

2. **What is the age group?**
   Usually 6 months to 10 years; however, also seen in adult age.
3. **How is it transmitted?**
   Usual mode of transmission is oro-oral or feco-oral route. It is transmitted by air droplet. Human is the only reservoir.
4. **Which is the common season?**
   It is most commonly seen in summer and monsoon season. It comes in epidemic form. However, sporadic cases are also seen.
5. **Which virus causes it?**
   Most frequently in large outbreak, it is caused by Coxsackie virus A16. It can be caused by Enterovirus 71; Coxsackie A virus 5,6,7,9 and 10; Coxsackie B virus 2 and 5, and some Echo virus.
6. **What are the clinical manifestations?**
   It presents with low- to high-grade fever. It is associated with irritability and pain during swallowing. On day 1, only complaints will be excessive salivation. Few palatal enanthem may be seen. On day 2, three ulcerative and vesicular eruptions are seen in oral cavity, and on hand, foot and buttocks. Eruptions may be variable in intensity. Fever subsides within 2–3 days. Lesions heal within 5–7 days. Disseminated rash may complicate preexisting eczema.
7. **What are the complications?**
   In milder form, difficulty in swallowing is main concern. Lesions may subside, but may leave scarring in few patients. Nail shedding may be seen after 20–30 days (onychomadesis). This is more common with Coxsackie A6 virus. Beau's line and desquamation of skin may be seen. These changes start appearing after 2–3 weeks or after 4–6 weeks. Middle finger and upper limb nails are more commonly affected. Number of affected nails range from 3 to 20. If it is caused by Enterovirus 71, chances of cardiac and neurological complications are very high. Even Coxsackie A16 virus may cause encephalitis, acute flaccid paralysis, myocarditis, pericarditis and shock. Coxsackie A6 is associated with atypical hand–foot–mouth disease. It may cause herpangina (only oral cavity affected) or generalized rash affecting whole body.
8. **What is the treatment?**
   It is usually symptomatic. Antipyretic and analgesic are the main treatment. No need of antibiotic as it is a viral disease.

Hunter's Disease

Chapter 49

Jagdish Chinnappa

CASE STUDY

An 8-year-old boy is brought with progressive hearing loss, behavioral abnormalities and cognitive decline since the age of 3 years.
On general examination, you find the following skin lesions on his back.

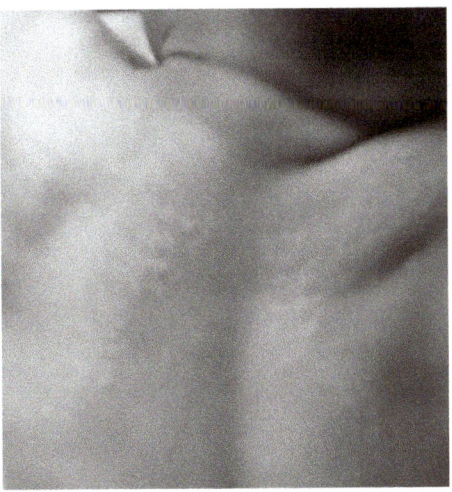

Fig. 1: Hunter's disease.
Courtesy: Jagdish Chinnappa

1. **What are the other findings you will expect?**
   These lesions are characteristic skin deposits of hunter disease which is an X-linked recessive mucopolysaccharidosis (MPS). It is not seen in other types of MPS.
   In addition, this child had coarse facial features, bony abnormalities and hepatosplenomegaly. There was no corneal clouding.

2. **How will you confirm the diagnosis?**
   - X-ray of the spine and skull
   - Urine for MPS
   - I2S Enzyme activity in serum and skin biopsy
   - Genetic analysis of the I2S gene.
3. **What are the treatment possibilities?**
   - Enzyme replacement therapy
   - Idursulfase is an enzyme that can arrest progress of the disease but cannot reverse existing disease
   - Bone marrow and stem cell transplantation
   - Gene therapy.

Hydrocele

Chapter 50

Amar Shah, Aniruddh Shah

CASE STUDY 1

A 5-month-old boy with a painless right scrotal swelling since birth. This was initially small to start and gradually, persistently and painlessly increased in size. The swelling does not change in size during the course of the day or night.

On examination, the child has a painless right scrotal swelling. It is possible to get above the swelling at the root of the scrotum. The swelling is not reducible. There is no impulse on crying. Transillumination is positive. The right testis cannot be palpated separately from the swelling. The left testis is normal.

CASE STUDY 2

A 4-year-old boy with a swelling over the left scrotum noted for the past 1 year. It was small, and gradually and painlessly increased in size.

On examination, the child has a painless cystic left scrotal swelling. The swelling is not reducible. There is no impulse on coughing. The left testis can be palpated separately from the swelling. Pulling the left testis fixes the left scrotal swelling. The right testis is normal.

The child in case 1 has got a right tunica vaginalis hydrocele (Fig. 1).

The child in case 2 has got a left encysted hydrocele of cord (Fig. 2).

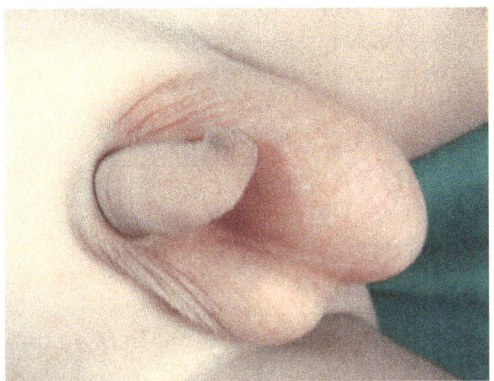

Fig. 1: Tunica vaginalis hydrocele.

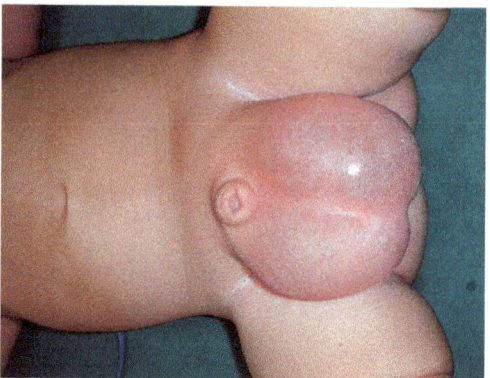

Fig. 2: Encysted cord hydrocele.

1. **What causes a hydrocele?**
   During the seventh month of fetal development, the testes move from the abdomen into the scrotum. During this course, it brings down a sac-like lining of the abdominal cavity with it. This is called "processus vaginalis." This causes peritoneal fluid to trickle down and collect around the testis in the scrotum. The processus vaginalis normally closes before birth, preventing additional fluid from going from the abdomen into the scrotum. The fluid around the testis gradually gets absorbed spontaneously.
   Hydroceles that occur in boys during their puberty are the adult-type hydroceles. This occurs simply by over production of fluid by the tissue surrounding the testis. Here there is no patent tract between the abdomen and the scrotum. If these hydroceles become large, surgery may be necessary. Sometimes, hydrocele may be the first and the earliest sign of a testicular tumor.

2. **What is a noncommunicating hydrocele?**
   When there is no connection (patent processus vaginalis) between the abdominal cavity and the scrotum, it is called a non-communicating hydrocele. These hydroceles are normally found in newborns and resolve over time and can be safely observed.

3. **What is a communicating hydrocele?**
   When there is a patency of the processus vaginalis, fluid around the testis may trickle back and forth from the abdomen to the testis and vice versa. In these cases, the parents may note changes in the size of the hydrocele over the course of the day. The size may reduce when the child is asleep or when the scrotum is pressed and it may increase over the course of the day or after the child has a phase of prolonged standing.

4. **What are the clinical features?**
   Hydrocele is a painless scrotal swelling. It is soft, cystic and transilluminant. Tense hydroceles may sometimes be painful.

5. **When is treatment required?**
   Most of the hydroceles resolve by the age of 2 years. Surgery is required if it persists beyond the age of 2 years or in the case of a large and tense hydrocele. Operation of the hydrocele is high ligation of the processus vaginalis (same as herniotomy). The distal sac is opened and the fluid emptied.

6. **How does a hydrocele differ from a hernia?**
   The pathophysiology of hydrocele and hernia is the same, i.e. patency of the processus vaginalis. If bowel comes down through the patent processus vaginalis, it is called hernia and if only fluid trickles down, it is termed hydrocele.

7. **In cases of bilateral hydroceles should Surgery be done simultaneously?**
   Yes, in bilateral hydroceles, simultaneous surgery should be done on either sides. However, in bilateral hydroceles, medical causes such as idiopathic scrotal edema, nephrotic syndrome, ascites, etc. need to be excluded before subjecting the child to surgery.

8. **Which surgery is better? Open or laparoscopic?**
   Surgery involves closure of the processus vaginalis only. This can be done open or laparoscopic. The only disadvantage of laparoscopic surgery is a high recurrence rate.

9. **Does ear piercing help to resolve hydroceles?**
   Ear piercing is commonly done for hydroceles and that it resolves hydroceles is a myth. Hydroceles are known to resolve spontaneously in the first 2 years of life. If ear piercing is done prior to this and the hydrocele resolves, undue credit is given to the ear piercing for resolution of the hydrocele.

10. **When should surgery be done for encysted hydroceles of cord?**
    Encysted hydrocele of cord does not resolve spontaneously. Surgery for the same should be done at the earliest after the diagnosis.

11. **What are the chances of a child developing contralateral hydrocele when operated on one side?**
    The chances of a contralateral patent processus vaginalis in a child with hydrocele is between 10% and 15%. This may/may not present as a clinical hernia/hydrocele. However, there is a theoretical possibility of the child developing a contralateral hydrocele/hernia due to it in the future.

Hypospadias

Chapter 51

Amar Shah, Aniruddh Shah

> **CASE STUDY**
>
> A child comes with a history of passing urine from an abnormal opening on the undersurface of the penis. The child's prepuce is also malformed. It is like a hood over the dorsal aspect penis and deficient over the ventral aspect. The urethral opening is not seen at the normal site at the tip of the glans, but instead is located at the undersurface of the penis.

1. **What is hypospadias?**

    Hypospadias is a congenital defect where the urethral opening is located on the undersurface of the penis instead of at the tip. This is always accompanied with an incomplete prepuce (hooded prepuce).

    Hypo in Greek means "Below," and Spadon in Greek means "Opening."

    Hypospadias is thought to result from failure of the urinary channel to completely tubularize to the end of the penis. The cause for the same is unknown. Hypospadias is most often the only abnormal finding. However, in about 10% of cases, hypospadias may be part of a syndrome with multiple abnormalities.

2. **What are the types of hypospadias?**

    The urethral opening may be located anywhere from the penoscrotal region to near the tip of the penis, and accordingly, hypospadias is classified as proximal (Fig. 1), mid (Fig. 2) and distal (Fig. 3) penile hypospadias.

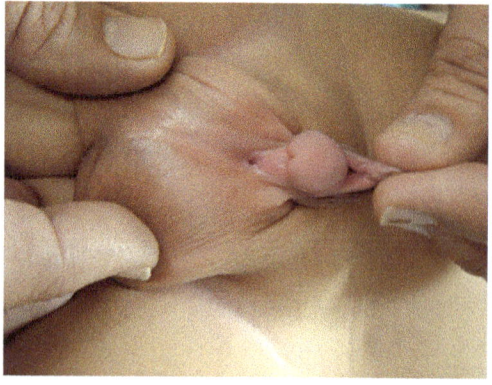

Fig. 1: Hypospadius proximal.

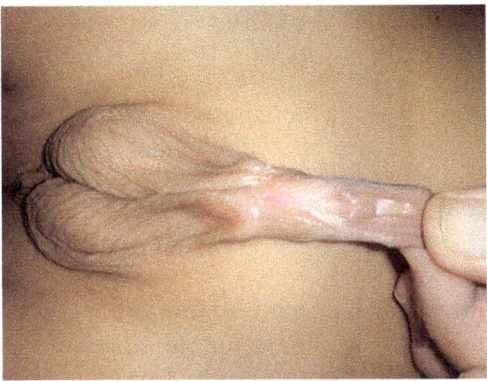

Fig. 2: Hypospadias mid.

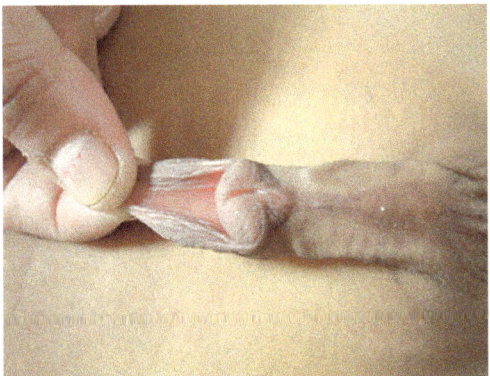

Fig. 3: Hypospadias distal.

3. **What associated anomalies should be looked for in a child with hypospadias?**
   Hypospadias may be associated with other anomalies like undescended testis, inguinal hernias, congenital renal anomalies and vesicoureteric reflux. Undescended testis is seen in almost 3% of the children with distal penile hypospadias and in 10% of the children with proximal penile hypospadias. In a child with proximal hypospadias with a unilateral or bilateral undescended testes, ambiguous genitalia should be suspected and detailed work-up for the same should be done.

4. **When should surgery be done for hypospadias?**
   Surgery for hypospadias should be done around 1.5 years of age. The goal should be for completion of treatment before the child is toilet trained. Most of the distal and mid penile hypospadias can be repaired in a single stage. However, for proximal and complex hypospadias, two or more stages of surgery may be necessary. If the penis is small, testosterone or human chorionic gonadotropin (hCG) injections may be given to enlarge it before surgery.
   The clinician should make sure that children with hypospadias do not get circumcised as the prepuceal skin will be helpful for the surgeon in the urethral reconstruction.

Some infants with hypospadias may have associated severe meatal stenosis. In these children, meatoplasty may need to be done as a primary procedure while waiting for the child to grow up.

Complications following surgery for hypospadias:
- Urethral fistula—most common complication. However, with experience, good instrumentation and newer techniques, the incidence is gradually reducing
- Meatal stenosis
- Urethral stricture
- Urethral diverticulum.

5. **What is the long-term outcome in children with hypospadias?**

   Children operated for hypospadias have a normal physical and mental development. They do not have long-term issues in the marital life or reproductive capabilities.

Infantile Hemangioma

Chapter 52

Upendra Kinjawadekar, Vipin Goyal

CASE STUDY

A 4-month-old female presented with bright red plaques over the right side of her face, which were progressively growing (Figs. 1A and B).

Patient underwent magnetic resonance imaging (MRI) scan since a significant portion of face was involved. As the lesion caused significant disfigurement, it was treated with oral propranolol at 1 mg/kg/day and later on topical tacrolimus was added for 3weeks. The patient responded well, and the lesions started regressing. After 4 months, the lesions decreased significantly. During the treatment, we monitored the patient's blood glucose, since she was on oral propranolol (Figs. 1C and D).

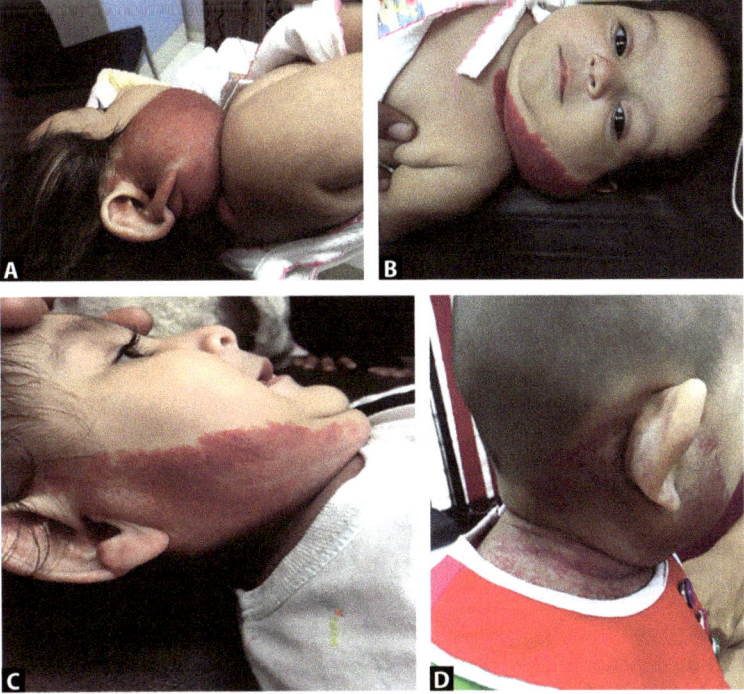

Figs. 1A to D: Infantile hemangioma. (A and B) A 4-month-old female presented with bright red plaques; (C and D) After 4 months follow-up.

1. **What is infantile hemangioma?**
   Infantile hemangiomas are proliferative, benign vascular tumors which originate from vascular endothelium. They may be present at birth, or more commonly, may become apparent in the first 2 weeks of life. They are the *most common tumors of infancy, occurring in 5% of newborns.*

2. **What are the risk factors for infantile hemangiomas?**
   The risk factors include prematurity, low birth weight, female gender and white race.

3. **How are infantile hemangiomas classified?**
   - *Superficial hemangiomas:* These are bright red, dome-shaped papules, plaques and tumors which are rubbery and may compress with palpation (as seen in the patient in this case study).
   - *Deep hemangiomas:* These are blue-purple subcutaneous nodules and tumors which may have prominent surface telangiectasias and may be warm to palpation.
   - *Combined hemangiomas:* These have both superficial and deep components. They have a bright red surface component, and a deeper blue nodular component.

4. **What is the typical natural course of infantile hemangiomas?**
   They typically become evident around 1–2 weeks of age. They generally go through the proliferative (growth) phase for the first year, followed by the plateau phase and the phase of spontaneous involution. Thirty percent involute by 3 years, 50% by 5 years, 70% by 7 years and 90% or more by 10 years. Involution may not lead to complete resolution of all skin changes.

5. **What are the complications and "Red Flags" associated with hemangiomas?**
   Complications include impairment of a vital function, ulceration, secondary infection and permanent disfigurement. Clinical findings that need to be further investigated, and can be called as "Red Flags" include:
   - Facial hemangioma involving significant areas of face—evaluate for PHACE syndrome. PHACE stands for Posterior fossa—brain malformations that are present at birth
   - Hemangioma—This usually covers a large area on the skin of the head or neck (greater than 5 cm). The term "segmental" is sometimes used to describe these hemangiomas.
   - Arterial lesions—abnormalities of the blood vessels in the neck or head
   - Cardiac abnormalities/aortic coarctation—abnormalities of the heart or the blood vessels that are attached to the heart
   - Eye abnormalities (MRI for orbital hemangioma and posterior fossa malformation, cardiac and ophthalmologic evaluation, and evaluation for midline anomalies)
   - Cutaneous hemangiomas in beard distribution—evaluate for airway hemangioma, especially if manifesting with stridor
   - Periocular hemangioma—MRI of orbit and ophthalmologic evaluation
   - Paraspinal midline vascular lesions—ultrasonography (USG) or MRI to evaluate for occult spinal dysraphism
   - Hemangiomatosis (multiple small cutaneous hemangiomas)—evaluate for parenchymal hemangiomas, especially hepatic and central nervous system (CNS)
   - Large hemangiomas, especially hepatic—USG with Doppler flow studies, MRI and thyroid function studies
   - Thrill and/or bruit associated with hemangiomas—cardiac evaluation and ECHO
   - Head tilting—evaluate for specific site of lesion and consider physical therapy evaluation

- Delayed milestones—consider side effect of corticosteroids or interferons
- Lumbar syndrome—MRI of spine and kidneys

6. **What are the look-alikes of infantile hemangioma?**
   Skin lesions that may imitate infantile hemangiomas during its various stages include port wine stain, venous malformations, lymphatic malformations, arteriovenous malformations, kaposiform hemangioendothelioma, pyogenic granuloma and soft tissue malignancy.

7. **How are they diagnosed?**
   Clinical examination and history usually suggest the diagnosis. USG and MRI are rarely indicated and should be done only when complications are suspected. Tissue biopsy is rarely necessary, and can be confirmed with immunostaining for glucose transporter 1, fcyRII, merosin and Lewis Y antigen.

8. **How are infantile hemangiomas treated?**
   In the usual patient with an infantile hemangiomas who has no serious complications or extensive growth resulting in tissue destruction and severe disfigurement, treatment consists of expectant observation, emotional support, education and referral to family support groups.
   Ulcerated lesions require local wound care with topical antibiotics (ex-bacitracin, mupirocin, metronidazole, etc.), nonstick wound dressings and compresses or becaplermin (recombinant platelet derived growth factor) and pain control with oral analgesics, topical anesthetics, pulsed dye laser therapy or rarely oral narcotic analgesics.
   Systemic antibiotic therapy may be used for moderate or severe secondary infection.
   Topical corticosteroids may be useful when applied nightly to localized, superficial lesions. Intralesional corticosteroids may be used for localized lesions.
   Oral corticosteroids form the traditional mainstay of therapy. Prednisolone or prednisone, 2-4 mg/kg/day with histamine 2 blocker like ranitidine for gastritis prophylaxis have a prompt response.
   Oral propranolol is an evolving therapy for infantile hemangiomas. It is started at 1 mg/kg/day and titrated up to 2 mg/kg/day, divided 2-3 times daily. Risks include hypoglycemia, hypotension, bradycardia, bronchospasm and hypothermia.
   Pulsed dye laser therapy is mainly useful for ulcerated lesions or early superficial hemangiomas.
   Recombinant interferon alpha is reserved for life-threatening and function-threatening hemangiomas, which are refractory to other treatments, since they have a risk of spastic diplegia.
   Vincristine is a chemotherapeutic agent beneficial for life-threatening lesions, including the risks of developing peripheral neuropathy.
   Surgical excision is useful in selected situations, including involuted lesions, residual scars, or fibrofatty redundant tissue.

Infective Endocarditis

Chapter 53

Ritesh Sukharamwala, Chintan Bhatt

CASE STUDY 1

A 12-year-old male presented with history of chronic fever for 3 weeks. He subsequently developed abscesses at multiple sites—subcutaneous, intramuscular and even bony lesions. His blood culture and pus culture grew methicillin sensitive *staphylococcus aureus*. Transesophageal echo was done to identify source of infection. It revealed bicuspid aortic valve with multiple small vegetation (Fig. 1) over aortic valve with aortic root abscess. He was treated in direction of infective endocarditis (IE) for 6 weeks with sensitive antibiotic. During the last follow-up, that is after 2 months, he was afebrile and there were no new lesions. Echo showed disappearance of vegetation (Fig. 2).

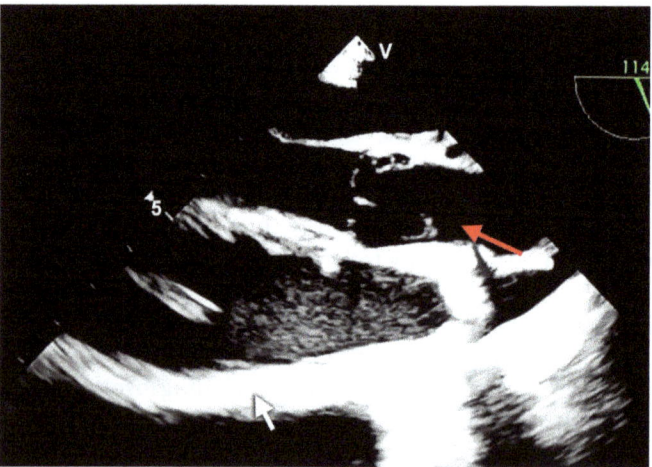

Fig. 1: Transesophageal long axis view of aorta with vegetation in aortic root.

Infective Endocarditis

Antibiotic sensitivity report (Manual and automated)			
Antibiotic	Result	MIC	ZOI
Staphylococcus aureus			
Benzylpenicillin	R	> =0.5	
Oxacillin	S	0.5	
Amikacin	S		18
Gentamicin	S	> =0.5	
Tobramycin	S		23
Ciprofloxacin	R	>=8	
Ciprofloxacin	R	4	
Azithromycin	R		<=13
Erythromycin	R	>=8	
Clindamycin	S	0.25	
Linezolid	S	2	
Daptomycin	S	0.5	
Teicoplanin	S	<=0.5	
Vancomych	S	1	

Fig. 2: Blood culture sensitivity report of the same patient.

CASE STUDY 2

A 21-day-old preterm baby was being treated for fever in the neonatal intensive care unit (NICU). The baby had relatively smooth course post-delivery and had only brief duration of ventilation. On the 18th day of life, the baby had started to spike fever and subsequently collapsed on the 21st day of life. Cardiac evaluation was ordered in view of sudden collapse. Two-dimensional (2D) echo revealed large vegetation (Fig. 3) over mitral valve causing obstruction of left inflow and severe pulmonary venous obstruction. Conventional blood culture revealed no growth, but in view of large globular vegetation (fungal balls) on echo, fungal culture was suggested which grew candida species. The source of infection is likely to be umbilical venous catheterization. Usually central venous line can cause involvement of tricuspid or pulmonary valve; in this case, mitral valve involvement is explained by presence of central line tip in left atrial (LA) through patent foramen ovale.

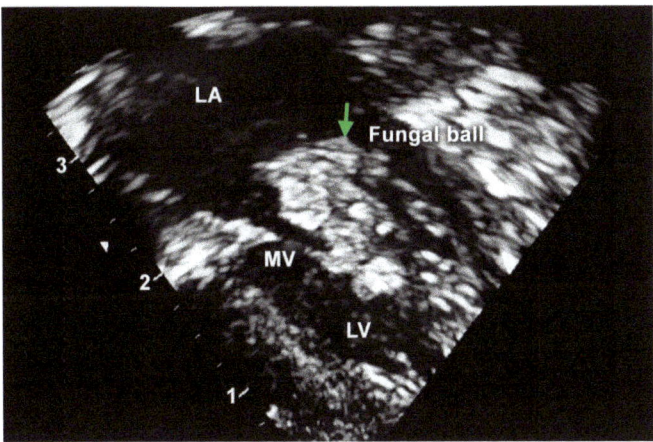

Fig.3: Large vegetation mass totally occluding mitral valve.

1. **What is the incidence of IE?**
   - Incidence—0.05 and 0.12 cases per 1,000 pediatric admissions
   - In the last two decades, coronary heart disease (CHD) is most the underlying condition—aortic valve abnormalities, ventricular septal defect (VSD), tetralogy of Fallot (TOF), etc. Earlier, rheumatic heart disease was the common underlying condition.

2. **When should one suspect IE on clinical grounds?**
   Modified Duke criteria is used to diagnose IE. It includes major criteria and minor criteria. Positive blood culture and evidence of endocardial involvement demonstrated by echocardiography are major criteria. Minor criteria include prolonged unexplained fever, vascular phenomena like major arterial emboli, septic pulmonary infarcts, mycotic aneurysm, intracranial hemorrhage, conjunctival hemorrhages, and immunologic phenomena like glomerulonephritis, Osler nodes, Roth's spots and positive rheumatoid factor.

3. **What is the association of IE in children with previous cardiac surgery or after placement of transcatheter devices?**
   - Corrective surgery with no residual defects eliminates risk for IE in children with VSD/atrial septal defect (ASD) and PDA after 6 months of endothelialization
   - Presence of murmur post cardiac surgery is a risk factor for IE and one should consider IE prophylaxis after consultation with cardiologist
   - In the current era, presence of prosthetic valve or conduit caries highest risk of IE
   - A long-term study of transcatheter device closure of ASD/PDA shows no cases of IE

4. **How common is IE in newborn infants?**
   - IE is more common in neonates than in general population (incidence 7.3%—AHA 2015 IE guidelines)
   - Commonest source if IE is central venous catheters more commonly affecting tricuspid valve
   - IE in newborn is more common among premature babies and those with underlying CHDs
   - The most common infecting organisms were *Staph aureus, coagulase* negative staphylococcus strains, Gram-negative bacterial species and *Candida species*
   - Clinical manifestations are non-specific, indistinguishable from sepsis or CHF
   - Neonates often present with feeding difficulties, respiratory distress, tachycardia and hypotension
   - Septic emboli are common compared to big children resulting in foci of infection outside the heart (osteomyelitis, pneumonia and meningitis/hemiparesis/apnea).

5. **How many blood cultures should be obtained in children with clinically suspected IE?**
   At least three separate blood cultures should be taken preferably 1 hour apart if the patient is stable irrespective of febrile status of the patient.

6. **What is the role of echocardiogram for the diagnosis of IE?**
   IE is a clinical- and laboratory-based diagnosis and not solely an echocardiographic diagnosis. Echo can diagnose certain cases having vegetation or mass over valves or congenital heart defect (i.e. PDA). Likelihood of positive finding on echo increases under certain conditions like indwelling catheters, prematurity, immunosuppression and evidence of peripheral embolization. A negative echo study does not rule out IE.

7. **What is different characteristic of vegetation depending upon organism?**
   Common organisms associated with native valve endocarditis in children are *Streptococcus viridans*, *Staphylococcus aureus*, and in neonatal age group, it is *Candida albicans*. Staphylococcus and candida related vegetations are usually large and can complicate early in spite of adequate treatment while vegetation related to *Streptococcus* are usually small and disappear with treatment.

8. **What are the common cardiac complications in relation to IE?**
   Cardiac complications include congestive heart failure, new or progressive valvular dysfunction that is usually seen as increased regurgitation, periannular extension of infection, sinus of Valsalva rupture, myocardial dysfunction, obstruction of conduits or shunts, prosthetic valve dysfunction including dehiscence, pericardial effusion, and less commonly, septic emboli to the coronary arteries.

9. **What are the indications for antibiotic prophylaxis for a dental procedure?**
   It is reasonable to shift the disproportionately large focus on antibiotic prophylaxis to an emphasis on oral hygiene and prevention of oral diseases. Current American Heart Association recommends the following indications:
   - Cardiac valve repair with a prosthetic valve or prosthetic material
   - Previous IE
   - Unrepaired cyanotic CHD
   - Repaired CHD with prosthetic material or device during the first 6 months after the procedure
   - Repaired CHD with residual defects
   - Recipients of cardiac transplants who develop cardiac valvulopathy

Iron Deficiency Anemia

Chapter 54

Nirav Buch

CASE STUDY

A 1-year old child was brought with increased respiratory effort and irritability and refusing to eat since last 15 days. Child had fever and running nose for 2 days. He was born prematurely at 32 weeks had turbulent in NICU stay and was transferred twice. He was discharged on oral colloidal iron that was given with milk so that the kid would not vomit. The child was given bottle feed as mother felt that she did not lactate adequately and choose advised commercial milk formula meaning of situated at 9 months but child refused to eat and preferred milk over other foods which he spat out.

1. **What are the signs and symptoms of iron deficiency anemia?**
    - Mechanical symptoms of iron deficiency anemia depend on is severity of anemia, the speed of onset, the age group and comorbidity.
    - Hematopoietic skin and CNS manifestations are often affected.
    - Very frequent:
        - Pallor (Fig.1) exhaustion, dyspnea and headache.

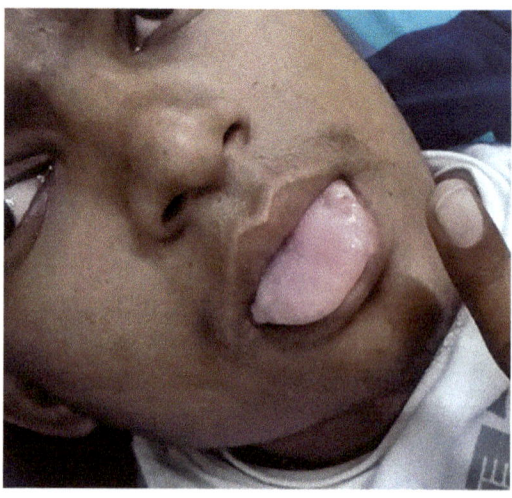

Fig. 1: Pale tongue.

- Frequent:
  - Diffuse and moderate alopecia, atrophic glossitis, koilonychia (Fig. 2) restless leg syndrome, dry and rough skin, dry and damaged hair, cardiac murmur, tachycardia, neurocognitive dysfunction, angina pectoris and vertigo.
- Rare
  - Hemodynamic instability, syncope, koilonychia, platy nychia plummer- vinson syndrome.

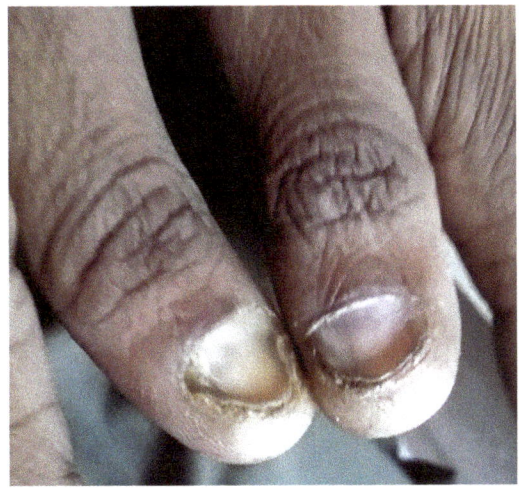

Fig. 2: Koilonychia (Spoon shaped nails)Drop Label A and B.

2. **What are the common causes of iron deficiency anemia?**
   - Blood loss
   - digestive tract carcinomas, ulcers, angiodysplasia and parasites
   - Gynecological loss
   - Surgery
   - Hematuria epistaxis, hemostasis, hemodialysis, nonsteroidal anti-inflammatory drugs.
   - Malabsorption
   - Disease gastrectomy, helicobacter pylori, gut resection, atrophic gastritis bypass surgery is bacterial overgrowth interaction with food elements for example; tea coffee, calcium, pica pagophagia, antacids and proton pump inhibitors H2 antagonists.
   - Anemia of chronic disease
   - Chronic heart failure, cancer, chronic kidney disease, rheumatoid arthritis, obesity, inflammatory bowel disease
   - Genetic forms
   - Metabolic defects like iron refractory and iron deficiency anemia.

3. **What are the hematological parameters used in management of iron deficiency anemia**
   - Hemoglobin   Low
   - MCV   Reduced
   - MCH   Low

- MCHC — Decreased
- RDW — Increased
- Reticulocyte count — Low — Useful in assessment of response
- Reticulocyte hemoglobin — Reduced — Useful in early diagnosis and assessment of content (CHr) response immature reticulocyte useful in response assessment fraction.
- Serum iron — Reduced — Affected by several factors ex. Therapy
- Total iron binding capacity — Increased
- Serum ferritin — Reduced — Increased in anemia of chronic inflammation
- Transferrin levels — Low
- Transferrin saturation — Increased
- Serum soluble transferrin — Increased — Useful in differentiating between iron receptor levels
- Hepcidin levels — Low — Useful in differentiation of anemia of chronic inflammation and IRIDA.
- Serum ceruloplasmin — Rare genetic cases with neurodegeneration — Deficiency and anemia of chronic inflammation
- Zinc protoporphyrin — Beta thalassemia trait iron deficiency and lead poisoning
- Bone marrow examination — Gold standard in diagnosis but invasive
- Other special tests:
  - Tissue biopsy MRI scan — Especially for iron overload
  - Endoscopy, tissue transglutaminase — Workup of etiology
  - RBC Tagged Scan, Meckel scan
  - Iron staining of bronchioalveolar aspirate
  - Gene sequencing etc.

4. **Treatment of iron deficiency anemia.**
   - Treatment of cause
   - Treatment of iron deficiency
   - Nutritional rehabilitation and prevention of recurrence
5. **What are the various oral iron preparations available?**
   - Ferrous salts, ferric salts and colloidal iron.
   - Ferric salts have no place in treatment of iron deficiency anemia
6. **Which salt of iron is preferable?**
   It is necessary to have a ferrous salt the type of salt does not matter.
7. **What are the types of intravenous iron preparations available for use?**
   Iron is available conjugated with following carbohydrate:
   Dextran polysaccharides, gluconate, sucrose, polyglucose sorbitol carboxymethyl ether, isomaltoside, carboxymaltose and ferumoxetol.

Chapter 55

Lamellar Ichthyosis

Vijay Shah, Upendra Chaudhari

CASE STUDY

A 7-year-old male child presented with ichthyotic lesion (Fig. 1) all over the skin since birth. There is no history of consanguinity in parents, he is the only child and no history of abortion in mother. He is full term, cried immediately after birth, was kept in neonatal intensive care unit (NICU) for 12 days as he was born as a collodion baby and had no history of frequent infections or hospitalization. His developmental milestones are normal. He has ectropion and eclabium.

The child is suffering from *lamellar ichthyosis*.

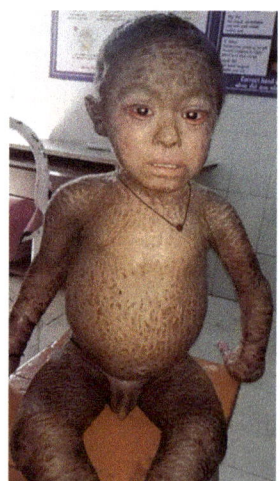

Fig. 1: Lamellar ichthyosis.

1. **What is ichthyosis?**
   Disorder of cornification is called ichthyosis (Fig. 1). It is an inherited condition in which scaling is present, and on histology hyperkeratosis.

2. **What is the characteristic of different types of ichthyosis?**
   They are differentiated on the basis of inheritance patterns, clinical features, associated defects and histological changes.
3. **What is lamellar ichthyosis?**
   A patient with lamellar ichthyosis presents with erythroderma and scaling. It is an autosomal recessive disorder. There is increased proliferation of epidermal cells. Prevalence is <1 per 3 lacs. Both sex and all population involved.
4. **Which are the genes responsible for lamellar ichthyosis?**
   There are three genes:
   - L I-1 (Transglutaminase 1)
   - L I-2 (ABCA 12)
   - L I-3 (CYP4F22)

   Transglutaminase 1 mutation leads to abnormality in cornified envelope.
   ABCA 12 mutation leads to abnormal lipid transport.
   CYP4F22 mutation leads to abnormal lamellar granules.
5. **What are the clinical features of ichthyosis?**
   At birth, collodion membrane is present which sheds within 10–14 days which is followed by large quadrilateral, dark scales (Hyperkeratosis) (Fig. 3) that are free of the edges and adherent at center, often involves entire body surface resembling fish skin (Figs. 2 and 5). Ectropion (Fig. 4), eclabium and bilateral conjunctivitis present, ears are small and crumpled, and hairs are sparse and thin. Entrapped hairs and nails growth is 2–3 times the normal rate. Palm and soles are also hyperkeratotic. Teeth and mucosal surface are normal. There is abnormal sweat gland function. There is mild erythema. This condition persists throughout life.

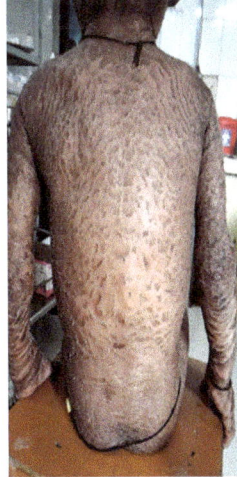

Fig. 2: Fish like scales on skin.

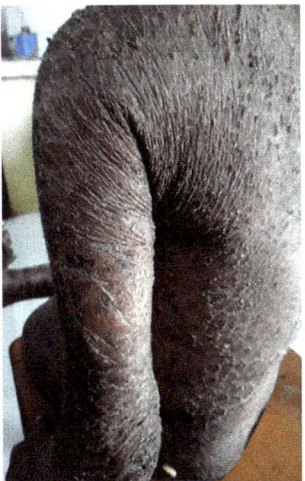

Fig. 3: Hyperkeratotic skin.

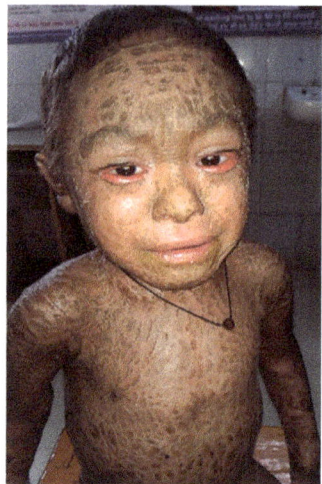
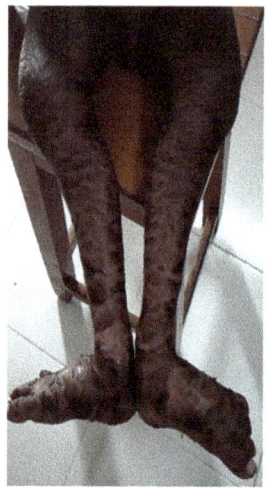

Fig. 4: Ectropion (outwardly turned lower eye lid
Eclabium: Outwardly turned lower lip.

Fig. 5: Fissuring over dorsum of feet and fish like scaling.

6. **What is the histological finding?**
   Markedly thicken stratum cornium and mild thickening of epidermal layer is characteristic.
7. **Is any test available for diagnosis?**
   Yes.
   - Transglutaminase deficiency in skin biopsy
   - Genetic study
   - Prenatal diagnosis by CVS or amniocentesis
8. **What is the treatment of lamellar ichthyosis?**
   High humidity during winter and cool environment during summer reduces discomfort.
   Removal of loose scales with soft moist cloth during bathing.
   Bad odor and unattractive appearance create psychological problems, and need psychological therapy.
   If bad odor, bathing in potassium permanganate solution.
   Soap is best avoided.
   Keratolytic agents are useful, and they are:
   - Urea 10–40%
   - Lactic or glycolic acid 5–12%
   - Salicylic acid 2–3%
   - Topical calcipotriol
   - Tazarotene 0.1% gel
   - Retinoic acid 0.1% cream reduces scaling

   Oral retinoids 1 mg/kg/day should be administered indefinitely.
   Methotrexate has variable results.
   Ectropion requires ophthalmological care.

9. **What are the complications with ichthyosis?**
   - Infection
   - Thermal regulation disturbance
   - Hypernatremic dehydration
   - Fissures on the skin
   - Exposure keratitis
   - Alopecia
   - Inflexible digits.
10. **What is risk to Life?**
    Risk of death is elevated during neonatal period.

Lymphangioma

Chapter 56

Aniruddh Shah, Amar Shah

CASE STUDY

A newborn child is brought with a swelling over the left side of the neck since birth. On examination, the child has a large ill-defined cystic mass (Fig. 1) over the left side of the neck. It is non-tender and has a slight bluish hue of the skin above it. The rest of the neck is normal.

This is a cystic hygroma/lymphangioma over the neck.

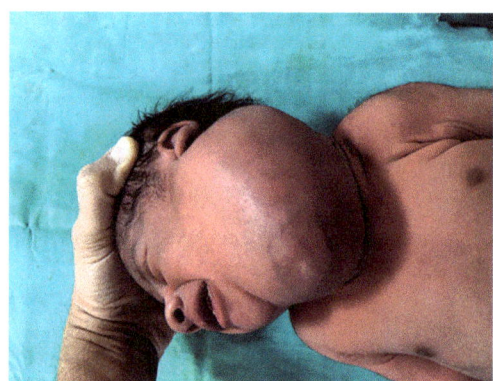

Fig. 1: Cystic selling in neck.

1. **What is a lymphangioma?**
    Lymphangiomas are benign hamartomatous tumors of the lymphatic system. They account for 4% of all vascular tumors in children. Almost 50% are seen at birth and 90% of them become evident by 2 years of age. Lymphangiomas lesions arise from sequestration of the lymphatic sacs/cells that form the lymphatic system.
2. **What are the types of lymphangiomas?**
    - Lymphangioma simplex—small, capillary sized lymphatic channels
    - Cavernous lymphangioma—dilated lymphatic channels with fibrous covering
    - Cystic lymphangioma—cystic hygromas
    - Lymphangio-hemangiomas—lymphangiomas with vascular component.

Lymphangiomas can also be classified according to the size of their cysts:
- *Microcystic:* Lymphangiomas composed of cysts which measure less than 2 cm^3 in volume
- *Macrocystic:* Lymphangiomas composed of cysts which measure more than 2 cm^3 in volume
- *Mixed:* Lymphangiomas which contain both microcystic and macrocystic components.

3. **What are the common sites of a lymphangioma?**
   They may be present anywhere over or even inside the body. However, the neck, abdomen and chest wall are the common sites. Large lymphangiomas may be present in the intrauterine life and antenatal ultrasound helps pick up these lesions.

4. **What syndromes are associated with cystic hygromas?**
   - Multiple pterygium syndrome
   - Turner's syndrome
   - Noonan's syndrome
   - Robert's syndrome
   - Pena-Shokeir syndrome.

5. **What is the natural progress of lymphangioma?**
   Unlike hemangiomas, lymphangiomas always grow and never regress.

6. **What are the treatment options for lymphangioma?**
   A child with an antenatally diagnosed cystic hygroma should be delivered at a center where neonatal intensive care unit (NICU) care is readily available as these children need to be closely monitored for airway obstruction. If the cystic hygroma is large, a cesarean section may be preferred by the obstetrician. In the event of an emergency, a thin needle may be used to reduce the volume of the cystic hygroma to prevent airway obstruction.
   - *Surgery:* Conservative excision of lymphangiomas should be done with due care to prevent damage to the normal neurovascular structures. Inadequately performed surgery may lead to recurrence.
   - *Sclerosants:* Sclerosants like bleomycin and OK-432 are also being used with good results. Treatment options vary from patient to patient and depend upon the site and the size of the lymphangioma.

Microtia

Chapter 57

Jagdish Chinnappa

1. **Describe the disorder?**
   - Microtia with congenital canal atresia (Fig. 1).
   - Seen in about 1:10,000 neonates.

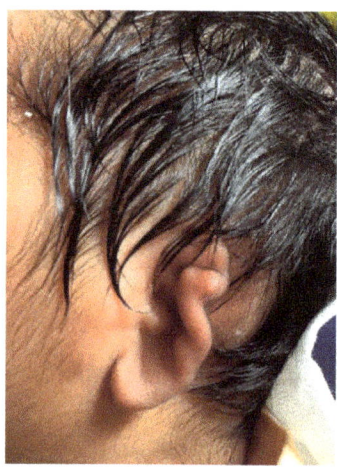

Fig. 1: Poorly formed ear (microtia) with Atretic ear canal.

2. **What else will you look for?**
   Contralateral ear, other anomalies and hearing evaluation.
3. **Should unilateral conductive hearing loss be treated?**
   Yes.
   With a bone conduction hearing device.
4. **Which syndromes are associated with this condition?**
   - Down's
   - Charge
   - Treacher Collins
   - Goldenhar
   - Branchio oto renal
5. **When should one plan surgery?**
   When adequate cartilage is available, about 8–10 years.

Mitral Stenosis

Chapter 58

Kewal Kishore Arora, Swati Mulye

CASE STUDY

An 11-year-old male child was brought to us with the complaint of breathlessness on exertion since 3–4 years, no weight gain, easy fatigability and palpitations (Fig. 1A).

The child was taking treatment from some physician, and was prescribed penicillin G as prophylaxis for rheumatic fever after two-dimensional (2D)-Echo was suggestive of rheumatic heart disease (RHD). Currently, the child came with chest pain on and off, and breathlessness on exertion.

On examination, the child's anthropometry was between the third and fifteenth percentile, had malar (Fig. 1) flush, pulse was 86 per minute, jugular veins were full thin built, apical impulse was in 5th intercostals space in mid clavicular line, tapping apex on palpation, systolic thrill present at apex, with a palpable right ventricular (RV) lift at left parasternal area on auscultation characteristic loud first heart sound, an opening snap and a diastolic rumble heard. The second heart sound was normally split with loud pulmonary component of second heart sound and a systolic murmur heard at mitral area. Clinical impression of MS with mitral regurgitation (MR) of rheumatic etiology was made.

X-ray Chest: Shows straightening (Fig. 2) of left cardiac border due to LA enlargement and LA appendage, and upward displacement of the main stem bronchi, prominent pulmonary vessels.

ECG: 12-lead electrocardiography (ECG) in this patient with mitral stenosis (MS) is showing evidence of—LA enlargement (inverted distal portion of P-wave in lead V1 and elongated P-wave in lead II)—increased right heart forces consistent with pulmonary hypertension and RV overload—tall R-waves in LV leads, deep S-waves in RV leads suggestive of LV hypertrophy (Fig. 3).

2D-Echo: Suggestive of RHD
- Moderate MS/moderate MR/mild aortic regurgitation (AR)
- Dilated Left atrial (LA) and left ventricular (LV)
- Mild pulmonary arterial hypertension (PAH)
- Good LV function [ejection fraction (EF) 65%]
- Right atrial (RA) and RV normal in size
- Intact interatrial septum (IAS)/intact ventricular septum (IVS)

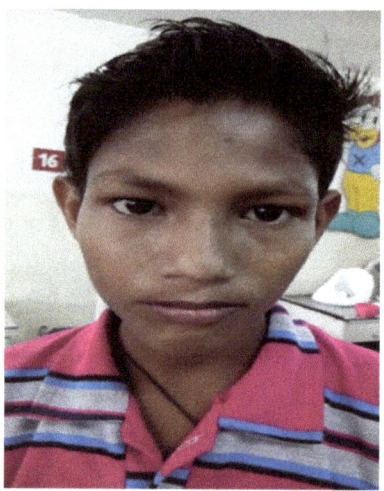

Fig. 1: Malar flush.

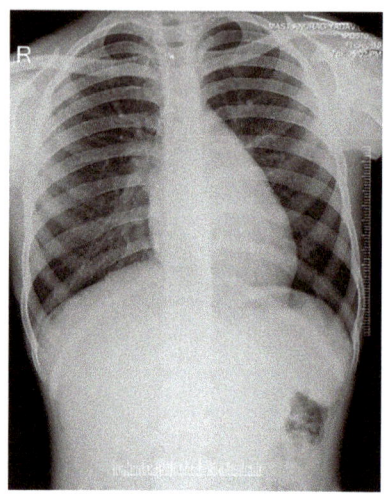

Fig. 2: Chest X-ray of same patient.

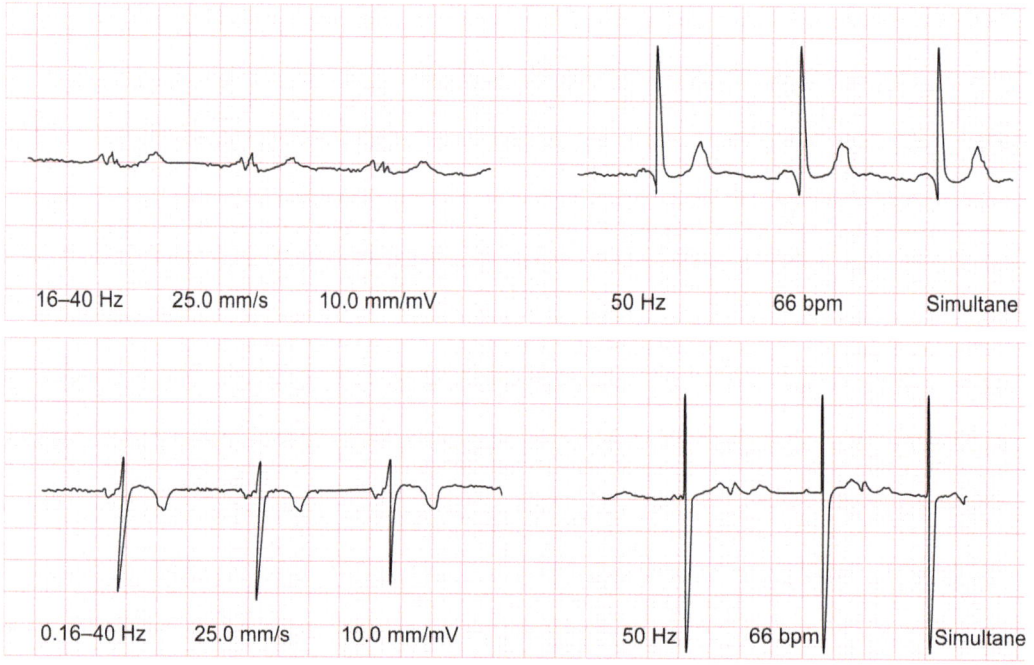

Fig. 3: Tall R-waves in LV leads, deep S-waves in RV.

Investigations

Complete blood count (CBC): hemoglobin (Hb)—10.9; total leukocyte count (TLC)—11,900 P63, L26, M8, E2; platelets—3.17; erythrocyte sedimentation rate (ESR)—14; C-reactive protein (CRP)—0.3; antistreptolysin O (ASO)—400.

1. **What is the prevalence of rheumatic heart disease and MS?**
   The prevalence of rheumatic disease with MS is higher in developing nations like, India; for example, the prevalence is approximately 100–150 cases per 100,000. MS occurs at earlier age in developing countries than developed countries.

2. **What are the symptoms of MS?**
   Shortness of breath, fatigue, swelling on feet, palpitations, dizziness or fainting, hemoptysis, and chest pain.

3. **What is Malar flush?**
   Malar flush is a plum-red discoloration of the high cheeks classically associated with *MS* due to the resulting CO_2 retention and its vasodilatory effects. It can also be associated with other conditions, such as systemic lupus erythematosus (SLE) or polycythemia rubra vera.

4. **What are the signs of MS?**
   The presence of mitral facies indicate chronic severe MS, jugular vein distension, often a RV lift is palpable in the left parasternal region in the patient with pulmonary hypertension. A P_2 may be palpable in the second left intercostal space.
   The auscultatory findings like a loud first heart sound, an opening snap, and a diastolic rumble, the second heart sound is normally split, and the pulmonic component is accentuated if pulmonary hypertension is present, the diastolic murmur is of low pitch, rumbling in character, and best heard at the apex, a high-pitched decrescendo diastolic murmur secondary to pulmonary regurgitation (Graham Steell murmur) may be audible at the upper sternal border, a pan systolic murmur of tricuspid regurgitation (TR) and an S3 originating from the right ventricle may be audible in the fourth left intercostal space (ICS) in the patient with RV dilatation.

5. **Which imaging studies are indicated in the work-up of MS?**
   - X-ray chest—Chest radiographic findings suggestive of MS include LA enlargement, prominent pulmonary vessels, redistribution of pulmonary vasculature to the upper lobes, mitral valve calcification and interstitial edema (Kerley A and B lines)
   - Echocardiography is the most specific and sensitive method of diagnosing and quantifying the severity of MS
   - Using a transthoracic 2D echocardiogram (TTE), Doppler study and color-flow Doppler imaging, the anatomic abnormalities of the stenotic valve, calcification, involvement of the sub-valvular apparatus and the characteristic fusion of the commissures can be well defined
   - Transesophageal echocardiography (TEE) provides better quality images than TTE and is more accurate in assessing the anatomic features of the valve and the presence of LA appendage thrombus.

6. **What is the role of ECG in the work-up of MS?**
   ECG is quite diagnostic, and in moderate-to-severe MS, the ECG can show signs of LA enlargement, and commonly, atrial fibrillation. A mean QRS axis in the frontal plane is greater than 80 and an R-to-S ratio greater than 1 in lead V_1 indicates the presence of RV hypertrophy. As the severity of the pulmonary hypertension increases, the mean QRS axis in the frontal plane moves toward the right.

7. **What are the goals of medical treatment for MS?**
   The goals of medical treatment for MS are:
   - To reduce recurrence of rheumatic fever

- Provide prophylaxis for infective endocarditis
- Reduce symptoms of pulmonary congestion (paroxysmal nocturnal dyspnea)
- Control the ventricular rate if atrial fibrillation is present
- Prevent thromboembolic complications
- Because rheumatic fever is the primary cause of MS, secondary prophylaxis against group A beta-hemolytic streptococci (GAS) is recommended.

8. **How is an MS patient treated?**
   The treatment includes:
   - Use anticoagulants to help prevent blood clots
   - A daily aspirin may be included
   - Beta blockers or *calcium channel blockers* to slow your heart rate and allow heart to fill more effectively
   - *Antiarrhythmics* to treat atrial fibrillation or other rhythm disturbances associated with mitral valve stenosis
   - Surgical management when indicated.

9. **What is the duration of secondary rheumatic fever prophylaxis?**
   - In rheumatic fever with carditis and residual heart disease (persistent valvular disease), it is 10 years or until age 40 (whichever is longer)
   - Rheumatic fever with carditis but no residual heart disease (no valvular disease)—10 years or until age 21 (whichever is longer)
   - Rheumatic fever without carditis—5 years or until age 21 (whichever is longer).

10. **What is the surgical care given to MS patients?**
    Surgical therapy for MS consists of mitral valvotomy (which can be either surgical or percutaneous) or mitral valve replacement.

11. **What is the prognosis of MS?**
    After percutaneous balloon valvotomy or surgical commissurotomy, the 5- to 7-year survival rate is 50–90%. After surgical commissurotomy, the reoperation rate is 5–7% and the 5-year complication-free survival rate 80–90%.

Molluscum Contagiosum

Chapter 59

Vijay Shah, Upendra Chaudhari

CASE STUDY

A 6-year-old female child presented with rounded 3 mm size, non-itchy, non-erythematous, umbilicated, pearly white lesion in front of right ear since 1 week (Figs. 1 and 2).

The child presented with the above-mentioned skin lesion without any abnormality in general and systemic examination. There was no fever, cough or cold. There was no involvement of mucosa and no drug exposure.

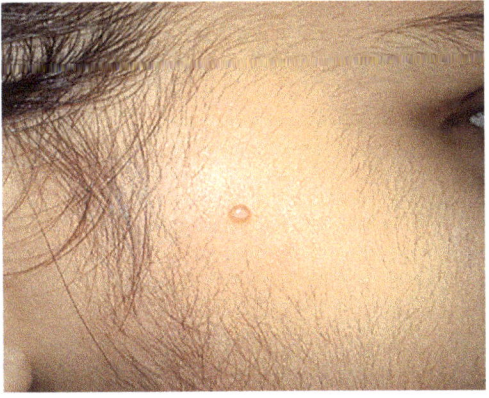

Fig. 1: Molluscum contagiosum.

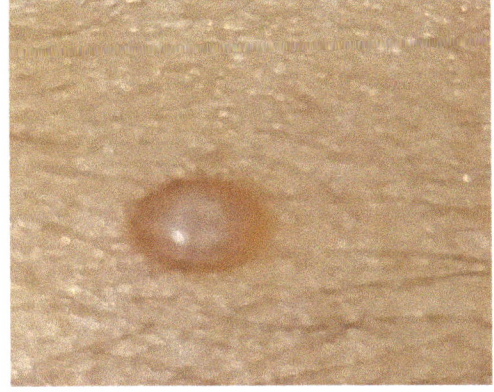

Fig. 2: Molluscum contagiosum macro look.

1. **What is molluscum contagiosum?**
   It belongs to the poxviridae family which presents as single or multiple umbilicated skin colored, opalescent smooth dome-shaped waxy papules.
2. **What is the hallmark character of molluscum contagiosum?**
   Pearly white umbilicated papules with central depression is the hallmark characteristic of molluscum contagiosum.
3. **Which is the commonest age of molluscum contagiosum and what is the incidence in general population?**
   Commonest age is 2–5 years and worldwide incidence is 2–8%.

4. **What differentiates molluscum contagiosum from chickenpox?**
   Though both are umbilicated, in molluscum contagiosum, primary skin lesion is papule, while in chicken pox, primary skin lesion is vesicle.
   Pleomorphism is present in chickenpox but absent in molluscum contagiosum.
   Papule: Elevated firm skin lesion <1 cm in diameter.
   Vesicle: Fluid filled elevated skin lesion <1 cm in diameter.
   Constitutional symptoms are present in chickenpox and herpes, which are fever, pain and burning sensation at site of lesion; they are absent in molluscum contagiosum.
5. **Is there any change of molluscum contagiosum in immunosuppressed patient?**
   Normally, molluscum contagiosum is 2–6 mm in diameter, but in immunosuppressed patient, it can be up to 1 cm or more.
6. **Which are the most common sites of molluscum contagiosum?**
   Face, axilla, antecubital and popliteal fossa are the most common sites.
7. **Which virus is responsible for molluscum contagiosum?**
   Molluscum contagiosum is caused by pox virus.
   Chicken pox is not caused by pox virus even though the name include pox (it is caused by varicella zoster HHV-3 virus).
8. **Which are the clinical differential diagnoses of molluscum contagiosum?**
   - Wart
   - Ectopic sebaceous gland
   - Millia
   - Acne
   - Milliria
   - Basal cell carcinoma.

   Classical pearly white umbilicated lesion usually differentiates the above condition from molluscum contagiosum.
   But in doubt an extraction of lesion there will be molluscum body.
   Henderson-Peterson body (molluscum contagiosum body) is 100% specific for molluscum contagiosum.
9. **Which are the predisposing factors for molluscum contagiosum?**
   - Poor hygiene
   - Over crowding
   - Humidity.

   All these predispose to molluscum contagiosum.
10. **What is prognosis of molluscum contagiosum?**
    Usually prognosis is good as it is self-limiting in 6–9 months, but recurrence can occur.
11. **What are diagnostic investigations of molluscum contagiosum?**
    - Biopsy showing the presence of *Henderson-Peterson* (intra cytoplasmic inclusion body) is diagnostic of molluscum contagiosum.
    - Molluscum contagiosum virus (MCV) deoxyribonucleic acid (DNA) has been recognized by in situ hybridization.
12. **What are therapeutic considerations?**
    It may subside on its own, but early treatment is necessary as it is contagious.
    Treatment options are curettage, topical tretinoin, topical imiquimod, topical 20% KOH application.
    Avoid sharing towels and bathing, and avoid use of swimming pools.

Moyamoya Disease

Chapter 60

Alok Gupta, Mohit Vhora

INTRODUCTION

1. **What is a Moyamoya disease?**
   Moyamoya disease is a rare progressive cerebrovascular disorder caused by blocked arteries at the base of brain in an area called basal ganglia. Blockade of vessels results into marked generation of collaterals. On angiography these collaterals produce an image of puffed smoke; appearance in Japanese is called as Moyamoya (Fig. 1).

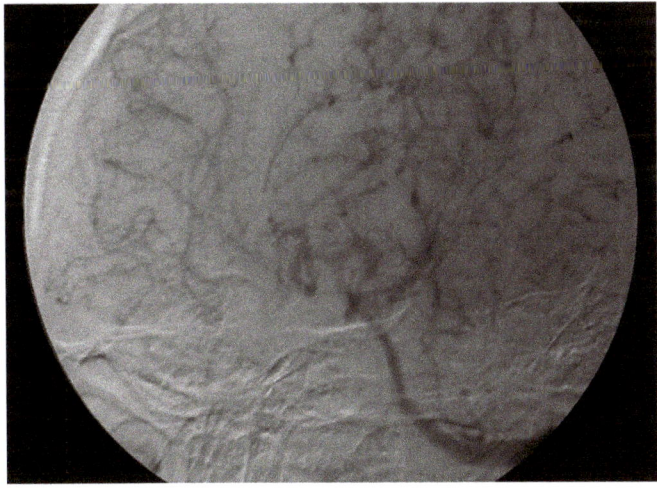

Fig. 1: Digital subtraction angiography showing narrowing of internal carotid artery and its branches with formation of collaterals. Findings are suggestive of moyamoya disease (puff of smoke).

2. **What are the symptoms of Moyamoya disease?**
   Moyamoya disease is often presented as stroke or recurrent transient ischemic attacks frequently accompanied by muscular weakness or paralysis affecting one side of the body or seizures.

3. **What causes Moyamoya disease in children?**
   There are a variety of factors ranging from genetic to traumatic. The most common cause remains idiopathic.
4. **What is the diagnostic modality for Moyamoya disease?**
   Cerebral angiogram remains the investigation modality of choice.
5. **How is Moyamoya treated?**
   There are various types of surgeries which can restore blood flow to the brain (revascularization) by opening narrowed blood vessel or by bypassing the blocked arteries. Drugs like aspirin and calcium channel blockers also have a role in managing complications.

Mucormycosis

Chapter 61

Vishal Gajimwar, Vasant Khalatkar

1. **Identify the abnormality in the Figure 1.**

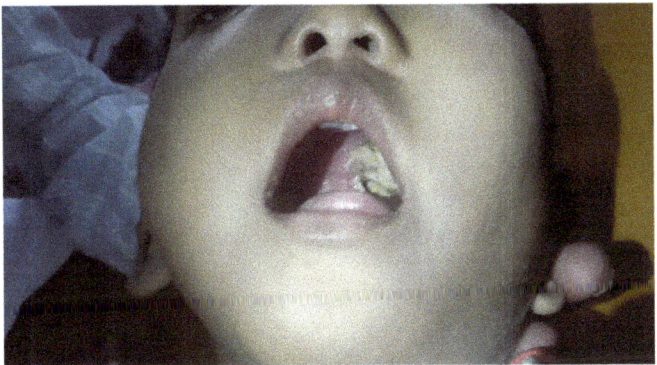

Fig. 1: Palatal fungal growth.

2. **Mention clinical differential diagnosis.**
   - Fungal infections like mucormycosis
   - Palatal abscess
   - Benign and malignant salivary gland neoplasms
   - Benign neural tumors
   - Traumatic or irritation fibroma
   - Carcinoma of palate
   - Chronic granulomatous infection such as tuberculosis and tertiary syphilis.

3. **What is mucormycosis?**
   - Mucormycosis is a rare, rapidly progressive, and often fatal opportunistic infection caused by fungi belonging to the class Zygomycetes order Mucorales.
   - It is the third most common angioinvasive fungal infection after candidiasis and aspergillosis.
   - Mucor are ubiquitous fungi, can be found on decaying vegetation and in the soil. They are usually harmless but can become pathogenic in humans under immunosuppression.
   - Most involved sites are nose and paranasal sinuses route of entry being through inhaled dust (Fig. 2).

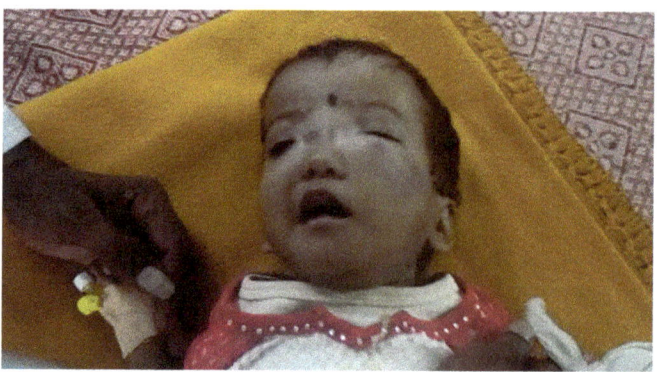

Fig. 2: Mucormycosis involving the nose and paranasal sinuses.

- The organisms proliferate in tissues, vessel walls, perineural spaces, and have a predilection for muscle layers of arteries, veins, and lymphatics, causing thrombosis and infarction.
- The fungus invades the orbit and cranial vault leading to meningoencephalitis and cavernous sinus thrombosis which affects cranial nerves III, IV, V, LMN VII, which may present as swelling, facial pain, orbital cellulitis, proptosis, loss of vision, ophthalmoplegia, necrosis of nasal turbinate and palate as well as osteomyelitis of facial bones.

4. **What are the common predisposing conditions causing mucormycosis?**
   - Uncontrolled diabetes mellitus
   - Hematological malignancies such as leukemia and lymphoma
   - Severe burns
   - Immunocompromised states such as deficient Tcell immunity, HIV/AIDS, bone marrow transplants or organ transplantations, prolonged use of drugs such as corticosteroids, Severe and prolonged neutropenia, immature babies or babies with low birth weight, renal failure, malnutrition
   - Iron overload and chelation therapy with deferroxamine
   - Patients on cytotoxic drugs
   - Contamination of traumatized mucosa such as ulcer or extraction socket by fungal spores.

5. **What are the signs and symptoms of palatal mucormycosis?**
   Patients with mucormycosis usually present with malaise, headache, facial pain, swelling, and low-grade fever. Many patients manifest signs and symptoms involving facial and oral tissues. A black necrotic eschar is the most characteristic and pathognomonic lesion. Other sites of oral lesions include gingiva, lips, alveolar ridge, cheeks, tongue, and mandible. Necrosis of the maxilla is usually rare due to its rich vascularity but it spreads rapidly, leading to necrosis of the palatal bone and palatal perforation.

6. **What are the clinical forms of mucormycosis?**
   Mucormycosis usually occurs in one of the following six clinical forms:
   1. Rhinocerebral
      a. Rhinoorbitocerebral - involves the ophthalmic and internal carotid arteries

b. Rhinomaxillary form - involves the sphenopalatine and greater palatine arteries, resulting in thrombosis of the turbinate and necrosis of the palate (Fig. 1).
2. Pulmonary
3. Cutaneous
4. Gastrointestinal
5. Disseminated, and
6. Uncommon rare forms, such as endocarditis, osteomyelitis, peritonitis, and renal infection.

7. **Mention histological features of mucormycosis.**

   Histopathological examination is done by using hematoxylin and eosin (H and E), PAS, and Grocott's Methenamine Silver (GSM) stains.

   Typical histopathological picture of mucormycosis shows the characteristic ribbonlike branching, smaller width nonseptate (aseptate) fungal hyphae which are prominent and have long, acuteangled, or rightangled branching varying from 45° to 90°.

   Being angioinvasive, the fungus is found in close proximity to necrotic vessel walls.

   Usually, tissue shows nonspecific inflammatory cell infiltrate, with necrosis and granulation tissue along with the hyphae.

8. **Mention the laboratory test to confirm mucormycosis.**
   - Microscopy:
     - KOH mount – KOH wet mount is very helpful for diagnosis of sample from tissue, show characteristic broad, non-septate, ribbon like hyphae.
     - Histopathological examination – H & E, PAS, GMS staining methods can be used.
   - Culture on Sabouraud's Dextrose Agar (SDA) shows unrestricted cottony mycelia mostly white to grey and black in color and confirming the growth by Lactophenol cotton blue staining which facilitates to view clear morphology of fungus for identification (Fig. 3).
   - Molecular confirmation by detection of fungal DNA in tissue samples by polymerase chain reaction (PCR) is a novel method. In particular, PCR with sequencing of the 18S ribosomal DNA of Mucorales species in order to diagnose this organism in clinical cases of invasive fungal infection can improve the diagnosis.

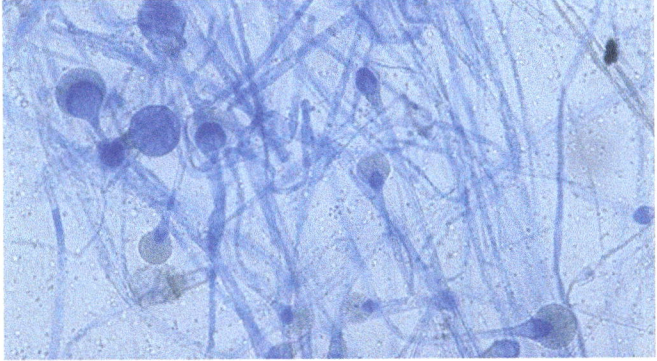

Fig. 3: Culture on Sabouraud's Dextrose Agar (SDA).

9. **What is the treatment of mucormycosis?**

   Treatment of mucormycosis involves a combination of aggressive and repeated surgical debridement of necrotic tissue, systemic antifungal therapy with Intravenous (IV) amphotericin B (lipid formulation) and immediate control of the underlying systemic diseases.

10. **What about mortality in mucormycosis despite early treatment?**

    Despite early treatment, the mortality rate of patients with mucormycosis is very high, ranging from 16% to 100%. Cutaneous mucormycosis has a mortality rate of 17%, whereas rhinocerebral, pulmonary, and gastrointestinal forms of mucormycosis have mortality rates of 67%, 83%, and 100%, respectively.

Necrotizing Fasciitis

Chapter 62

Atul Kulkarni

CASE STUDY

A 2-year-old male child with history of fever for 6 days vomiting, irritability, not taking orally—tachycardia, tachypneic, febrile, hypotensive, skin lesions right groin, right supraclavicular region (Fig. 1). The child had history of chickenpox 12 days back.

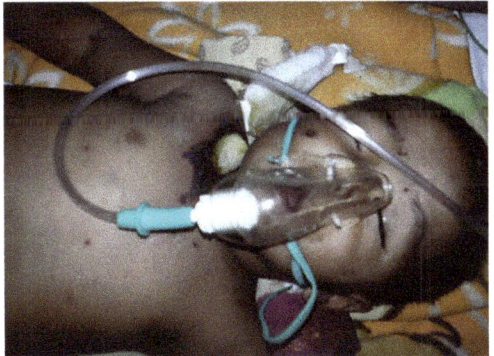

Fig. 1: Chickenpox marks, hypoxia.

1. **What is necrotizing soft tissue infection?**
   Necrotizing soft tissue infections (NSTI) are characterized by fulminant tissue destructions, with systemic signs of toxicity and high mortality.
2. **What are the types of necrotizing soft tissue infections?**
   - Necrotizing fasciitis
   - Necrotizing myositis
   - Necrotizing cellulitis.
3. **What is necrotizing fasciitis?**
   It is an infection of the deep soft tissues, which results in progressive destruction of the muscle fascia and over lying subcutaneous fat. The infection typically spreads along the

muscle fascia due to relatively poor blood supply. The tissues involved are epidermis, dermis, subcutaneous tissue, fascia and muscle.

4. **What are the types of necrotizing fasciitis?**
   - Polymicrobial (type 1)
   - Monomicrobial (type2).

5. **What are the organisms causing necrotizing fasciitis?**
   Staph aureaus, group A *Streptococcus*, B Haemolytic streptococci, *Streptococcus pyogens*, *Aerophilic streptococcus*, bacteroids, clostridium, peptosteptococcus, enterobacteriaceae, klebsiella, proteus, *Enterococcus, fusobacteria,* spirochetes, *Vibrio vulnificus, Aeromonas hydrophilia, Streptococcus pneumonia* and *H. influenza* type B.

6. **What are the risk factors causing necrotizing fasciitis?**
   - Major penetrating trauma
   - Minor lacerations or blunt trauma
   - Skin breach (varicella lesion, insect bite, injection drug use)
   - Recent surgery (colonic, urologic, gastro intestinal, gynecologic, perineum, neonatal circumcision, omphalitis, balanitis, etc.)
   - Mucosal breach (hemorrhoids, rectal fissures, episiotomy, etc.)
   - Immunosuppressions [diabetes, cirrhosis, neutropenia, human immunodeficiency virus (HIV), Primary immune deficiency (PID), etc.]
   - Malignancy, intravenous (IV) drugs, hypodermic needle injections
   - Obesity and alcoholism
   - Use of nonsteroidal anti-inflammatory drugs (NSAIDs) and corticosteroids.

7. **What are the clinical manifestations of necrotizing fasciitis?**
   Local swelling, heat, erythema (sharp margins), tenderness, edema, severe pain, fever, crepitus, skin bullae, necrosis and ecchymosis. In surgical wound infection, NSTI is characterized by copious drainage, dusky and friable subcutaneous and pale devitalized fascia. Subcutaneous gas is often present in polymicrobial type particularly in diabetes.

8. **What is the pathogenesis of necrotizing fasciitis?**
   Infection advances along superficial plane and extent to subcutaneous tissue firm and indurated. Skin changes in 24–48 hours. Nutrient vessels are thrombosed and cutaneous ischemia develops. This causes skin anesthesia later frank tissue gangrene, slough develop owing to ischemia and necrosis.
   Vesiculation/bullae formation->ecchymosis->crepitus->anesthesia->necrosis.
   Bullae fluid->straw colored->bluish hemorrhagic->red to purple to blue.

9. **What are the common sites involved?**
   - Perineum (Fourniers gangrene)—polymicrobial type, involvement of ant abdominal wall and gluteal muscle
   - Head and neck region—breach in oropharynx following instrumentation or odontogenic infection, Ludwigs angina and Lemierre syndrome sometimes progress to NF
   - Mediastinum—prior corticosteroid use, infection by gas producing bacteria
   - Neonatal infection—abdominal or perineal often due to B haemolytic, omphalitis and balanitis.

10. **What are the lab diagnosis of necrotizing fasciitis?**
    C-reactive protein (CRP), complete blood count (CBC), erythrocyte sedimentation rate (ESR), serum creatinine, serum lactate, creatinine kinase, aspartate aminotransferase

(AST), blood culture, magnetic resonance imaging (MRI), frozen section incisional biopsy and ultrasound.

11. **What are the complications?**
    Edema may develop in the extremity, which leads to compartment syndrome causing surgical emergency—fasciotomy, systemic toxicity—shock, organ failure and death.

12. **What are the treatment modalities of necrotizing fasciitis?**
    - Surgical debridement
    - Antibiotic therapy—carbapenems, beta lactams, vancomycin, clindamycin, etc.
    - Hemodynamic support—IV fluids.

13. **What are the differential diagnosis of necrotizing fasciitis?**
    - Cellulitis
    - Pyoderma gangrenosum
    - Gas gangrene
    - Pyomyositis
    - Deep venous thrombosis.

Chapter 63: Neonatal Post-pyrexial Hyperpigmentation

Indra M Shekhar Rao

CASE STUDY 1

A term, appropriate for gestational age (AGA), girl baby was admitted at 2 days of life with fever and suspected sepsis. The baby had shock requiring inotropes. C-reactive protein (CRP) was positive and thrombocytopenia was present. Vesicular rash (Fig. 1) developed on day 10 of life followed by desquamation and later hyperpigmentation (Fig. 2).

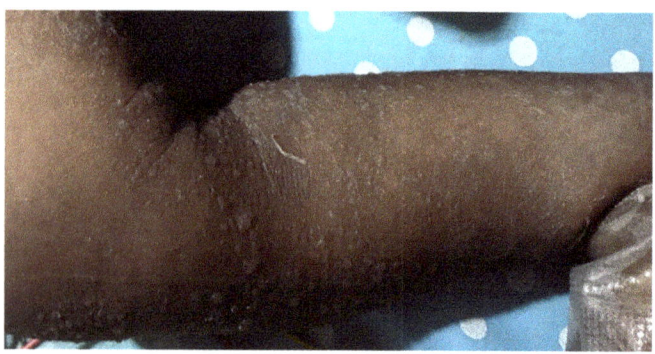

Fig. 1: Vesicular rash.

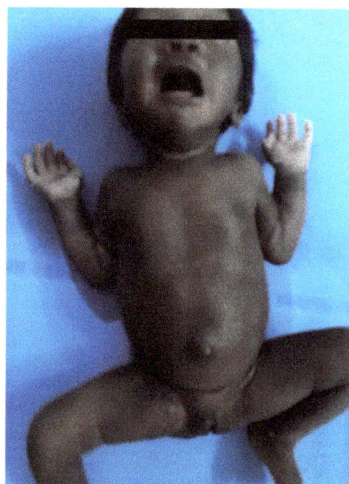

Fig. 2: Blackish hyperpigmentation.

CASE STUDY 2

A term baby born to a mother with fever for 3 days before delivery was admitted for dullness and decreased acceptance of feeds on day 2 of life. At admission, she had fever, fine erythematous rash over extremities, CRP was 20 mg/L and white blood cell (WBC) counts were normal, and first-line antibiotics were started. The baby went into shock on day 4 of life. The baby had thrombocytopenia (45,000), positive CRP (50 mg/L) and leucocytosis. Antibiotics were escalated and inotropes started. Blood (bacterial and fungal) and urine culture were sterile. On the 10th day of life, she had vesicular rash followed by desquamation and hyperpigmentation all over the body. The baby had inguinal and axillary lymphadenopathy. NS1 antigen and dengue immunoglobulin M (IgM) were negative. Suspecting chikungunya infection, work-up was done. Chikungunya IgM was positive in both mothers and babies.
Mother had arthralgia for few weeks after delivery.

1. **What are the differential diagnoses of neonatal skin rash and hyperpigmentation?**
   Drug rash (imipenem), neonatal chikungunya, fungal sepsis (candida), bacterial (Listeria, S. epidermidis), viral infections (HHV—6 and enterovirus), congenital lupus and familial glucocorticoid deficiency.
2. **What is the most common dermatological feature of neonatal chikungunya?**
   Hyperpigmentation over nose (Brownie nose or chik sign). Rash can be varied from maculopapular to vesicular.
3. **What causes chikungunya infection, and how is it spread?**
   It is caused by chikungunya virus, an alpha virus. It is spread by a mosquito bite (Aedes aegypti).
4. **What is the fate of maternal to fetal or neonatal transmission of chikungunya?**
   Higher risk for abortion in the first trimester compared to when the disease was acquired in last trimester.
   Neonatal infection transmitted vertically, and has multisystem involvement with less mortality.
5. **What are the manifestations of neonatal chikungunya?**
   Fever, poor feeding, unexplained apnea
   Dermatological—macular erythematous rash, vesicular rash, hyperpigmentation. Hyperpigmentation is more prominent over the tip of nose in most of the babies
   Hematological—thrombocytopenia, leukocytosis, etc.
   Neurological—irritability, encephalopathy, seizures, etc.
   Joints—arthritis and arthralgia (manifested as paradoxical cry).
6. **How is this condition diagnosed?**
   In acute stage, diagnosis can be made by reverse transcription (RT)—polymerase chain reaction (PCR).
   Chikungunya IgM antibodies are detectable usually by day 5 of illness and remained positive for several weeks to 3 months.
   IgG antibodies can be detected in convalescent samples done a few weeks later and persist for years.
7. **How is this condition managed?**
   No specific antiviral medication. The baby should be managed conservatively.
8. **What is the prognosis of this condition?**
   Mortality is rare in neonates. Usually they have a good outcome. Dermatological changes and paradoxical cry due to arthralgia may remain for a few months.

Neonatal Purpura Fulminans

Chapter 64

Narendra Rathi

CASE STUDY

A newborn, born out of consanguineous marriage, delivered by lower segment cesarean section (LSCS), was brought at the age of 12 hours with the complaints of dark red spots on lower limb and buttocks since 7 hours of age. On examination, purple black spots (necrotic purpura) were noted which were indurated, having sharp borders and necrotic (Fig. 1). Routine investigations like hemoglobin, total leucocyte count (TLC), c-reactive protein (CRP), serum creatinine, blood sugar, serum sodium, potassium, calcium and cerebrospinal fluid (CSF) were normal. Blood culture was sent. Previous two siblings were normal. Platelet count was 50,000 per cubic millimeter.

Considering hemorrhagic skin necrosis occurring in early neonatal period, a diagnosis of purpura fulminans (PF) was considered and further investigations were sent. Prothrombin time (PT) and partial thromboplastin time with kaolin (PTTK) were prolonged. Fibrin degradation products (FDP) and d-dimer were raised. Serum fibrinogen and protein C were very low. Ophthalmological examination was normal. Blood culture came negative. A diagnosis of PF due to protein C deficiency was made.

The baby was put on platelet transfusion and fresh frozen plasma (FFP) was given 12 hourly. Low molecular weight heparin was started. After 7 days, oral warfarin therapy was started to keep international normalized ratio (INR) at around 3. Skin lesions started improving with local surgical treatment. Condition of the baby gradually improved.

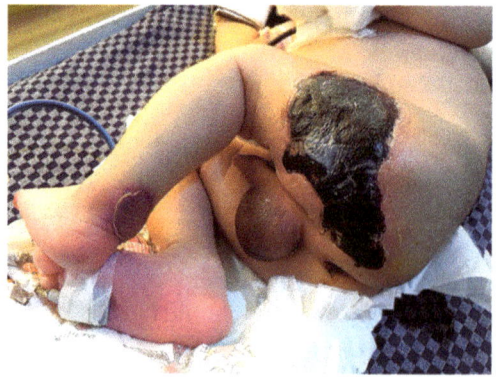

Fig. 1: Necrotic purpura.

1. **What is PF?**
   PF is a syndrome of hemorrhagic skin infarction associated with intravascular thrombosis. It is a rapidly progressive condition.

2. **What are the types of PF?**
   PF is of three types: neonatal, idiopathic and acute infectious. Idiopathic PF develops 7–10 days after precipitating infection while acute infectious PF occurs during the course of infection and is associated with fever. Acute infectious PF needs empiric broad-spectrum antibiotic therapy along with intravenous immunoglobulin (IVIG).

3. **What is the basic pathophysiology of PF?**
   PF basically has microvascular thrombosis associated with perivascular hemorrhage. It is due to qualitative or quantitative deficiency in protein C or protein S or anti-thrombin III, all of which are anticoagulants. Due to the deficiency of natural anti-coagulant factors in blood, intravascular thrombosis occurs and leads to skin necrosis.

4. **What is the etiology of PF?**
   PF can occur due to congenital or acquired causes. Congenital causes are protein C and protein S deficiency. Acquired causes are due to increased consumption of anticoagulant proteins due to infections, disseminated intravascular coagulation (DIC), anti-phospholipid antibodies, etc. and due to decreased synthesis of anticoagulant proteins due to galactosemia, hepatic dysfunction or congenital heart disease. Sometimes repeat testing of protein C levels at 3 months and parental testing is needed to differentiate between congenital and acquired PF.

5. **What are the clinical features of PF?**
   Non-blanching purpura, sharply demarcated skin necrotic lesions, hemorrhage bullae, multiorgan failure, stroke, bleeding diathesis and respiratory failure.

6. **What investigation should be done in PF?**
   Basic metabolic panel, septic screen and coagulation profile. Investigations basically reveal DIC.

7. **What is the management of neonatal PF?**
   Immediate treatment is with platelets, FFP and low molecular weight heparin, followed by oral anticoagulation with warfarin, debridement of necrotic tissue and proteins C supplement if available. Acute phase treatment should be given till skin (and CNS and ocular, if present) lesions resolve. Periodic monitoring with INR and d-dimer levels should be done. Rising d-dimer levels herald PF. Liver transplant can be done for homozygous protein C deficiency.

8. **What are the prognostic factors?**
   Failure to diagnose early and failure to initiate early replacement therapy with FFP are poor prognostic factors.

9. **What are the complications of neonatal PF?**
   Cerebral thrombosis, renal vein thrombosis, vitreous hemorrhage and retinal detachment are various complications seen in neonatal PF.

10. **What about prenatal diagnosis of PF?**
    Prenatal diagnosis of PF can be done by mutation studies on chorionic villous sampling and by assessing levels of protein C or S in fetal blood.

Nephrotic Syndrome

Chapter 65

Fagun Shah

CASE STUDY 1

Three years old male child presented with generalized body edema gradually increasing since 7 days. Typically, the edema is more when child gets up in morning and decreases in the evening. The child has decreased urine output but no gross hematuria, and on examination, the child is normal hemodynamically without hypertension.

Picture depicts the classic presentation of patient with idiopathic nephrotic syndrome having periorbital (Fig. 3) puffiness, lower limb edema (Fig. 1) and ascites (Fig. 2). The edema appears more in morning and reduces gradually by evening.

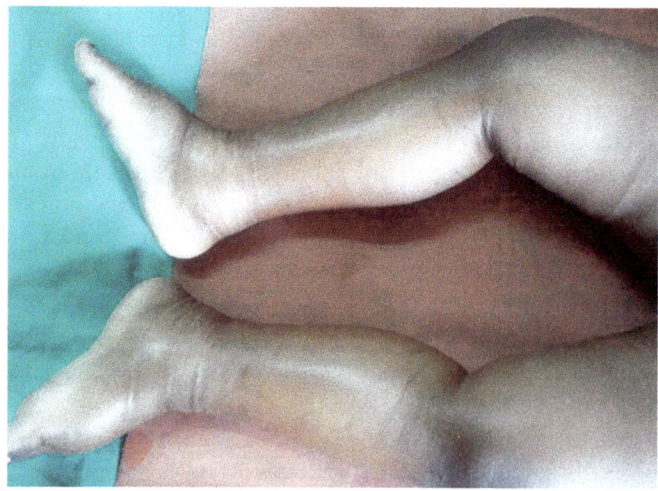

Fig. 1: Lower limb edema.

Nephrotic Syndrome

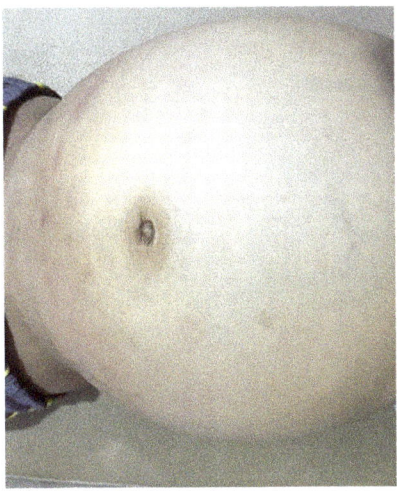

Fig. 2: Ascitis.

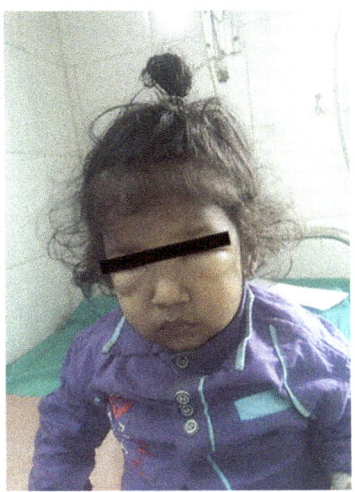

Fig. 3: Periorbital edema.

1. **What is idiopathic nephrotic syndrome?**
   Idiopathic nephrotic syndrome is a common disease involving kidneys in pediatric population. Ninety percent of the patients have idiopathic (primary) nephrotic syndrome. It occurs due to altered perm selectivity of glomerular basement membrane leading to massive proteinuria, hypoalbuminemia, hypercholesteremia and generalized edema.

2. **How do we investigate these patients?**
   The investigations may be divided into those required for diagnosis and those required to rule out other infections and atypical causes.
   The basic investigations include a renal function test (RFT), serum cholesterol, serum albumin and urine analysis. The patients with nephrotic syndrome have a normal serum creatinine, hypercholesteremia (>200 mg/dL), hypoalbuminemia (<2.5 mg/dL) and proteinuria. It is necessary to quantify proteins in urine by doing either 24-hour urinary protein estimation (>40 mg/kg/hour) or an urine protein creatinine ratio (>2 mg/mg).
   In addition, a Mantoux test and chest X-ray to rule out tuberculosis (TB) and tests to rule out infections at any other site are imperative.

3. **How to treat these patients?**
   It is imperative to rule out TB and any infection before starting the treatment. Majority of these patients respond to treatment with corticosteroids, and hence are steroids responsive. First episode of nephrotic syndrome is treated with steroids (prednisolone) for total duration of 12 weeks—2 mg/kg/day in divided doses for 6 weeks followed by 1.5 mg/kg/day for 6 weeks. Diuresis starts after 7–10 days of initiating steroids. The child depicted in Figure 4 has gone into remission after commencing steroids, during recovery he lost edema fluid from all over the body.

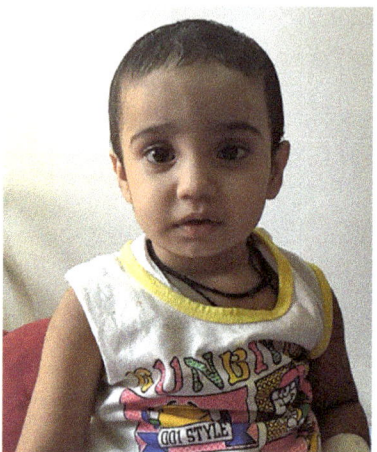

Fig. 4: Facial look during recovery.

4. **Do all patients respond to steroids?**
   Yes, 90% are steroid responsive, meaning persistent absence of proteinuria within 4 weeks of commencing treatment. If the child has persistence of proteinuria despite giving adequate dose of steroids (2 mg/kg/day) for 4 weeks, it is considered steroid resistant. These children need to be under care of pediatric nephrologist and managed with renal biopsy and higher immunosuppression.

CASE STUDY 2

Second patient is a steroid-dependent case of nephrotic syndrome on prolonged course of steroids along with cyclophosphamide. The child is stunted (Fig. 5) with cushingoid features due to long-term use of steroids.

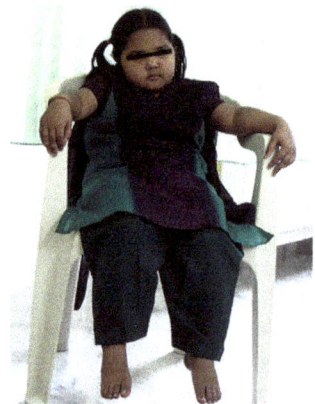

Fig. 5: Stunted child with cushingoid features.

5. **What are the clinical classifications of nephrotic syndrome depending upon the steroid responsiveness?**
   Infrequent relapse—less than or equal to three relapses in 1 year or less than two relapses in 6 months. The relapse is treated with prednisolone at 2 mg/kg/day till urine albumin becomes nil for three consecutive days and then shifted to 1.5 mg/kg/day for 4 weeks followed by abrupt discontinuation.
   Frequent relapse—more than three relapses in 1 year or two or more relapses in 6 months. It is treated with low-dose steroids for long duration or steroids plus levamisole.
   Steroid dependence—relapse on tapering doses of steroids or relapse within 2 weeks of completely stopping steroids. It is treated with low-dose steroid plus addition of either levamisole or cyclophosphamide.

6. **Which are the other drugs used for treatment?**
   Mycophenolate mofetil, calcineurin inhibitors like cyclosporine and tacrolimus, and anti CD 20 monoclonal antibody—rituximab is also used for treatment. These drugs are prescribed under strict supervision of pediatric nephrologist only.

7. **What should be diet in these patients?**
   The patients of nephrotic syndrome should be regular diet and normal fluid intake baring periods of relapse and edema when salt restriction is necessary. Calcium and Vitamin D has to be supplemented in children on steroids for more than three months.

8. **Can we immunize child on steroids?**
   A child on 2 mg/kg/day or more than 20 mg daily steroids for more than 2 weeks is immunosuppressed. Killed vaccines or toxoids can be safely given. However, live attenuated vaccines are avoided till the child is off steroids and all immunosuppressive agents for at least 4 weeks. Pneumococcal vaccine is mandatory.

9. **Can we start steroids in patients with Koch's?**
   Patients with asymptomatic Mantoux positive or with active Koch's need to be started on adequate AKT as per Revised National Tuberculosis Control Program (RNTCP) recommendations. Steroids are added after 2 weeks of therapy with AKT.

10. **What are the complications of nephrotic syndrome?**
    The most common complication is edema. Other common complications include infections, dyselectrolytemia, thromboembolic phenomenon, acute kidney injury and drug complications. Since steroid is the most common immunosuppression used, all patients on steroids for more than 6 months should be screened for steroid toxicity, namely impaired growth, risk of infections, bone demineralization, cataracts and hypertension.

11. **What are the indications of biopsy?**
    Steroid-resistant cases, children less than 1 year or more than 8 years with first episode, children with gross hematuria, hypertension, altered renal parameters right from onset and before commencing therapy with drugs like cyclosporine or tacrolimus.

Neurocysticercosis

Chapter 66

Ritesh Shah

CASE STUDY

A 7-year-old boy presented with episodes of sudden tingling in left hand followed by clonic movement of left upper limb with twitching of mouth to left side and episode subsided in 3–4 min with preserved consciousness. Such multiple episodes over last 2 months. His general and neurological examination is normal. His magnetic resonance imaging (MRI) findings are shown in (Figs. 1 to 3).

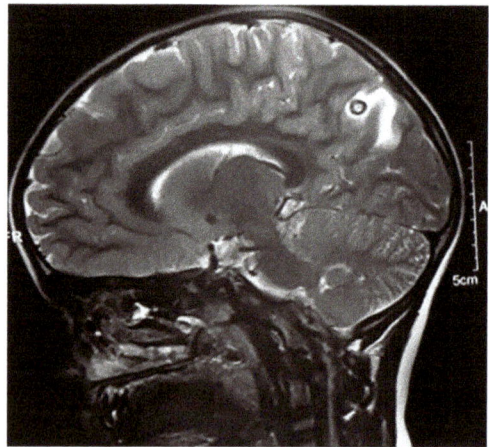

Fig. 1: T2w sagittal image showing central lesion with surrounding perilesional edema.

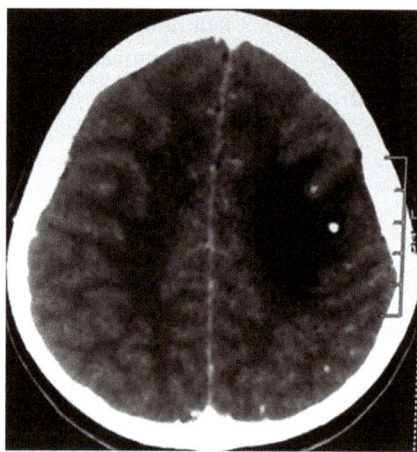

Fig. 2: Contrast enhanced T1 coronal image showing regular thin ring enhancement.

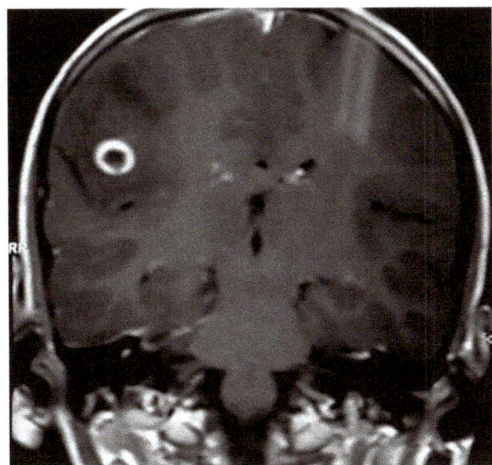

Fig. 3: Plain computed tomography showing central scolex with surrounding edema.

1. **What are the common causes of focal seizure in children?**
   Focal seizure may be symptomatic (21.7% of all epilepsies), cryptogenic (21.8%) or idiopathic. *In children, it is much more common for foal epileptic seizure to be idiopathic than symptomatic.* Few most common causes of focal seizures are central nervous system (CNS) infection [which include neurocysticercosis (NCC)], trauma, antenatal and perinatal risk factors, cerebrovascular accidents and malformation of cortical developments.

2. **How to decide about choice of first investigation between electroencephalography (EEG) and MRI in focal seizures?**
   If focal seizure has classical phenotype of idiopathic focal epilepsy (age between 4 and 12 year, seizures soon after sleep onset, and lots of drooling and unilateral facial sensory motor symptoms, oropharyngolarygeal manifestations, short lasting (1–4 min) and infrequent occurrence) then first investigation of choice is EEG, and if EEG is showing classical centerotemporal spikes then neuroimaging may not be needed. For rest of the focal seizure patients, neuroimaging (preferably MRI) is recommended to find out the cause of seizures.

3. **What are the different causes of ring enhancing lesion on MRI?**
   Few common causes of ring enhancing lesions are granulomatous lesions (like NCC, tuberculoma), brain abscess, fungal infections, demyelination, metastasis and sub-acute infarcts.

4. **What is NCC?**
   NCC is CNS parasitic infection caused by larval form of *Taenia solium*. It happens due to ingestion of undercooked meat—pork that contain larval cyst—and ingestion of contaminated food with eggs of *T. Solium* (feco-oral route); hence, NCC is seen in vegetarians as frequently as it is seen in non-vegetarians.

5. **What are the types of NCC based on anatomical location?**
   NCC can be broadly classified as parenchymal and extraparenchymal (which include intraventricular, subarachnoid, spinal and ocular). The clinical presentation and management differ in extraparenchymal types.

6. **How NCC usually presents?**
   Seizures are the most common presentations of NCC and occur in over 90% of cases. Most of this is partial seizures depending on location of lesion. It is seen in otherwise normal children and either singly or in clusters. They are generally brief (<5 min). Status epilpeticus is seen in about one third of the cases. NCC can also present with headache and vomiting only without seizures. Rarely it may present as encephalitic picture.

7. **What is the most useful diagnostic study for NCC?**
   MRI and computed tomography (CT) scans are the most useful studies for diagnosis of NCC. MRI provides most information about cyst location, viability, associated inflammation and sometimes scolex visible within cyst. CT scan is useful for identifying calcification. None of the serological test has good sensitivity and specificity for the diagnosis of NCC, particularly for single lesions, and so is not recommended.

8. **What are the characteristic features of NCC on MRI?**
   On MRI, NCC looks cystic, round, <2cm in diameter, isointense (vesicular stage) to hyperintense (colloidal stage) on T1W, T2W and flair with ring enhancement on contrast with or without perilesional edema (Figs. 1 to 3).

9. **How to differentiate NCC from tuberculoma on MRI?**

NCC	Tuberculoma
Small (<20 mm), single or multiple	Larger (>20 mm), single or multiple
Smooth margin	Irregular margin
Cystic	Solid
Less edema	More edema
Mural nodule present	Mural nodule absent
Present at gray–white matter junction	More common in posterior fossa
Not associated with meningitis	Associated with meningitis

10. **What are the different stages of NCC?**
    There are four pathological stages—vesicular, colloidal, granular–nodular and calcified stage. The different stages of cyst have different MRI/CT appearance, and current recommendations about use of cysticidal drug also vary according to different stages.

11. **How to treat NCC?**
    NCC is treated with anti-convulsants, anti-parasitic (cysticidal) and anti-inflammatory (steroids). Appropriate treatment of NCC is a matter of debate. There are different views about the use of anticonvulsants, cysticidal drugs and steroids. We will try to present the best suggestions based on currently available evidence.

12. **How to treat seizures in NCC?**
    Seizures should be treated like any other symptomatic focal epilepsy. Carbamazepine should be used as a first choice of antiepileptic drug. Phenytoin is also commonly used, but due to association with serious side effects, carbamazepine is preferred over it. Regarding duration of anticonvulsants, shorter duration (1 year) may be enough as long as the neuroimaging abnormalities have disappeared. Refractory seizures are rare in NCC, but in few such cases epilepsy surgery evaluations are recommended.

13. Should the cysticidal be used?
Cysticidal treatment aims to destroy live cysts on the assumption that once inactive they will cause fewer symptoms. Faster resolution of neuroimaging lesion is proven in many studies and beneficial effect in terms of seizure control is reported in some studies. Although both albendazole and praziquantel have been found effective in NCC, albendazole is better tolerated and less expensive. The usual regime of albendazole is 15 mg/kg/day divided into two doses for 7–28 days. Both short (7 days) and long (28 days) duration therapies were found to be equally effective for parenchymal NCC.

14. How to go about steroids?
Steroids are generally given to reduce the perilesional edema. They are started 1-2 days before starting albendazole and continued for the next 2-3 days with the objective of minimizing any inflammatory response that might be flared up by cysticidal therapy. Usually, prednisolone 2 mg/kg/day is used, and in children with raised ICT, intravenous dexamethasone may be used.

15. What are the contraindications of cysticidal drugs?
Cysticidal drugs should not be used in cases with markedly raised intracranial pressure (ICP), particularly in disseminated NCC as sudden elevation of ICP may occur secondary to host immune responses. Inappropriate use of albendazole in calcified NCC should be avoided.

16. What is the overall prognosis in NCC?
Prognosis depends on the type of NCC, cyst location and numbers. Cases of NCC who present with seizure and single lesion generally have good prognosis, seizure are controlled in most cases and lesion disappears within 6 months in 60% of cases. Cases with calcifications and disseminated NCC have frequent seizure recurrence.

Neurofibromatosis

Chapter 67

Vijay Shah, Upendra Chaudhari

CASE STUDY

Two male children, 1- and 3-year-old, 36-year-old father, and grandfather.

A 1-year-old male child presented with multiple black color spots of various sizes on the body since birth.

A child has history of brownish black colored spots of different sizes all over the body since birth which is stationary and non-fading. Similar types of lesions are present in elder brother since birth, who is 3 years old. The father also has similar lesions and nodular swelling of different sizes all over the body. There is history of similar type of lesions to paternal grandfather who expired before 10 years.

Both children and father are developmentally normal and without any complications.

All three family members have neurofibromatosis type 1.

1. **What is neurocutaneous syndrome?**
   It is a congenital defect with the involvement of skin and nervous tissue.
2. **What is neurofibromatosis (NF)?**
   A distinct genetic disorder with benign growth of peripheral nerve sheaths, neurofibroma1 and café au lait macules. It may be associated with various other skin and generalized manifestations.
3. **What is the hallmark character of NF?**
   Diagnosed when two out of seven features present:
   1. Six or more café au lait macules more than 5 mm in prepubertal more than 15 mm in postpubertal (Figs. 1 and 2).
   2. Axillary or inguinal freckling consisting of hyperpigmented area 2–3 mm in diameter
   3. Two or more iris Lisch nodules
   4. Two or more neurofibroma or one plexiform neurofibroma
   5. A distinctive lesion such as sphenoid dysplasia or cortical thinning of long bones
   6. Optic gliomas
   7. A first degree relative with NF-1.

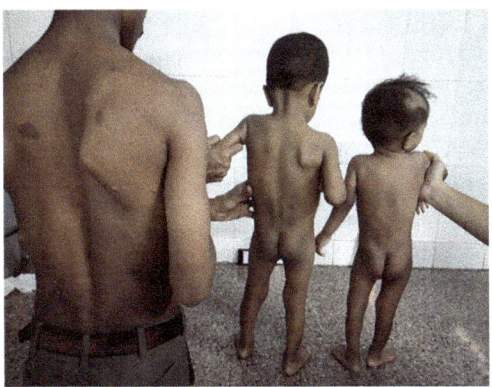

Fig. 1: Brown black spots (café au lait) over back of children and their father.

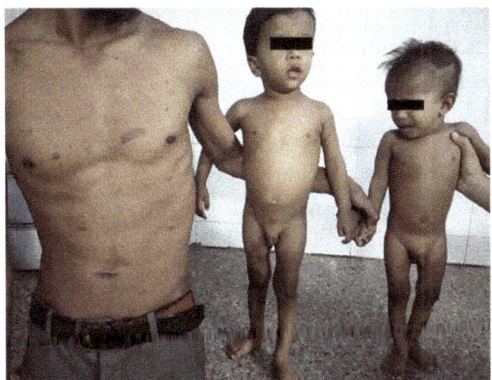

Fig. 2: Brown black spots over chest of children and their father.

4. **Can Café au Lait spot normally be present?**
   Yes, it can be present. 1–3 café au lait spots are common in 10% of normal children.
5. **Can Café au Lait spot be present in conditions other than NF?**
   Yes, like ataxia telangiectasia, basal cell nevus syndrome, tuberous sclerosis, Gaucher disease, Fanconi anemia, and Russell-Silver syndrome.
6. **How can you differentiate the above condition from NF?**
   Each condition has typical clinical features by which they can be differentiated from NF.
   - Ataxia telangiectasia—have progressive ataxia
   - Basal cell nevus syndrome—characterized by jaw cyst and skeletal anomaly
   - Bloom syndrome—short stature, photosensitive
   - Fanconi anemia—limb anomalies, pancytopenia
   - Tuberous sclerosis—white macules, multiple hamartomas.
7. **Is NF-1 and NF-2 part of a single entity?**
   No, previously it was believed that it was single entity, but now it is recognized that they are clinically and genetically distinct diseases and should be considered separate entities.

8. **Which are the other features and complications of NF?**
   Learning disability seizure disorder, cerebral vessel aneurysms or stenosis resulting in moyamoya syndrome, cerebrovascular ischemic attacks, hemiparesis, cognitive defect, precocious puberty, malignant neoplasms, and scoliosis. There can be other mucosal ocular skeletal central nervous system (CNS) and endocrinal manifestations.
9. **What is the mode of transmission?**
   It is an autosomal dominant disorder. More than 50% are de novo sporadic mutation in gene on chromosome region 17q11.2.
10. **What is pathogenesis?**
    Normal neurofibroma gene produces neurofibromin which inhibits oncogene. Mutation of this gene leads to non-formation of neurofibromin and thereby non-inhibition of oncogene.
11. **Is there any role of oncogene?**
    Yes, as mentioned above oncogenes are not inhibited so give rise to abnormal tissue proliferation.
12. **Is there any role of any infectious agent in pathogenesis of NF?**
    No, it is purely genetic disorder.
13. **What is treatment of NF?**
    It is supportive, psychological. If neurofibroma is big and causing pressure symptoms it should be removed. Gene therapy is curative. Regular multidisciplinary follow-up is required as they increase in size and can get converted in malignancy. Prenatal diagnosis is available and genetic counseling should be done.

Chapter 68

Nutritional Rickets

Meenakshi Girish

CASE STUDY 1

A 1-year-old child, exclusively breastfed till 6 months and still on breast feed along with solid foods, presents with inability to get up to standing position and delayed walking. She is found to have widened wrist (Fig. 1), rachitic rosary (Fig. 2), genu varus (Fig. 3), and caput quadratum (Fig. 4). Her X-ray wrist showed cupping and fraying of the lower ends of radius and ulna (Fig. 5). Laboratory biochemistry showed normal calcium, low phosphorus, and increased alkaline phosphatase (AP). The child was treated with oral vitamin D and calcium, and improved biochemically and radiologically over a period of few weeks.

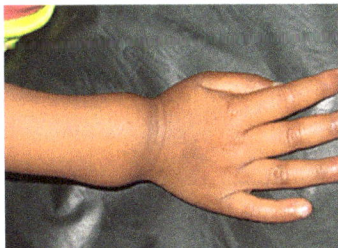

Fig. 1: Widened wrist.

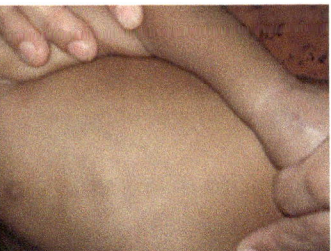

Fig. 2: Rachitic rosary.

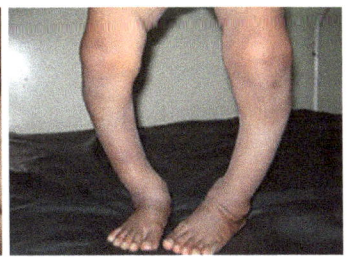

Fig. 3: Genu varus.

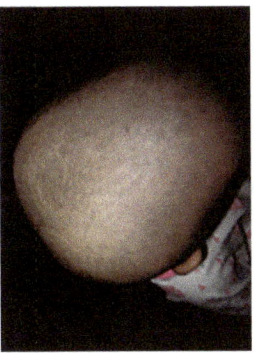

Fig. 4: Caput quadratum.

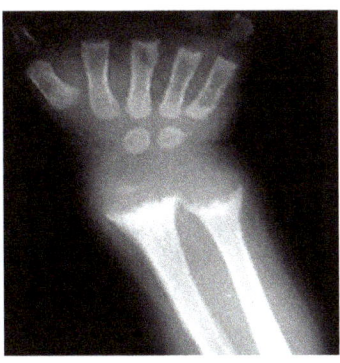

Fig. 5: Cupping and fraying of radius and ulna.

CASE STUDY 2

An 8-year-old boy presented with short stature and progressive bowing of legs (genu varus) since infancy. His X-ray was suggestive of rickets. Biochemistry showed normal calcium, low phosphorus, and increased AP.

1. **Both the cases have rickets. what is the difference?**
   The difference is in the mechanism of development of rickets. Based on the mechanism, rickets is broadly classified into two types:
   - Calcipenic rickets (↓ 1,25 (OH)$_2$ Vit D3)
   - Phosphopenic rickets

   Case 1 is suffering from calcipenic rickets and Case 2 has phosphopenic rickets.

2. **The phosphorus value in both cases have been reported to be low. Then why is type 1 not phosphopenic rickets?**
   A classic triad of normal or low serum calcium, low phosphorus and an increased AP characterizes rickets. In calcipenic rickets (Case 1), phosphorus levels are low due to secondary hyperparathyroidism, whereas in phosphopenic rickets, phosphorus is low because of primary renal phosphate wasting as illustrated in the following:

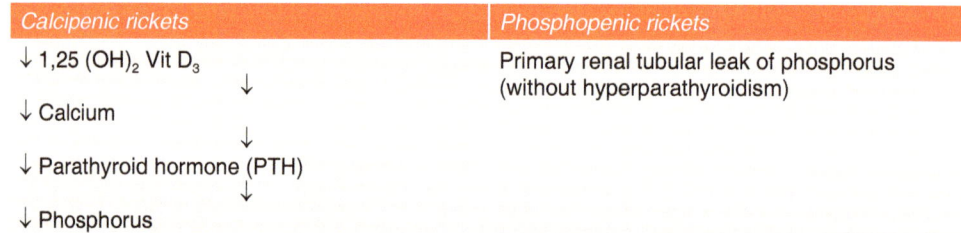

Calcipenic rickets	Phosphopenic rickets
↓ 1,25 (OH)$_2$ Vit D$_3$ ↓ ↓ Calcium ↓ ↓ Parathyroid hormone (PTH) ↓ ↓ Phosphorus	Primary renal tubular leak of phosphorus (without hyperparathyroidism)

Thus, low phosphorus is seen in both types of rickets; serum parathormone (PTH) levels differentiate the two types.

3. **Why is calcium normal in calcipenic rickets?**
   Rickets can be conceptually understood as poor mineralization of growth plate cartilage. This process depends on adequate balance of calcium and phosphorus in blood; thus, the two types, calcipenic and phosphopenic rickets, occur due to deficiency of the former and latter, respectively. In calcipenic rickets, the primary event is a decrease in vitamin D in the body. This leads to decreased absorption of calcium from the gut, decreased reabsorption from the kidney and from bones, and thus hypocalcemia. Parathormone, which is extremely sensitive to fall in serum calcium, increases, thereby restoring normocalcemia by the same mechanism as vitamin D (but unlike vitamin D, parathyroid hormone increases phosphate excretion from the kidney).
   It is important to note that occasionally this compensatory mechanism is inadequate and hypocalcemia may be observed in calcipenic rickets. This is the reason why children with rickets often present with seizures due to transient hypocalcemia.

4. **What are the common sources of vitamin D?**
   Sunlight is an important source of UV rays (290–315 nm) which converts 7-dehydrocholesterol found in human skin to cholecalciferol. Dietary sources are few and inadequate. Animal sources rich in vitamin D are salmon, cod, and mushroom. Vegetables constitute plant sources and are considered inadequate.

5. **Calcipenic rickets should be very uncommon in India as we have abundant sunshine, and consume diet rich in dairy products?**
   Unfortunately, that is not true. The reasons why calcipenic rickets is common in India are:
   - Too much sunshine, but too little sun exposure!
     Babies are not exposed to sunlight for a duration considered ideal for our geographic region—approximately 30–60 minutes per day
   - Pigmented skin
     Melanin impairs conversion of dehydrocholesterol to cholecalciferol
   - Dairy products: It is a myth that dairy products are rich in vitamin D. They are rich in calcium not vitamin D. In breast milk, vitamin D is inadequate (hence rickets in Case 1).

6. **Other than poor exposure to sunlight and inadequate intake, what are the other causes for calcipenic rickets?**
   Calcipenic rickets can also occur because of the following reasons:
   - Failure in conversion of cholecalciferol to 25-hydroxy cholecalciferol (by enzyme 25 hydroxylase in liver)—chronic liver disease
   - Failure in conversion of 25-hydroxy cholecalciferol to 1,25-dihydroxycholecalciferol, (by enzyme 1α-dihydroxylase in kidney)—chronic renal failure and 1α-hydroxylase deficiency, a rare genetic disorder
   - Failure of action of 1,25-dihydroxycholecalciferol on end organs—hereditary resistance to vitamin D
   - Malabsorption syndromes.

7. **When should we suspect calcipenic rickets due to reasons other than inadequate intake?**
   While calcipenic rickets due to inadequate intake is commonly suspected in toddlers who have not been supplemented with vitamin D or have received unfortified milk and especially if born preterm, other causes can be suspected when there are additional clinical clues indicating chronic liver disease, malabsorption or kidney disease. Anemia and short stature may be the only clues in chronic kidney disease, but a diagnostic clue is the presence of *hyperphosphatemia* rather than hypophosphatemia.
   Absence of end organ receptor and hereditary resistance to vitamin D are suspected in children who also have alopecia totalis (Fig. 6) and are born of consanguineous marriage 1α-hydroxylase deficiency and hereditary resistance to vitamin D (formerly known as vitamin D type I and type II rickets, respectively) are always associated with hypocalcemia and suspected when rickets persists with hypocalcemia and secondary hyperparathyroidism.

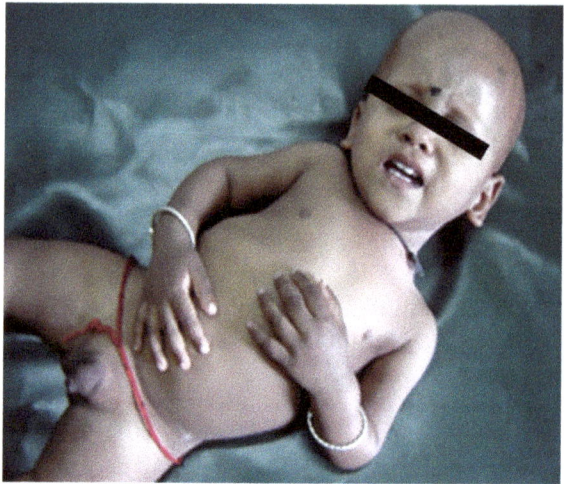

Fig. 6: Alopecia totalis, with signs of rickets.

8. **Why does phosphorus loss occur in phosphopenic rickets?**

   Majority of renal phosphate load is handled by proximal tubules. Several conditions can lead to phosphate wasting through the tubules. These conditions were originally termed as vitamin D resistant rickets that resembled vitamin D deficiency but did not respond to pharmacologic doses of vitamin D.
   - X-linked dominant hypophosphatemia (XLH) is the most important cause of phosphopenic rickets and occurs because of a mutation in the *PHEX* gene. The clue is to look for some evidence of lower limb deformity in mother (Fig. 7). Case 2 had XLH.
   - Fanconi syndrome refers to a generalized impairment in proximal tubular function leading to urinary wasting of compounds normally reabsorbed in the proximal tubule. The most common causes in children are cystinosis and Wilson's disease.
   - *Oncogenic rickets*: Some tumors secrete phosphatonins which increase tubular secretion of phosphates, e.g., hemangiopericytoma, epidermal nevus, etc. (Fig. 8).

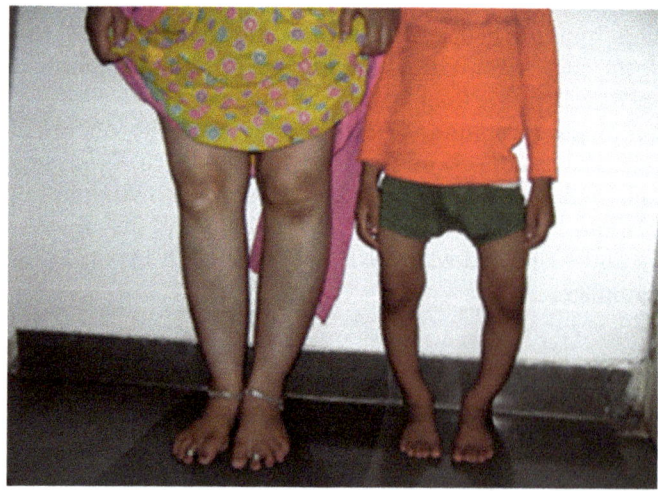

Fig. 7: Bowing of legs in child and mother.

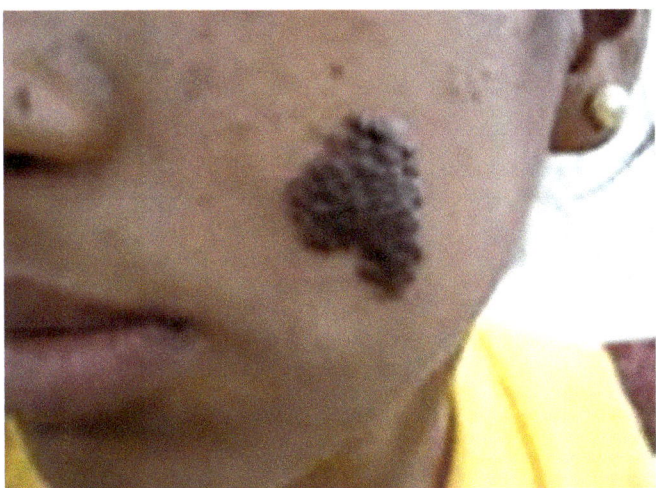

Fig. 8: Epidermal nevus.

9. **As hypovitaminosis D is not the causative factor in phosphopenic rickets, does vitamin D supplementation have any role?**

   Most of the conditions in phosphopenic rickets cause increase in phosphatonins (a regulatory protein), which promote phosphate excretion and impair bone mineralization. These phosphatonins also suppress calcitriol synthesis. Hence, apart from phosphate supplementation, calcitriol therapy is necessary for healing of rickets.

10. **If you encounter a child with rickets, what should be your approach?**

    The most important investigation to confirm that clinical suspicion of rickets is raised serum AP. Though radiology is important, metaphyseal dysostosis may mimic rickets radiologically. All children with rickets thus confirmed should be initiated on one of the following regimens:
    - Intramuscular (IM) dose of vitamin D (IU)
    - More than 12 years—300,000
    - 1–12 years—150,000
    - 3–12 months—50,000
    - Daily oral dose for 3 months (IU)
    - More than 12 years—6,000
    - 1–12 years—3,000 to 6,000
    - 3–12 months—2,000

    If no healing is observed during the course of therapy, then refractory rickets should be considered and further evaluation should proceed as per the algorithm given in Flowchart 1.

Flowchart 1: Evaluation of refractory rickets.

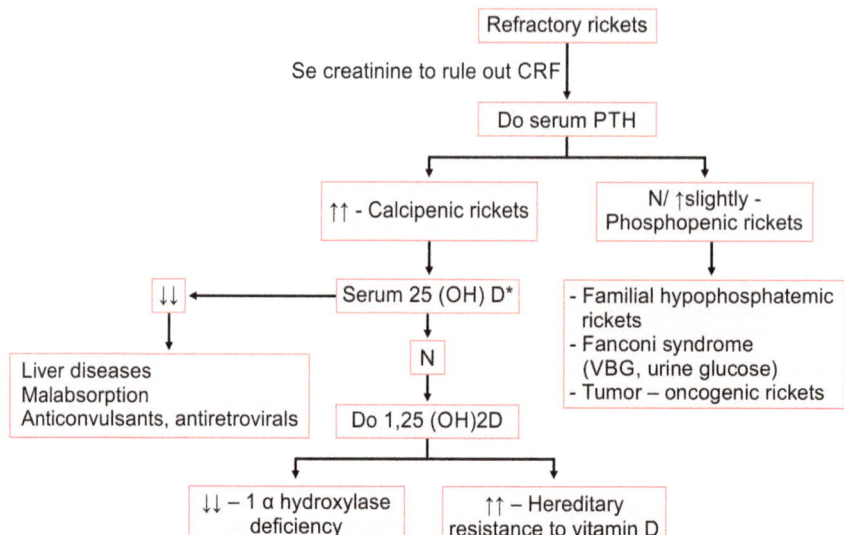

*In vitamin D deficiency conditions, 25 (OH) D is low but 1, 25 $(OH)_2$ D is normal or elevated, hence not used as a test for diagnosis of vitamin D deficiency.

Phimosis

Chapter 69

Aniruddh Shah, Amar Shah

CASE STUDY

A 3-year-old child comes with a history of ballooning of prepuce at micturition. On examination, there is no swelling or redness over the penis. The prepuce is not retractile and the urethral meatus is not visible from outside (Figs. 1 and 2).

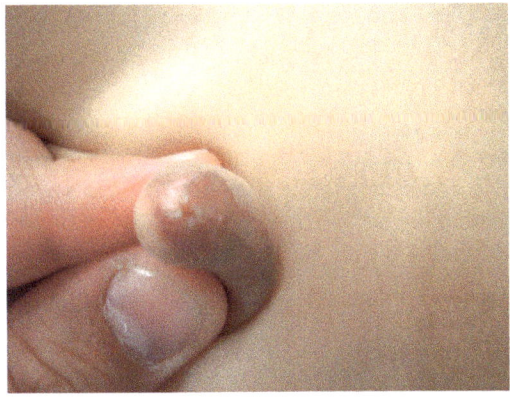
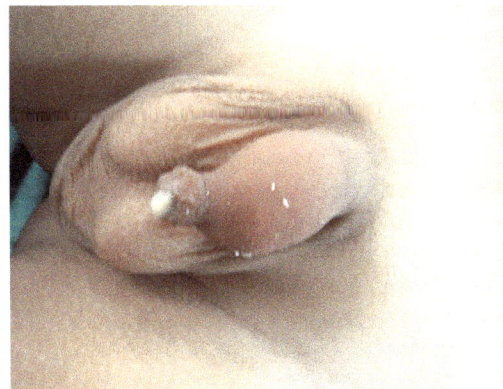

Fig. 1: Ballooning of prepuce front view.   **Fig. 2:** Ballooning of prepuce side view.

1. **What is phimosis?**
   Phimosis is the inability to retract the foreskin (prepuce/skin over the penis) over the glans.
2. **What is the natural process of preputial skin retraction/what is physiological phimosis?**
   The prepuce is normally not retractile at birth and gradually separates, and begins to retract by the age of 1–1.5 years. The prepuce is nature's way to protect the urethral meatus from the ammonia in the urine especially in the infancy when the children are not toilet-trained and are in diapers when the penis is in constant contact with urine.
3. **What is smegma?**
   Smegma is a collection of skin cells from the glans penis and inner foreskin that is often noted with retraction of the foreskin. This natural skin shedding helps to separate the

foreskin from the head of the penis. Smegma may appear as white pearls underneath the skin, which can easily be washed off once the foreskin is retracted. This is sometimes misinterpreted as pus formation under the foreskin.

4. **When does phimosis need medical attention?**
   In children whom the prepuce does not retract beyond 1.5–2 years of age, the child needs medical attention.

5. **What are the complications that phimosis can cause?**
   Phimosis may lead to complications like balanitis, balanoposthitis, and urinary tract infections (UTIs). The most acute complication is paraphimosis. Here, the foreskin is immobilized by swelling in a partially retracted position. This causes the glans to become swollen and painful. This may result in excruciating pain and also cause acute urinary retention in the child.

6. **What are the surgical options for a child with phimosis?**
   Circumcision is required for a child with phimosis. Parents sometimes are hesitant to get their child circumcised for phimosis. For such children, a surgery called "prepuceplasty" is available where the opening of the prepuce is surgically widened in such a way that it looks like a normal foreskin, but becomes easily retractile. Both circumcision and prepuceplasty do not have long-term issues in the marital life or reproductive capabilities.

7. **What are the non-surgical options for a child phimosis?**
   Tropic steroid creams such as betamethasone, mometasone furoate, and cortisone are effective in treating phimosis and may provide an alternative modality of treatment in selected cases by reducing the inflammatory and immune responses and thin out the skin. Mechanical stretching of the skin with forceps, balloons, etc. may show a transient response. However, this is quite painful for the child and trivial trauma caused by it may cause fibrosis and may further potentiate the problem.

8. **When is circumcision indicated for children who do not have phimosis?**
   In children who are on expectant treatment for vesicoureteric reflux, circumcision has been shown to prevent breakthrough UTI. For lesions like sebaceous cysts over the prepuce, small hemangiomas over the prepuce or traumatic injuries like zip injuries circumcision may be necessary.

9. **What is the absolute contraindication for circumcision?**
   A child with hypospadias should never be circumcised.

10. **When should a child with balanoposthitis undergo circumcision?**
    Any child with acute balanoposthitis should be managed with oral analgesics, local antibiotic ointments and also worked up and treated for UTI. Once the swelling and redness subsides, the child can undergo a planned circumcision.

Post Kala-Azar Dermal Leishmaniasis

Chapter 70

Arun Shah

CASE STUDY 1

A 12-year-old female patient named Kajal Kumari, with a no past history of visceral leishmaniasis, with hypopigmented lesions since 2016 and small nodules since 2017. Post kala-azar dermal leishmaniasis (PKDL) was suspected, and she was referred to Kala Azar Medical Research Centre (KAMRC), a specialized referral institute for visceral leishmaniasis, for confirmation of diagnosis. She had multiple small nodules on chin and macular lesions on whole of the body, and these lesions were non-anesthetic to touch and pain. On palpation, the ulnar and common peroneal nerves were not thickened, thus ruling out leprosy (Fig. 1).

The rapid diagnostic test rk39 gave a positive result. Microscopy of skin snip smear on Giemsa staining demonstrated Leishman-Donavani (LD) bodies and polymerase chain reaction (PCR) confirming PKDL. She was treated with combination therapy with liposomal amphotericin-B (1 mg/kg/wt × 5 days) with miltefosine (150 mg × 21 days) and needed four courses at 7-day intervals for complete disappearance of lesions. Skin snip at day 30 was negative for LD bodies. She was followed up after 3 and 6 months, and has remained symptom-free with no recurrence of skin lesions.

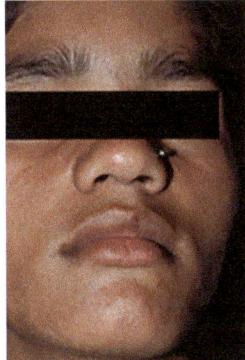
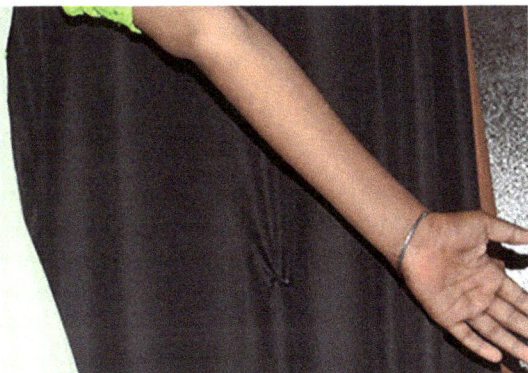
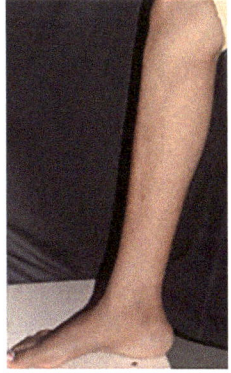

Fig. 1: Case Study 1. A 12-year-old patient with multiple small nodules on chin and macular lesions on whole of the body.

CASE STUDY 2

A 10-year-old male Anshu Kumar with a past history of visceral leishmaniasis (VL) presented in March 2015 with hypopigmented patches. He had multiple maculopapular lesions on the upper and lower limbs, progressive in nature, and these lesions were non-anesthetic to touch and pain (Fig. 2). On palpation, the ulnar and common peroneal nerves were not thickened, thus ruling out leprosy. He reported to have suffered from VL in March 2015 and was treated with a liposomal amphotericin-B (AmBisome) 10 mg/kg/wt. single dose.

The diagnostic test rk39 gave a positive result, and his routine hematology and biochemistry tests were within the normal range. PCR demonstrated LD bodies confirming PKDL. He was treated with liposomal amphotericin-B (3 mg/kg/wt., 5 days). Skin snip after three courses was negative for LD bodies.

He was followed up after 3 and 6 months, and has remained symptom-free with no recurrence of skin lesions. Each case has PKDL; the first patient has nodules and hypopigmented patches (macular), while the second patient has only macular.

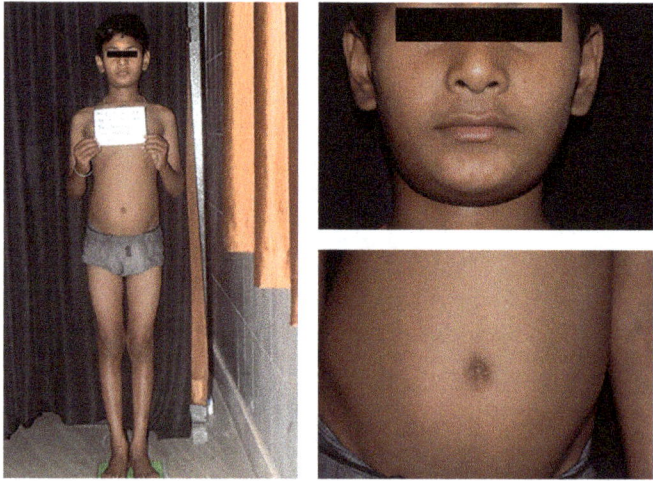

Fig. 2: A 10-year-old male with multiple maculopapular lesions on the face, abdomen and limbs.

1. **What is PKDL?**
   Post-kala azar dermal leishmaniasis may follow after treatment of VL (kala-azar). It is an intermediate disease state before full recovery from VL and is characterized by a skin rash around persisting parasites in the absence of systemic parasitemia. Alternatively, reinfection after VL may be considered. It is thought that these patients may play a role in the transmission of VL.
   After infection with leishmanial parasites through the bite of the sand fly, individuals may develop VL with fever, hepatosplenomegaly, weight loss and pancytopenia; typically with high levels of antibodies and absent cellular immunity against the leishmania parasites. After successful treatment with anti-leishmanial drugs, the patient becomes immune, as can be demonstrated in vitro by the cellular immune responses and in vivo by the leishmanin skin test (LST) that becomes positive in 80% of the patients.

A proportion of treated VL patients may develop PKDL; these patients are not ill, usually do not have hepatosplenomegaly and have recovered from the malnourished state. PKDL is mainly restricted to follow VL caused by *Leishmania donovani*; hence, it occurs in Africa and Asia. There are, however, important epidemiological and clinical differences.

2. **What is the hallmark character of PKDL?**
   A hallmark of many infectious diseases is persistence of the pathogen after clinical cure, as in tuberculosis, viral infections (e.g., herpes), and protozoan diseases (e.g., trypanosomiasis). In leishmaniasis, evidence of parasite persistence after clinical cure exists, and in areas where leishmaniasis is endemic, recurrence has been attributed to parasite persistence and/or reinfection.

3. **What are the other features of PKDL?**
   The main differential diagnosis is with leprosy and vitiligo, but many other skin conditions can be mistaken for PKDL and vice versa, thus complicating case finding and management. A clinical algorithm for diagnosis under field conditions has been proposed, but confirmation is often necessary. Parasitological diagnosis can be done by slit-skin smear or by biopsy. In slit-skin smears, macular lesions will often fail to show parasites, while nodular lesions will be positive in 20–40%. The yield is higher in a biopsy (imprint smears): 91% of nodular lesions and 40% of macular lesions will show parasites. Culture and immunohistochemical (IHC) staining improve routine hematoxylin–eosin staining

   PCR has been demonstrated to be sensitive and can be done in material obtained by a slit-skin smear. Quantitative PCR (qPCR) is sensitive (96–100%) and allows monitoring of parasite reduction as a result of treatment.

4. **What are the common drugs which can cause PKDL?**
   Epidemiological data and clinical reports have strongly suggested a link between administration of sodium antimony gluconate (SAG) and subsequent development of PKDL. In India, 73% of the patients with PKDL who were followed up for 9 years after cure from VL were treated with SAG for VL. A minority 27% developed PKDL after being treated for VL with amphotericin B, AmBisome miltefosine, miltefosine–amphotericin or paromomycin. In Sudan, Bangladesh and Nepal, 100% of PKDL patients received SAG.

5. **Which investigation is helpful in diagnosing PKDL?**
   Microscopy and PCR were compared for use in the diagnosis of PKDL in 63 patients. Aspirates of lymph nodes (samples from 52 patients), skin (23 samples) and bone marrow (18 samples) were used. For 11 patients, lymph node aspiration could be repeated 6 months after they recovered from PKDL. During active PKDL, PCR was positive for 42 of 52 (80.8%) lymph node aspirates and 19 of 23 (82.7%) skin aspirates, whereas microscopy was positive for only 9 of 52 (17.3%) lymph node aspirates and 7 of 23 (30.4%) skin aspirates. PCR was always positive when parasites were seen by microscopy.

6. **Which histologic findings are characteristic of PKDL?**
   A past history of kala-azar was present in 64 (72.7%) patients and PKDL developed a mean of 6.2 years after visceral leishmaniasis. Of the biopsies studied, the clinical lesions were macular in 14 (15.9%), papulo-nodular in 32 (36.3%), and showed both macules and papulo-nodules in 42 (47.8%). Follicular plugging was a common epidermal finding. A clear grenz zone was frequently noted. The dermal infiltrates were arranged mainly in three patterns: superficial perivascular infiltrates in 16 (18.1%), perivascular and perifollicular infiltrates in 24 (27.3%), and diffuse infiltrates in 41 (46.6%) biopsies. LD bodies were noted

in 13 (44.9%) of 69 cases on slit-skin smear and in 25 (28.4%) of 88 biopsies. In 16 patients, where both skin and mucosal biopsies were available, LD bodies were identified in 10 (62.5%) mucosal biopsies as compared to 3 (18.7%) skin biopsies.

The various histomorphological patterns of PKDL are a useful clue to the diagnosis even when LD bodies have not been detected. The study also suggests that LD bodies are more frequently seen in mucosal biopsies in comparison to cutaneous biopsies.

7. **How should the PKDL be treated?**
    Miltefosine is a relatively safe oral drug for the treatment of PKDL. Miltefosine is the preferred first-line drug. The inclusion, exclusion, and withdrawal criteria for use of miltefosine are available in the NVBDCP Guidelines on the Use of Miltefosine. *Dosage schedule:* After enrolment, miltefosine will be given at 2.5 mg/kg once daily after meals for 12 weeks The drug is not to be used in the case of children below 2 years of age, pregnant and lactating women, and women of reproductive age who refuse to use contraceptives during the treatment period and 2 months after completion of treatment and in human immunodeficiency virus (HIV) positive patients. *Duration of treatment:* For the treatment of PKDL, miltefosine is given in the dosages given above for a period of 12 weeks. *Adverse reaction:* Adverse reactions to miltefosine are mostly mild. The treating physician should monitor and watch for any adverse reactions. However, 98% of the patients are not likely to present with any adverse drug reaction. Even of those who report gastrointestinal reactions, 90% will have vomiting. A monitoring of renal and hepatic functions is recommended wherever feasible as about 1% patients may develop nephrotoxicity or hepatotoxicity. The second-line drug amphotericin B is recommended in the following cases: Patient not responding to the first-line of drug or the drug was discontinued due to toxic effect children of less than 2 years of age and patients with liver or kidney disease. *Dosage:* 1 mg/kg/body weight/day. *Route:* Through intravenous infusion in 5% dextrose after mixing the drug in water for injection, very slowly in 6–8 hours. *Contraindications:* Kidney disease, severe liver and heart disease. *Precautions:* Stop the drug when signs of renal failure and those of hypokalemia appear. Therefore, the treatment of the patients should be undertaken on indoor basis under strict supervision. For the treatment of PKDL, amphotericin B is given in the above dose for up to 60–80 doses over 4 months.

Pulled Elbow

Chapter 71

Chetan Trivedi

> **CASE STUDY**
>
> A 2-year-old child was not able to move the left upper limb since he was lifted by his father with his right arm few hours ago. The child is playful but does not allow anyone to touch or move his right upper limb (Fig. 1).

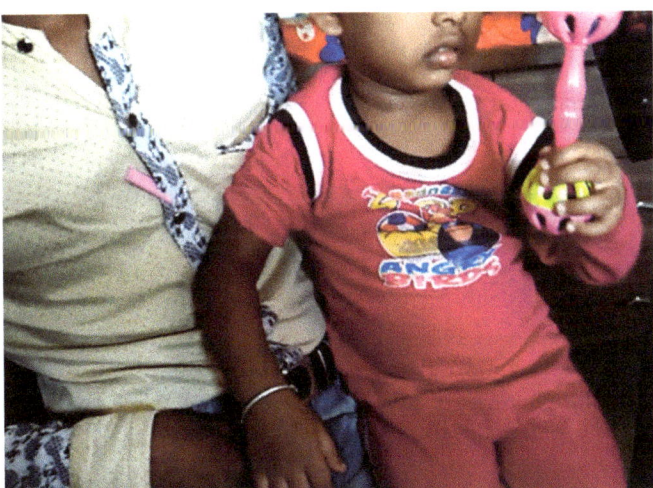

Fig. 1: Limp right upper limb.

1. **What would be the differential diagnosis in a patient not moving one upper limb?**
   Dislocation of elbow, fractured bones, osteomyelitis, septic arthritis, etc.
2. **What history would you like to ask?**
   The history of fall or injury, fever, painful movement, restriction of movement and since when the complaint started.
3. **What would you like to look?**
   Sick looking or non-sick-looking child, playful or irritable child, localized swelling over limb, bruise and injury to other parts of body.

4. **What would you like to feel?**
   Temperature, tenderness localized or painful/restricted movement of that limb.
5. **What should be the approach?**
   An algorithmic approach for a child who is unable to use upper limb is given in Flowchart 1.
   - This patient had no history of fall or injury, but history of lifting of child by his right upper limb by attendant
   - No fever
   - Child cries when tried to move his right upper limb particularly supination of forearm.

   Provisional diagnosis: Dislocation of elbow (pulled elbow).

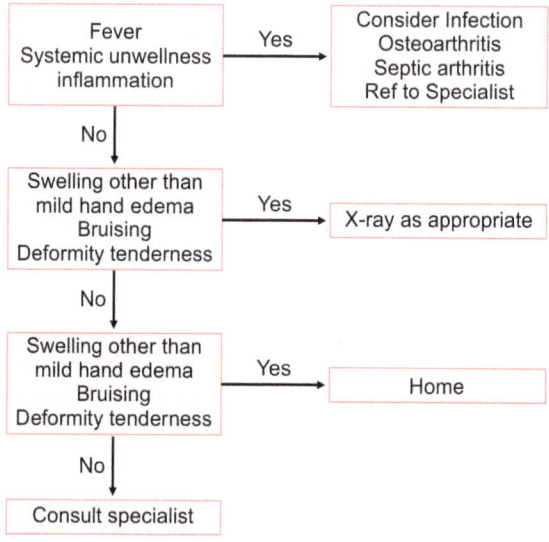

Flowchart 1: Algorithm for a child who is unable to use upper limb.

6. **Do we need to take an X-ray?**
   No, it is purely a clinical diagnosis.
7. **What is pulled elbow?**
   It is one of the most common subluxation seen in children. The most common mechanism is a fall on an outstretched hand. Subluxation of the radial head occurs after a pull on the forearm in a young toddler, mainly 1–3 years of age (but it can occur from as young as 3 months to 5 years of age).
8. **How to reduce it?**
   The reduction of pulled elbow can be done (Fig. 2) without any sedation analgesia by the pediatricians in their offices. Make the child to sit on the lap of mother with elbow held posteriorly, to prevent the child from running away during the reduction. The child's hand is grasped in a hand-shaking gesture, apply longitudinal traction, and then rapidly rotated externally and flexed simultaneously. There is often a palpable "click" or "pop" as the radial head reduces, accompanied by a sharp cry from the infant. If a pop is not felt, the maneuver may be repeated once. If still unsuccessful, a radiograph of the forearm should be obtained. If there has been a palpable pop, the child should have a return to normal movement in 5–15 minutes. If unsuccessful and subsequent radiographs are negative, the arm should

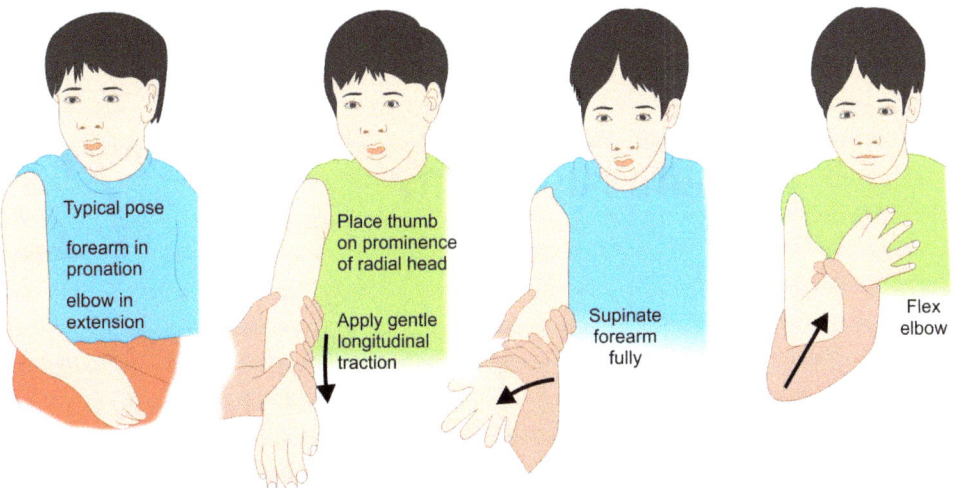

Fig. 2: Technique for reduction of pulled elbow.

be placed in a sling, and parents instructed to follow-up the next day with their primary care provider or orthopedist.

9. **Is recurrence possible?**
   Yes, it can recur few times. For recurrent dislocation of elbow sling can be used for few days after reduction.

Purpura Fulminans

Chapter 72

Mehul Gosai

CASE STUDY

A previously healthy 10-year-old girl presented to the emergency department with high fever, cough, shortness of breath and lobar pneumonia on chest radiograph. She had extensive purpura with hemorrhagic bullae on her feet and hands (Fig. 1). The patient was very ill-appearing with hypotension, tachycardia, tachypnea and oliguria. There was no other bleeding. Hemogram showed leukocytosis (13,000/mm$^{3)}$ with 35% bands, platelets 70,000/mL and sedimentation rate of 112 mm. The prothrombin time and partial thromboplastin time were prolonged and the fibrin degradation products were grossly elevated. Blood culture grew Group A *Streptococcus*.

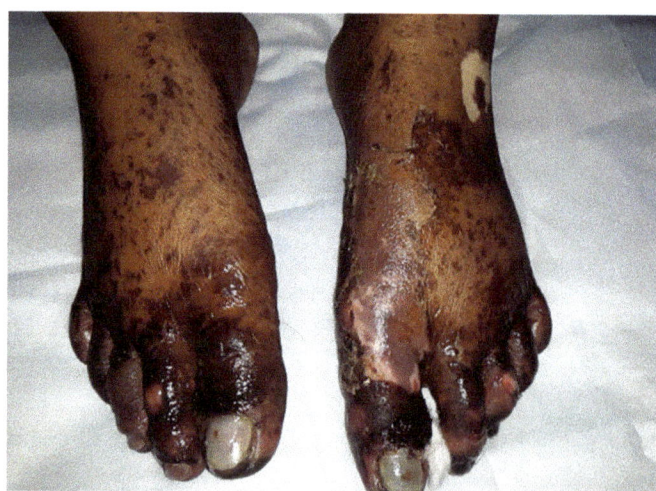

Fig. 1: Image showing extensive areas of purpura, ecchymosis and skin necrosis with hemorrhagic blebs and disrupted bullae, involving the upper and lower extremity.

Diagnosis: Purpura fulminans.

1. **What is purpura fulminans?**
   Rare hematological emergency presenting with rapidly progressive intravascular thrombosis, vascular collapse, and disseminated intravascular coagulation. It is in three forms:

- Neonatal purpura fulminans
- Idiopathic purpura fulminans
- Acute infectious purpura fulminans.

2. **Describe the forms of purpura fulminans?**
   - Neonatal purpura fulminans generally presents within the first 72 hours after birth, with purpuric lesions mainly over the perineal region, flexor of thighs and abdomen. Protein C mutations, inherited deficiency of protein S or antithrombin III may lead to neonatal purpura fulminans.
   - Idiopathic purpura fulminans follows a bacterial or viral illness and usually begins 7-10 days after the onset of the infection. Most cases occur in children. Varicella and streptococcal infections are most common. The pathogenesis involves acute transient decreases in protein C, protein S or antithrombin III levels.
   - The most common form, acute infectious purpura fulminans, occurs superimposed on a bacterial infection. In this illness, the balance of anticoagulant and procoagulant endothelial cell activity is disturbed. This disturbance is precipitated by bacterial endotoxin which consumes antithrombin III as well as proteins C and S.

3. **What are the causes of purpura fulminans?**
   - Congenital or acquired protein C deficiency
   - Severe acute sepsis—mostly *Streptococcus*, *Neisseria meningitidis*, Group A beta-hemolytic *Streptococcus*, varicella, *Haemophilus influenzae* type b (HIB) and *Staphylococcus aureus*.

4. **How does the lesion appear like?**
   It is a well-demarcated, non-blanchable erythematous lesion which progresses to irregular central areas of bluish-black necrosis.
   The early lesions are reversible, which appear like "Lakes" of confluent ecchymosis visible without petechiae.
   A thin border of erythema that fades into adjacent uninvolved skin typically surrounds advancing areas of central necrosis (Fig. 1).

5. **How to diagnose it?**
   During the acute phase, the laboratory findings are that of disseminated intravascular coagulation (DIC): Thrombocytopenia, hypofibrinogenemia, increased fibrin degradation products, and prolonged prothrombin (PT) and activated partial thromboplastin (aPTT) time and microangiopathic anemia. Genetic testing of the child and family members can be useful to confirm the diagnosis. Testing of a citrated plasma sample, collected prior to initiation of treatment is therefore crucial for accurate diagnosis. Functional (activity) assays are recommended for initial screening.

6. **What is the management protocol of purpura fulminans?**
   In acute infectious purpura fulminans, aggressive resuscitation, antibiotics and volume expansion are important.
   Correction of acid–base and electrolyte abnormalities is helpful.
   Prompt excision of necrotic tissue is recommended and escharotomies may be indicated. Heparin bonds with antithrombin III to inhibit thrombus formation and may reverse the development of skin necrosis. Protein C has got anticoagulant and anti-inflammatory properties, which contribute to improved survival. In homozygous protein C deficiency, fresh frozen plasma (8–12 mL/kg) can give effective replacement therapy.

Antithrombin III replacement has been shown to normalize levels and reverse disseminated intravascular coagulation.

Recombinant tissue plasminogen activator (rtPA) induces fibrinolysis and improves peripheral perfusion in doses of 0.25–0.5 mg/kg/hour.

Intravenous epoprostenol is a powerful vasodilator and has been used at doses of 5–20 ng/kg/min.

Plasmapheresis removes circulating endotoxin and assists in the control of fluid balance. Fresh frozen plasma and cryoprecipitate as replacement fluids increase fibrinogen concentrations.

Other therapies used include topical nitroglycerine, intravenous (IV) dextran and leech saliva.

7. **What is the prognosis in purpura fulminans?**

This is a hematological emergency. If not diagnosed and treated, mortality rate is as high as 80–90%.

Renal Osteodystrophy

Chapter 73

Fagun Shah

CASE STUDY 1

A 6-year-old boy was brought with severe bony deformities (Fig. 1), failure to thrive, polyuria and polydipsia. He was anemic and hypertensive on examination.

The investigations revealed elevated serum creatinine, severe metabolic acidosis with high anion gap, hypocalcemia and hyperphosphatemia.

The boy is a classic case of renal osteodystrophy that occurs in patients with chronic kidney disease when glomerular filtration rate (GFR) falls below 50 mL/min/1.73 m^2.

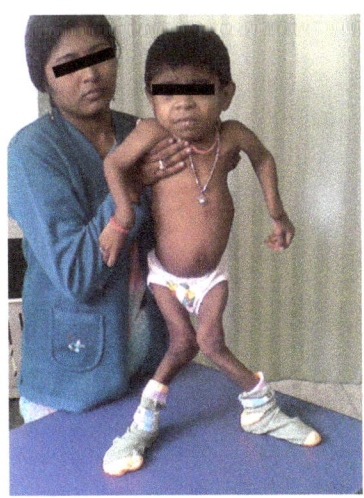

Fig. 1: A 6-year-old boy with severe bone deformities.

1. **What is renal osteodystrophy?**
   Renal osteodystrophy occurs primarily due to failure of conversion of 25-hydroxy vitamin D to 1,25-dihydroxy vitamin D by renal tubules leading to deficiency of 1,25-dihydroxy vitamin D and hypocalcemia.

2. **What other metabolic derangements are associated with it?**
   Other important features include retention of phosphates due to reduced renal excretion. The decreased serum calcium and increased phosphate levels stimulate parathyroid hormone (PTH) secretion, and thereby secondary hyperparathyroidism compounding the bone disease.

3. **When to suspect it?**
   All patients with resistant rickets should undergo evaluation for renal tubular functions to pick up the condition earlier and prevent worsening of the bony deformities.

4. **How to treat this condition?**
   Treatment includes supplementation with calcium, phosphate binders, and 1,25-dihydroxy vitamin D under supervision of pediatric nephrologist with proper monitoring of metabolic parameters periodically.

CASE STUDY 2

Eighteen months old boy presented with stunting (Fig. 2) resistant rickets, failure to thrive, polyuria and polydipsia. The investigation revealed normal renal functions and normal anion gap metabolic acidosis with hyperchloremia. The metabolic parameters revealed hypocalcemia and hypophosphatemia with phosphaturia.

This is resistant rickets in patients with Fanconi syndrome and proximal renal tubular acidosis (RTA).

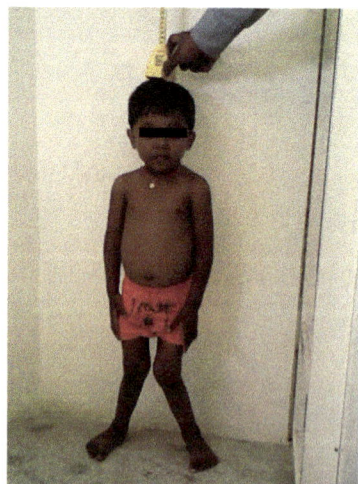

Fig. 2: Stunting and deformed bones.

5. **How to diagnose RTA?**
   As denoted earlier, all patients with resistance should undergo renal functions tests, venous blood gas and electrolytes. Normal renal functions with normal anion gap metabolic acidosis and hyperchloremia suggests RTA.
6. **Why does RTA cause rickets?**
   The primary cause of rickets is persistent acidosis. Hence, correction of acidosis by alkali supplementation is a must.
7. **What is the primary treatment for RTA?**
   Correction of acidosis will promote bone healing and obviates the need of vitamin and calcium supplementation. Inadvertent use of vitamin D and calcium supplements may lead to nephrocalcinosis as these patients might have hypercalciuria. If rickets persists despite adequate correction of acidosis, vitamin D may be tried with strict monitoring for hypercalciuria and nephrocalcinosis.
8. **Does this patient require phosphate supplementation?**
   In patients with proximal RTA due to Fanconi syndrome, phosphaturia contributes to severe rickets as well. Hence, all patients with proximal RTA need to be evaluated for phosphate levels and urinary phosphate excretion. If suggestive of phosphaturia, they require supplementation with oral phosphates and vitamin D for correction of bony deformities.

Chapter 74

Renal Tubular Disorders

Fagun Shah

CASE STUDY

Eighteen months old boy, weighing 5 kg, was brought with severe failure to thrive (Fig. 1), recurrent episodes of dehydration requiring frequent admissions and with polyuria. The child had severe dehydration, emaciated look and had constant craving for water. The child had full-term intrauterine growth restriction (IUGR), weighing 2 kg at birth and had history of polyhydramnios.

Investigations revealed metabolic acidosis with normal anion gap, hyperchloremia and normal creatinine. This was a case of renal tubular acidosis (RTA).

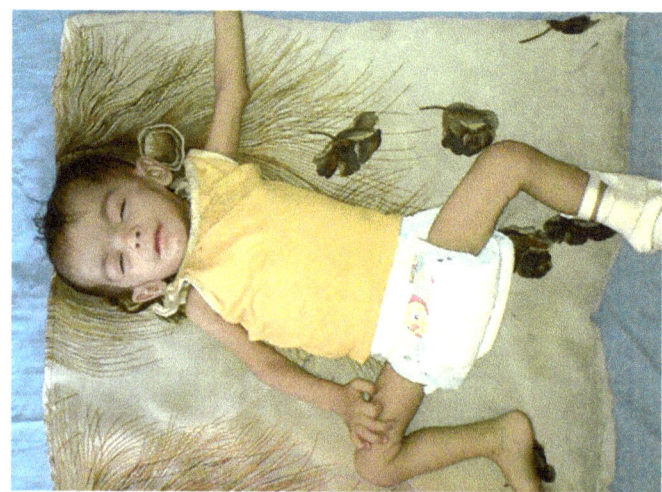

Fig. 1: Undernourished, dehydrated child.

1. **What are renal tubular disorders?**
   Enormous amount of ultrafiltrate is produced by the glomerulus which is similar to plasma in its solute content. If all is excreted without modification, it will lead to loss of catastrophic amount of fluid and electrolyte losses that is incompatible with life. Hence,

the different segments of tubules function to reabsorb this fluid, solutes and secretions of others to maintain homeostasis. Loss of function of these tubules at various segments leads to disorders classified as renal tubular disorders.

2. **What are the common renal tubular problems encountered?**
   The common disorders include: RTA, Bartter's syndrome and diabetes insipidus (DI).

3. **How will you suspect a child with renal tubular problem?**
   Milder variants present primarily with failure to thrive, polyuria, polydipsia, nocturia, bony deformities, etc.
   Severe life-threatening presentations include severe dehydration with electrolyte disturbances and acid–base disorders out of proportion of degree of fluid losses.

4. **How will you proceed with investigations in such children?**
   Three basic investigations are must in a child with suspected renal tubular disorder: serum creatinine, venous blood gas, and serum electrolytes.
   Children with normal serum creatinine, metabolic acidosis with normal anion gap and hyperchloremia suggest RTA which needs to be further classified into proximal RTA or distal RTA on further investigations.
   Children with metabolic alkalosis, hyponatremia, hypokalemia and hypochloremia classify into Bartter's syndrome and Bartter like other syndromes.
   Children with normal blood gas and hypernatremia or high serum osmolality and low urine osmolality suggest DI which has to be further differentiated into central or nephrogenic DI.

5. **How will you treat these patients?**
   Adequate hydration and proper nutrition is very important. Care must be taken and parents must be advised accordingly to prevent recurrent episodes of dehydration.
   Specific treatment involves alkali supplementation for RTA, potassium supplementation and prostaglandin inhibitors for Bartter's syndrome. Patients with central DI require intranasal desmopressin and with nephrogenic DI treated with thiazides or amiloride.

Rickettsial Fever

Chapter 75

Atul Kulkarni

CASE STUDY

A 9-year-old male child presented with high fever for 6 days, rash since 2 days, headache, altered sensorium, vomiting since 1 day, hepatomegaly splenomegaly and rash maculopapular all over the body including the soles and palms.
- The child had history of contact with cattle.
- On complete blood count (CBC)—leukopenia; thrombocytopenia
- Weil Felix test positive—1:80
- Spotted fever immunoglobulin M (IgM) positive

1. **What is rickettsial fever?**
   Rickettsial infections are a group of infections caused by obligate intracellular bacteria rickettsia.
2. **What is the history of rickettsial fever?**
   The genus rickettsia is named after Howard Taylor Ricketts (1871-1910), who described Rocky Mountain spotted fever (RMSF) in the Bitterroot Valley of Montana, and eventually died of typhus fever.
3. **What is the etiology?**
   Rickettsia is a group of motile, Gram-negative, non-spore forming highly pleomorphic bacteria that present as cocci (0.1 micron), rods (1–4 micron) or thread-like (10 micron), obligate, intracellular parasites. To survive, these have to enter, grow, and replicate in the cytoplasm or within the nucleus of the cell that they invade.
4. **What is the method of transmission?**
   Tick, mite, flea and louse are the natural hosts, reservoirs and vectors of rickettsial organisms (except Q fever). These maintain the infection naturally by transovarial transmission (passage of the organism from infected ticks to their progeny) and trans-stadial passage. Ticks transmit the infectious agent to mammalian hosts (including humans) by regurgitation of infected saliva during feeding. Dogs and rodents serve as reservoir hosts for these vectors.
5. **What are the types of rickettsial diseases?**
   The types of rickettsial diseases are discussed in Table 1.

TABLE 1: Classification of rickettsial diseases.

S. no	Disease	Rickettsial agent	Insect vector	Mammalian reservoir
1	**Typhus group**			
A	Epidemic typhus	R. prowazekii	Louse	Humans
B	Murine typhus	R. typhi	Flea	Rodent
2	Scrub typhus	R. tsutsugamushi	Mite	Rodent
3	**Spotted fever group***			
A	Indian tick typhus	R. conorii	Tick	Dog/rodents
B	Rocky Mountain spotted fever	R. rickettsii	Tick	Dogs/rodents
C	Tick born lymphadenopathy (TIBOLA)	R. slovaca	Tick	Wild boar
4	**Transitional group**			
A	Q fever	Coxiellaburnetti	Nil	Cattle/sheep/goat
B	Trench fever	Rochalimaea Quintana	Louse	Humans
C	Ehrlichiosis	Ehrlichia	Tick	Deer/dog
D	Anaplasmosis	Anaplasma phagocytophilum	Tick	Deer/dog

6. **What is the epidemiology of rickettsial fever?**
   Scrub typhus broke out in an epidemic form in Assam and West Bengal during World War II. It was later found that scrub typhus was prevalent throughout India in humans, trombiculid mites, and rodents. Recently, scrub typhus has been reported from Delhi, Himachal Pradesh, Haryana, Karnataka, Kerala, and Tamil Nadu.
   Spotted fevers and typhus fever has been reported from southern regions of India. Recent reports state that immune thrombocytopenic purpura (Itt) is prevalent in many districts of Maharashtra (e.g., Solapur, Osmanabad, Latur, Ahmadnagar, Beed, Aurangabad, Nanded, Akola, Hingoli, Parbhani, Raigad, Pune, Mumbai, etc.), Karnataka (e.g., Bijapur, Gulbarga, Hubli, Raichur, etc.), Tamil Nadu and Kerala. Itt is endemic in rural part of these areas. Serological surveys indicate that Q fever is present in animal as well as human populations in Haryana, Punjab, Delhi, Rajasthan and various other places in India.

7. **What are the clinical manifestations?**
   Incubation period 2–14 days, may extend up to 28 days. History of exposure to tick bite or close contact with an infected pet animal. Headache, fever, anorexia, myalgias, restlessness, calf muscle pain, tenderness, nausea, vomiting, diarrhea, and abdominal pain. Typical triad of—fever, headache, rash, edema (Fig. 1) over dorsum of the hand or foot, periorbital edema, hepatosplenomegaly, and generalized lymphadenopathy.

8. **What are the characteristics of rickettsial rash?**
   Rash appears after 2–4 days, initially discrete, pale rose red blanching macules or maculopapules appear on extremities, ankles, wrist or lower limbs (Fig. 2).
   Later rash spreads all over the body including palms and soles.
   After several days, rash becomes more petechial (Fig. 3), hemorrhagic sometimes with palpable purpura (Fig. 4).

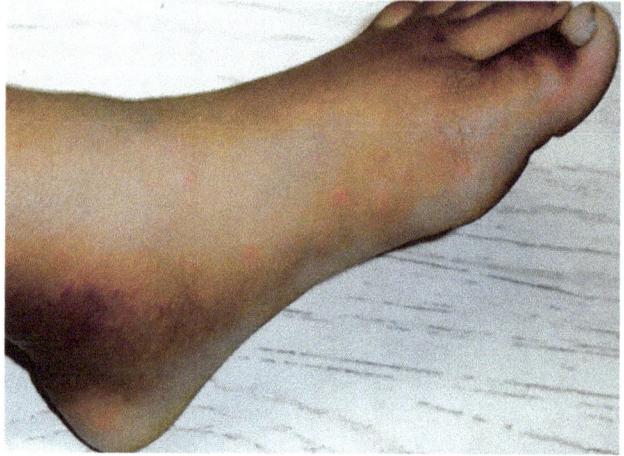

Fig. 1: Edema over feet with petechial rash.

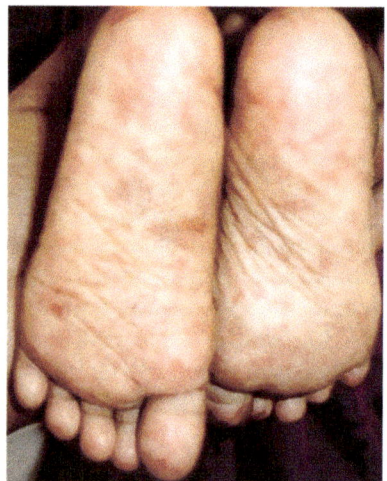

Fig. 2: Rash on sole.

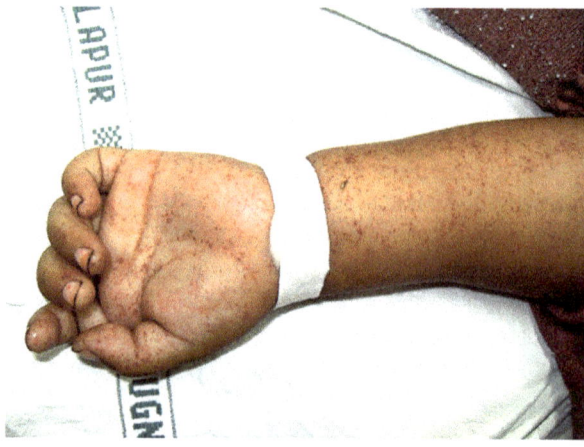

Fig. 3: Petechial rash.

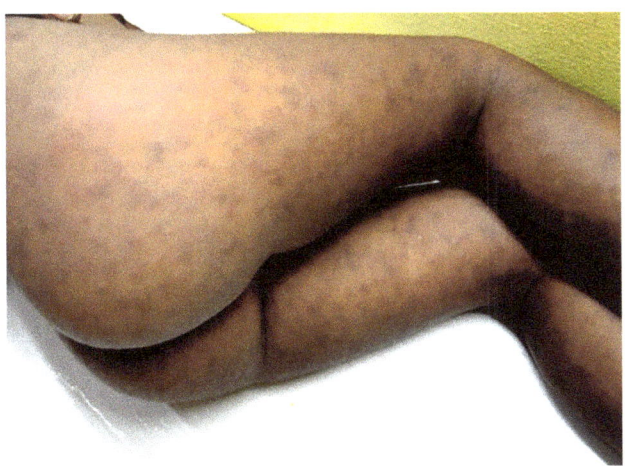

Fig. 4: Palpable purpura.

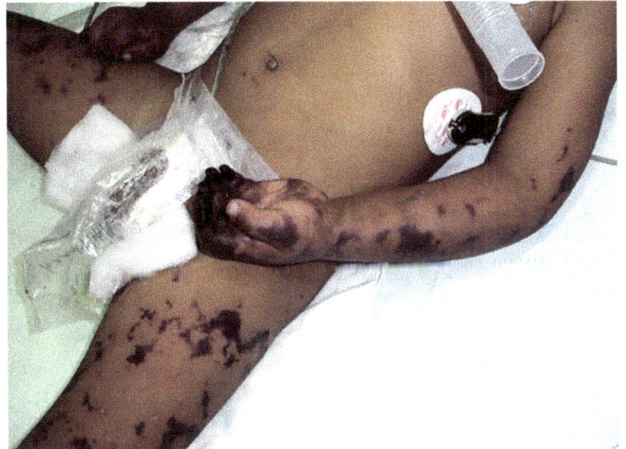

Fig. 5: Gangrene of digits and necrotic rash.

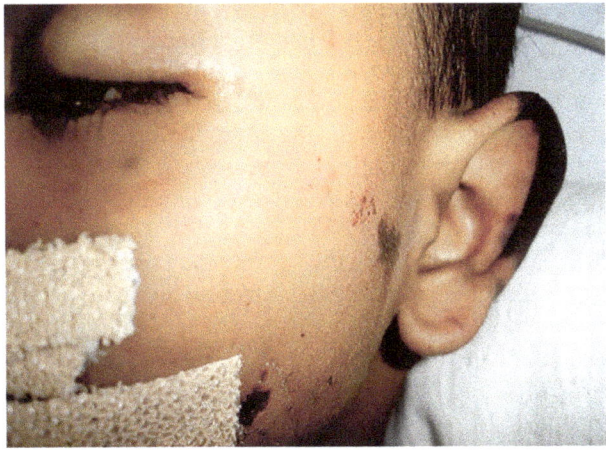

Fig. 6: Gangrene of ear lobe (Kan kapy).

In severe disease, petechiae may enlarge into ecchymosis which can become necrotic (Fig. 5). Severe vaso-occlusive disease secondary to rickettsial vasculitis and thrombosis is infrequent but can result in gangrene of the digits, toes, earlobes (Fig. 6), scrotum, nose or entire limbs. Painless eschar, the tache noire, may be seen at the initial site of tick attachment and regional lymphadenopathy.

9. **What are the complications of rickettsial fever?**
   Neurological involvement: Confusion or lethargy, stupor, delirium, ataxia, coma, deafness, seizures, encephalitis, etc.
   Pulmonary involvement: Pulmonary edema, interstitial pneumonitis, alveolar edema, acute respiratory distress syndrome (ARDS), etc.
   Others: Myocarditis, acute renal failure, disseminated intravascular coagulation (DIC), hepatitis, vascular collapse, etc.

10. **What are the laboratory findings?**
    There is no widely available laboratory assay that provides rapid confirmation of early rickettsial fever. Treatment decisions must be based on epidemiologic and clinical clues, and should never be delayed while waiting for confirmation by laboratory results.
    Laboratory findings are usually nonspecific. Total leukocyte count may be initially normal or low but leukocytosis develops as the disease progresses. Anemia, thrombocytopenia, hyponatremia, hypoproteinemia and elevated serum aminotransferases are some other features. Cerebrospinal fluid (CSF) findings are usually normal but occasionally mononuclear pleocytosis (<10–300 cell/µL) may be found.

11. **What are the serological test for the diagnosis of rickettsial infection?**
    Serological specific tests are the mainstay for diagnosis. As these may not be consistently positive during the first 2 weeks of illness, suspected patients should be treated immediately. Serologic tests are delayed until both acute and convalescent serum specimens are available. The following tests are used for diagnosis:
    Similarity of Proteus antigens OX 19, OX 2, OX K with rickettsial antigens is the principle of this heterophile antibody agglutination test. The test is usually positive after 5–7 days and 1:80 or rising titers are suggestive of rickettsial infections. This test has low sensitivity and specificity due to which its use has been discouraged in evidence-based practice. However, since it shows good correlation with IgM by indirect immunofluorescent assay (IFA) and since it is easily available in many cities and laboratories, it has been a popular screening test and a useful diagnostic tool in the developing countries. Single titer of more than 1:320 or fourfold rise of titer in paired sera is highly suggestive and specific.
    - *Enzyme-linked immunosorbent assay (ELISA):*
      IgM ELISA is one of the more sensitive tests which is available at few selected laboratories and some tertiary care hospitals in the developing world. Its sensitivity and specificity reaches almost 90%. A significant IgM titer is seen at the end of 6-7 days suggestive of acute infection, and immunoglobulin G (IgG) antibodies appear after 2-3 weeks.
    - *Polymerase chain reaction (PCR):*
      Rickettsial DNA can be detected by PCR, from blood or eschar sample. This is the most definitive test for diagnosis of rickettsial infection and can be positive within the first week itself of the illness.
    - *Immunoflurescent assay (IFA):*
      Indirect IFA is considered as Gold Standard Test for diagnosis of rickettsial fever. Antibody titers IgM >1:640 and IgG >1:254 suggest acute infection, while IgG >64 but

<124 is suggestive of past infection. The antibody titers rise after 5–7 days of the infection and peak at third week. These tests are available at selected advanced centers and are utilized for research purpose.
- *Indirect immunoperoxidase assay (IPA):*
This test is also a standard test, comparable with IFA but available at only few research centers.

12. **What is the treatment of rickettsial fever?**
Drug of choice: (1) doxycycline—2.2 mg/kg/dose BID or (2) tetracycline—25 to 50 mg/kg/dose QID or (3) chloramphenicol—50 to 100 mg/kg/day QID for 5–7 days or 3 days until the patient is afebrile. *Other:* (4) azithromycin 10 mg/kg/day OD for 3 days or (5) clarithromycin 15 mg/kg/day BD for 7 days.

Chapter 76

Roseola Infantum

Bakul Jayant Parekh

> **CASE STUDY**
>
> - An 8-month-old female with fever for the past 4 days
> - Baby does not look unwell
> - On examination, reveals no source of fever
> - White blood cells (WBC) mildly elevated; mostly lymphocytes
> - Advised to take acetaminophen
> - Next day mother calls to say baby has a rash.

1. **What is roseola infantum?**
   Roseola is a mild febrile exanthematous illness occurring almost exclusively during infancy.
2. **What are the other names?**
   It is also known as sixth disease and exanthem sabitum.
3. **What is the etiology?**
   Most commonly human herpes 6 virus (HSV 6), sometimes HSV 7.
4. **What is the mode of transmission?**
   Transplacental route.
5. **What is the incubation period?**
   5 to 15 days.
6. **What are the clinical manifestations of roseola?**
   Prodromal period—asymptomatic, may include upper respiratory tract infection, rhinorrhea, pharyngitis, mild conjunctival redness, cervical or occipital lymphadenopathy, mild palpebral edema, high grade fever. Others—seizures, irritability, anorexia, abdominal pain and vomiting. The child is active in intrafebrile period. Fever persists for 3–5 days. Rose colored rash appears within 12–24 hours of fever resolution (Fig. 1).
   Rash begins as discrete, small, slightly pink raised lesions over trunk and spreads over face, neck and proximal extremities. Rash fades after 1–3 days. Ulcers at uvulo palatoglossal junction (Nagayama spots) are common.

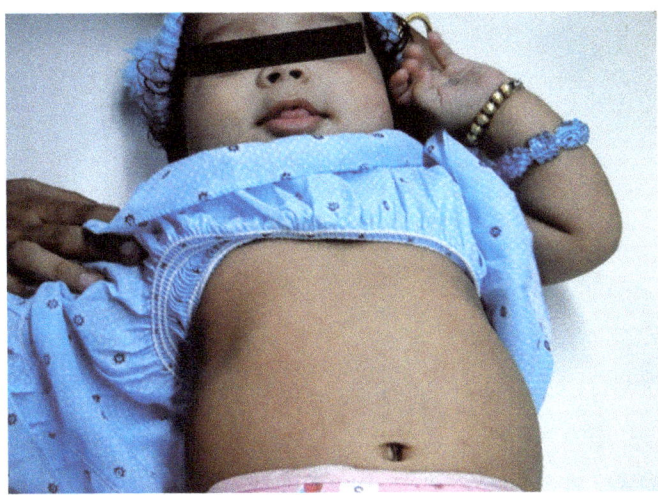

Fig. 1: Rose colored macular rash all over body.

7. **What are the investigations done?**
   - Complete blood count (CBC)—relative lymphocytosis
   - Cerebrospinal fluid (CSF)—herpes simplex virus (HSV) polymerase chain reaction (PCR).
8. **What is the treatment of roseola infantum?**
   Antipyretics and adequate hydration.
9. **What is the prognosis of roseola infantum?**
   Prognosis is excellent. Morbidity rates are in immunocompromised children.
10. **What are the complications of roseola infantum?**
    Hepatitis, encephalitis, pneumonitis, disseminated disease, and hemophagocytosis syndrome.

Spina Bifida

Chapter 77

Mehul Gosai

CASE STUDY

A 4-day-old full-term patient came to sick newborn care unit (SNCU) for not taking breastfeeding well and with tuft of hair in the lower back (Fig. 1). Patient was on expressed breast milk with top feeding with lethargy. Ultrasonography (USG) of local part was suggestive of the absence of dura mater and out-pouching of meninges locally, and absence of posterior segment of vertebra.

USG anterior fontanelle was suggestive of dilated ventricles confirmed with magnetic resonance imaging (MRI) as the patient had Arnold Chiari malformation type 2.

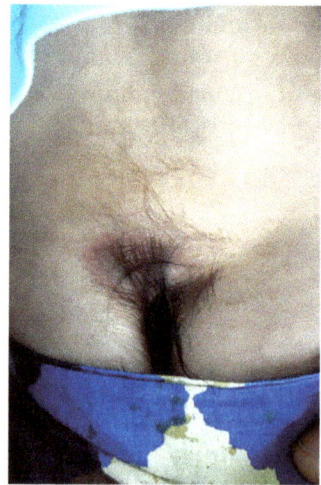

Fig. 1: Tuft of hair in the lower back.

1. **What does the tuft of hair in sacral dimple indicate?**
   Sacral dimple with tuft of hair is at times associated with a serious underlying abnormality of the spine or spinal cord.

2. **What is spina bifida?**
   Spina bifida is a treatable spinal cord malformation due to neural tube defects. It occurs in varying degrees of severity.
3. **What are the types of spina bifida?**
   - Spina bifida cystic
   - Spina bifida occulta
   - Syringomeningocele
   - Syringomyelocele and syringomyelia.
4. **What is the pathophysiology of spina bifida?**
   Neural tube defects result from a teratogenic process that causes failed closure and abnormal differentiation of the embryonic neural tube.
5. **What is the etiology of spina bifida?**
   The etiology in most cases of myelomeningocele is multifactorial, involving genetic, racial and environmental factors, in which nutrition, particularly folic acid intake, is the key. Cytoplasmic factors, polygenic inheritance, chromosomal aberrations and environmental influences (e.g. teratogens) have all been considered as possible causes.
6. **What is the epidemiology of spina bifida?**
   The incidence of spina bifida has been estimated at 1–2 cases per 1,000 population, with certain populations having a significantly greater incidence based on genetic predilection.
7. **What are the differential diagnoses of spina bifida?**
   - Mass lesions of the cord
   - Diastematomyelia
   - Cord cavitation and narrowing
   - Adhesions
   - Dural bands.
8. **What are the enzyme studies used in spina bifida?**
   Alpha-fetoprotein and acetylcholinesterase.
9. **What is the role of fetal USG in spina bifida?**
   Fetal USG can be used as the primary screening tool for neural tube defects, usually at approximately 18 weeks' gestational age. The procedure avoids roughly 1% risk of abortion following amniocentesis, but accurate diagnosis depends on the skill and experience of the operator and the quality of the equipment.
10. **What is the management of spina bifida?**
    Patients with spina bifida require extensive, active, interdisciplinary treatment by a trained and coordinated team. Antibiotics, sac closure and ventriculo-peritoneal shunt placement are the standard of care for spina bifida.
11. **What are the complications of spina bifida?**
    Complications of spina bifida can range from minor physical problems with little functional impairment to severe physical and mental disabilities. It is important to note, however, that most people with spina bifida are of normal intelligence. Spina bifida's impact is determined by the size and location of the malformation, whether it is covered, and which spinal nerves are involved. All nerves located below the malformation are affected to some degree. Therefore, the higher the malformation occurs on the back, the greater the amount of nerve damage and loss of muscle function and sensation.

12. **What is the prognosis of spina bifida?**

 The extent of disability and other continuing issues are basically linked to the following factors:
 - The site along the spine where the nerves were damaged
 - The size of the lesion
 - The timing and type of treatment
 - The presence of any other birth defects

 If the lesion is high up in the spine, the child may have paraplegia (inability to move the legs from the hips down) and will require a wheelchair for mobility. However, if the thigh muscles have movement and there is sensation in the legs below the knees, then the child probably will be able to walk with the aid of braces.

 The majority of children with spina bifida are able to manage their bladder and bowel output by doing regular self-catheterization (using a tube to drain urine from the bladder) and a bowel program so that they are fully continent.

Sacral Agenesis

Chapter 78

Pramod Jog

CASE STUDY

A three and a half year old male child presented with bladder and bowel incontinence with persistent dribbling of small quantities of urine (Figs. 1 and 2).

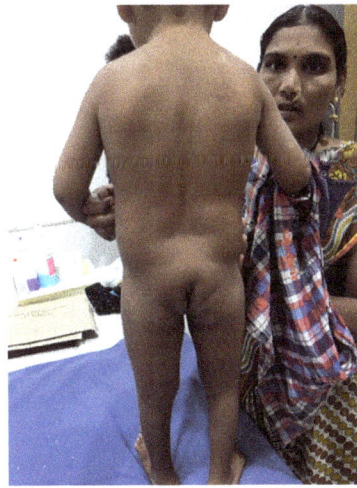

Fig. 1: Clinical photograph of the back showing short, flat gluteal cleft

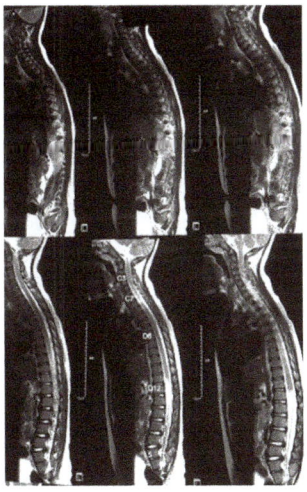

Fig 2: Magnetic resonance imaging spine T2 image showing wedge-shaped feature.

1. **What were the clinical features?**
   Clinical features are:
   - Inability to sense the urge to urinate
   - Dribbling of small quantities of urine
   - Persistent passing of small quantities of stools
   - Lower limb weakness (B/L lower limb hypotonia with power 4/5)
   - Wasting of gluteal muscles (Fig. 3)
   - Pes planus.

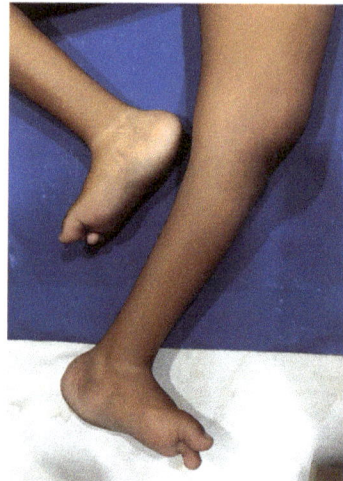

Fig 3: Clinical photograph showing lower limb wasting and weakness.

2. **What is the diagnosis?**
   Caudal regression syndrome or sacral agenesis (or hypoplasia of sacrum)(Fig. 4). It is a neural tube defect in which there is abnormal fetal development of the caudal part of the spine.

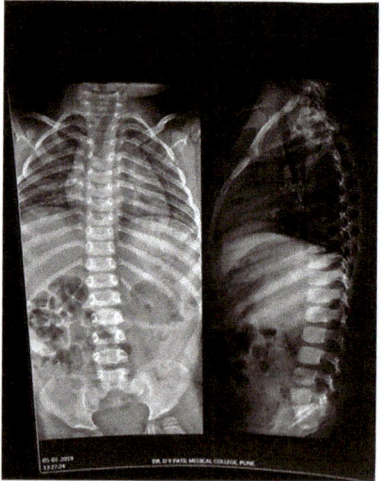

Fig 4: MRI showing sacral agenesis.

3. **What is the etiology?**
   Maternal diabetes mellitus is the most common cause.
4. **What are the important features?**
   This condition presents with a LMN type of bladder with absence of urge to urinate since the detrusor is relaxed.

- The urinary retention causes overflow incontinence
- There is inability to initiate urination
- Large post-void retention of urine
- Tonic, large bladder.

5. **What is the treatment?**
    - *Medical:* Cholinergic agents to increase the contractility of the detrusor (Bethanechol) and an alpha blocker to relax the sphincter (Tamsulosin).
    - *Short term:* Intermittent passage of Foley's to drain urine, colostomy opening.
    - *Long term:* Bladder strengthening surgery to reinforce the detrusor.

Scarlet Fever

Chapter 79

Aniruddha Ghosh, Ritabrata Kundu

CASE STUDY

A 6-year-old boy presented with high-grade (102–103°F) fever, 2–3 spikes/day along with sore throat for the last 4 days. Since the 2nd day of fever, diffuse blanchable erythematous rash (Fig. 1) was noticed on the trunk which was dark red in color around flexures of skin folds. Culture from throat swab yielded group A *Streptococcus* (GAS) which was sensitive to amoxicillin. Diagnosis of scarlet fever was made. Fever subsided after 2 days of starting oral amoxicillin. The rash gradually started to fade and dark punctate discoloration appeared near axilla, shoulders and back (Fig. 2). Peeling of skin was noted around the face, chest and back (Fig. 3) while the child was recovering.

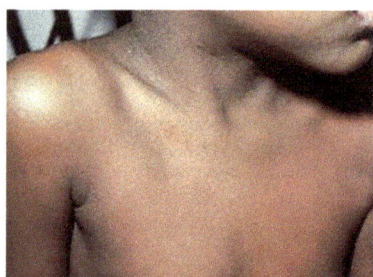

Fig. 1: Red erythematous rash.

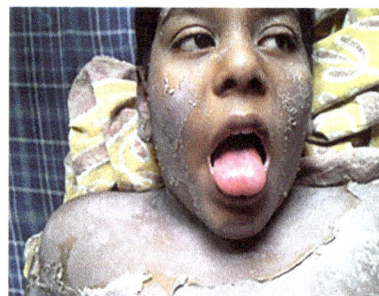

Fig. 3: Skin peeling

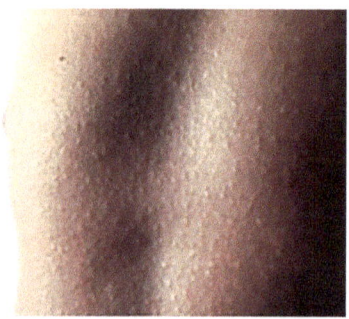

Fig. 2: Punctate erythema (Sand paper rash)

1. **What is the causative organism of scarlet fever?**
   Group A *Streptococcus* or in other terms *Streptococcus pyogenes*. It secretes pyrogenic exotoxin or erythrotoxin which causes disease in individuals who do not have antitoxin-antibodies. At times it may also follow staphylococcal infection where sore throat is not a usual presentation.
2. **Who suffer the common sufferers from scarlet fever?**
   Incidence is highest in 5–15 years age group, especially the school-going children.
3. **What is the mode of transmission of the infection?**
   Humans are natural reservoirs for GAS. GAS is a highly communicable organism which spreads via airborne salivary droplets and nasal secretion. Close proximity with other children with untreated acute GAS pharyngotonsillitis favors transmission. Food contaminated with GAS has the potential to cause outbreaks in daycare centers or schools. Chronic pharyngeal carriers rarely spread infection. 24 hours of antibiotic therapy is sufficient to make a patient non-infectious to other children.
4. **What is the incubation period?**
   The incubation period is 2–5 days for GAS pharyngitis as well as scarlet fever.
5. **What are the symptoms and signs of scarlet fever?**
   - Fever.
   - Sore throat due to upper respiratory tract infection.
   - *Rash:* Rash starts after 24–48 hours of fever but sometimes it may be the presenting symptom. It looks like diffuse, finely papular, blanching erythematous eruption producing bright red discoloration of the skin. It is often accentuated in the creases of the elbows, axillae and groin known as Pastia's lines. The skin has a goose-pimple appearance and feels rough (known as sand paper appearance). The cheeks are often erythematous with pallor around the mouth.
     After 3–4 days, rash starts to fade away and desquamation follows involving first the face and then gradually progressing downward. Sheet-like desquamation may occur in the palms, soles, and periungual regions.
   - Pharynx may be congested along with the tonsils.
   - Eyes may have mild watering.
   - Tongue is usually coated with enlarged papillae. Once desquamation subsides, inflamed and swollen papillae become prominent giving it a strawberry appearance.
6. **What are the differential diagnoses of scarlet fever?**
   - Viral exanthems
   - Kawasaki disease
   - Drug rashes
   - Scrub typhus
   - Staphylococcal infections.
7. **What are the complications of scarlet fever?**
   Like other streptococcal infections, the delayed/long-term complications are:
   - Acute rheumatic fever
   - Post-streptococcal glomerulonephritis
   - Post-streptococcal reactive arthritis.

8. **How to diagnose scarlet fever?**
   Diagnosis is mostly clinical. A history of GAS pharyngitis and the typical rash along with a high antistreptolysin-O titer (in low endemic regions) helps in diagnosis. Culture from throat swab often isolates the organism but it has got little role in confirming the diagnosis in highly endemic regions as GAS is a common colonizer of the upper airway in humans.

9. **How to treat scarlet fever?**
   For classic scarlet fever, antibiotic therapy should start immediately.
   GAS is exquisitely sensitive to penicillin and cephalosporins, and resistance is rarely seen. Recommended treatments are:
   - *Oral penicillin V:* 250 mg/dose bid-tid children weighing less than or equal to 60 lb and 500 mg/dose bid-tid for children weighing more than 60 lb for a 10-day course
   - *Parenteral therapy:* Single intramuscular injection of benzathine penicillin G (600,000 IU for children weighing less than or equal to 60 lb and 1.2 million IU for children weighing more than 60 lb)
   - Oral amoxicillin once daily 50 mg/kg (max 1 g) for 10 days has been demonstrated to be effective in several comparative clinical trials.

   However, it has also been documented that for the vast majority of patients with much less distinctive findings, treatment should be withheld without concrete microbiological confirmation by throat culture or specific rapid antigen detection test.

Scarlet Fever

Chapter 80

S Balasubramanian, Sumanth Amperayani

CASE STUDY

A 7-year-old child presented with fever of 3 days' duration (102–103°F). He had a sandpaper type of rash first appearing in the nape of neck and then it spread downwards.

The child also had other features like strawberry tongue, absence of cough and pain in the back of throat (Figs. 1 to 5).

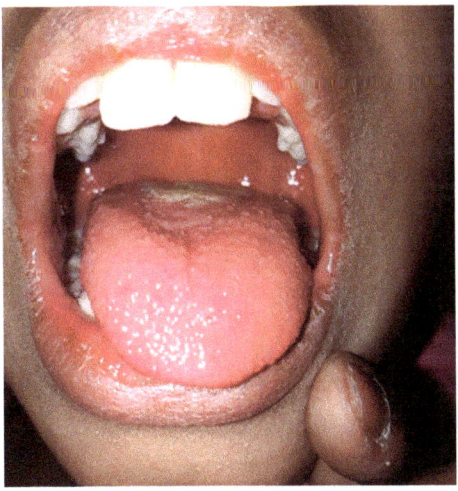

Fig. 1: Palatal erythema, strawberry tongue.

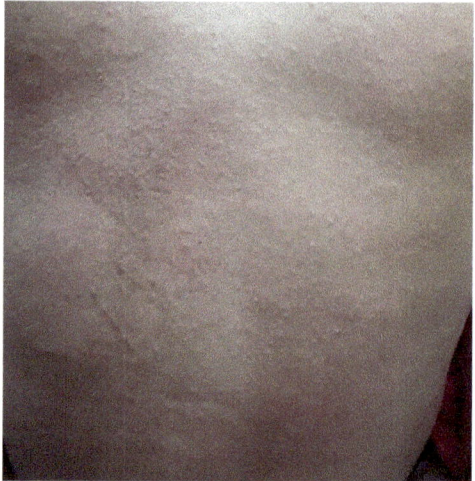

Fig. 2: Typical sandpaper rash.

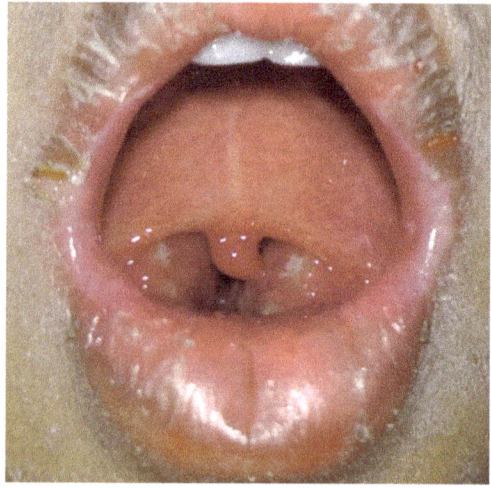

Fig. 3: Perioral pallor, exudative tonsillitis, cheilitis.

Scarlet Fever

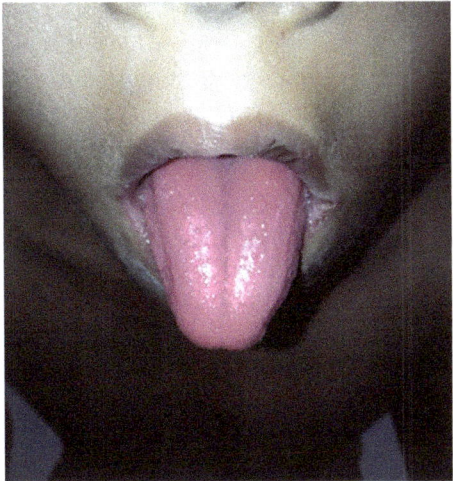

Fig. 4: Strawberry tongue.

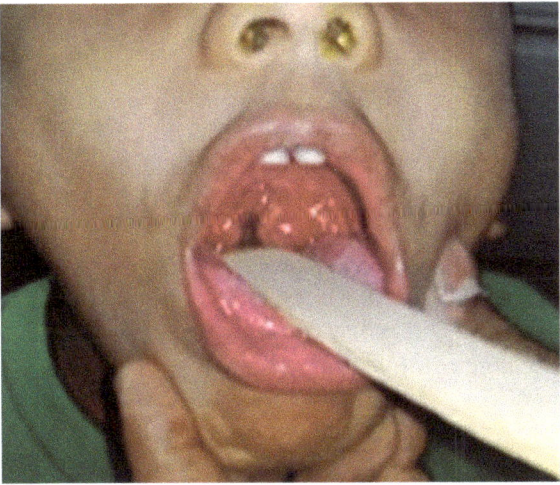

Fig. 5: Edema of uvula with pharyngitis.

1. **What is scarlet fever?**
   Scarlet fever (also known as "scarlatina") is a diffuse erythematous eruption that generally occurs in association with pharyngitis due to Group A β-hemolytic *Streptococcus*.
2. **What is the Hallmark feature of scarlet fever?**
   The classic presentation consists of rapid onset of fever, chills, malaise, headache, sore throat and vomiting with or without abdominal pain. Within 12–48 hours, an exanthem appears and rapidly generalizes, usually beginning on the trunk and spreading peripherally, but sometimes spreading cephalocaudally, mimicking measles. The face is flushed with perioral pallor.

Examination of the oropharynx usually shows large, erythematous and exudative tonsils, along with palatal erythema and petechiae. The uvula may be erythematous and edematous as well. The tongue also shows characteristic findings during the first 2 days, with a white coating through which erythematous papillae project ("white" strawberry tongue). The white coat subsequently peels, leaving a glistening red surface with prominent papillae ("red" strawberry tongue).

The rash of scarlet fever is a diffuse erythema that blanches with pressure, with numerous small (1–2 mm) papular elevations, giving a "sandpaper" quality to the skin. Later, the rash expands rapidly to cover the trunk, followed by the extremities, and ultimately, desquamates with sapring of the palms and soles. The rash is most marked in the skin folds of the inguinal, axillary, antecubital and abdominal areas and about pressure points. It often exhibits a linear petechial character in the antecubital fossae and axillary folds, known as Pastia's lines. This may be accompanied by diffuse petechiae. Few cases may present with fever or nasopharyngitis and urticaria as their initial manifestations. In dark-skinned children, erythema and perioral pallor may not be obvious and the papules may be larger, thus producing a texture like sandpaper.

Tender cervical adenopathy is noted in 30–60% of patients. Without treatment, the rash, fever and pharyngitis resolve within 1 week; with treatment, improvement is more rapid within days.

3. **What is the causative agent?**
Development of the scarlet fever rash requires prior exposure to S. *pyogenes* and occurs as a result of delayed-type skin reactivity to pyrogenic exotoxin (erythrogenic toxin, usually types A, B or C) produced by the organism. Staphylococcal infection can produce a scarlatiniform exanthem that is initially indistinguishable from group A β-hemolytic streptococcal infection.

4. **How is the diagnosis established?**
The diagnosis is established based on clinical manifestations. Apart from rapid streptococcal antigen testing and throat culture, there is no role for additional testing. Rise in antistreptolysin O (ASO) titers may confirm the diagnosis retrospectively only.

5. **What are the associated complications?**
Complications are rare. Most cases may recover even without treatment.
Peritonsillar abscess, mastoiditis, otitis media, pneumonia, sepsis and distant foci of infection. Acute rheumatic fever and inability to swallow liquids or upper airway obstruction requiring hospitalization are some complications that can occur rarely.

6. **How is it treated?**
Penicillin is the treatment of choice for Group A *Streptococcus* (GAS) pharyngitis due to its efficacy, safety, narrow spectrum and low cost. Resistance to penicillin among clinical GAS isolates has not been documented. Penicillin is the only antibiotic that has been studied and shown to reduce rates of acute rheumatic fever. Amoxicillin is often preferred for young children because the taste of the amoxicillin suspension is more palatable than that of penicillin and also because of non-availability of oral and parenteral preparations of penicillin. Amoxicillin can also be given once daily, either immediate release or as an extended-release tablet. In several randomized trials, standard-dose and once-daily dosing of amoxicillin appeared to have equivalent efficacy as oral penicillin.

Treatment with a 10-day course of penicillin or clindamycin (in penicillin-allergic children) helps reduce the risk of transmission and preventing rheumatic fever and pyogenic complications. In patients with fever or nasopharyngitis and urticaria and in children with scarlatiniform eruptions, a rapid streptococcal antigen testing/screening throat culture for *S. pyogenes* should be obtained. Failure to respond to amoxicillin should raise doubt about the diagnosis because the rapid test positivity or culture positivity may be due to carrier state.

7. **What is the duration of treatment?**
   The duration of therapy for oral penicillin or amoxicillin is 10 days. Although symptoms typically improve within the first few days of treatment, treating for 10 days appears to enhance the rate of GAS eradication from the oropharynx when compared with 5 or 7 days. Complications can be severe and are likely related to the presence of the organism in the oropharynx; therefore, treatment with a 10-day course seems prudent.

8. **What are the alternative drugs?**
   Cephalosporins, clindamycin and macrolides are alternatives for patients who are allergic to penicillin or who cannot otherwise tolerate penicillin. Selection of an agent depends on the type of allergy, local antibiotic resistance rates, and patient values and preferences.

9. **How is the skin rash treated?**
   The approach to treatment of scarlet fever is the same as that of streptococcal pharyngitis; no additional treatment is warranted for the skin rash.

10. **Does the case need isolation?**
    Children may return to school or day-care 24 hours after initiation of antibiotics. No additional monitoring for such patients is required.

Staphylococcal Scalding Skin Syndrome

Chapter 81

Kewal Kishore Arora, Swati Mulye

CASE STUDY

A 3.4 kg, male child, appropriate for gestational age (AGA) born to primigravida via normal vaginal delivery at a hospital in Indore, and discharged on the second day. History of massaging with (mustard) sarso oil after adding lahsun (garlic) and ajwain on 3rd–4th day. Massaging done for 3 days. After that, they noticed small skin lesions filled with fluid (blisterous lesions) (Fig. 1), which ruptured and was spread all over the body (groin/limbs/neck/scalp), associated with redness and discharge, and the baby was brought to our institution; based on clinical picture, a diagnosis of staphylococcal scalding skin syndrome (SSSS) was made and the skin scraping smear was send for Gram's stain which showed cocci and cells with multiple neutrophils. Local antibacterial in the form of mupirocin was started; being a newborn baby, systemic antibiotics by intravenous route was started, and ampicillin and cloxacillin combination(being cloxa alone not available) was started after sending the sample for complete blood count (CBC), C-reactive protein (CRP), and blood culture sensitivity. Antibiotic was upgraded to vancomycin on the third day due to poor feeding and baby improved remarkably in the next 2 days.

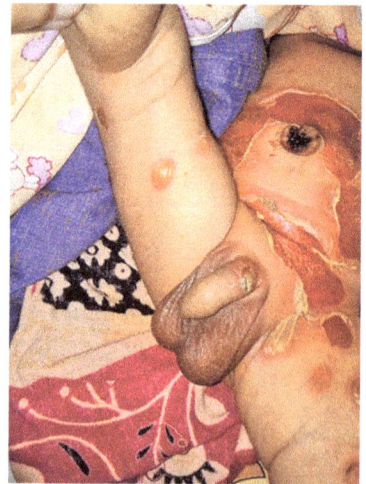

Fig. 1: Blisterous lesions.

Investigations

CBC: Hemoglobin (Hb)—17.5; red blood cells (RBC)—5.43; packed cell volume (PCV)—53.5; total leukocyte count (TLC)—17,800 P72, L26, M2; platelets—1.92; CRP—0.5.
Gram stain—Gram-positive cocci (*Staphylococcus*)
Tzank smear—acanthocytic cells with multiple neutrophils
Swab culture—coagulase negative staph
Blood culture sensitivity test—*Staphylococcus aureus* grown.

1. **What is staphylococcal scalded skin syndrome?**
   Staphylococcal scalded skin syndrome is an illness characterized by red blistering skin that looks like a burn or scald, hence its name SSSS.
2. **What causes staphylococcal scalded skin syndrome?**
   Staphylococcal scalded skin syndrome is caused by the release of two exotoxins (epidermolytic toxins A and B) from toxigenic strains of the bacteria *Staphylococcus aureus*. Desmosomes are the part of the skin cell responsible for adhering to the adjacent skin cell. The toxins bind to a molecule within the desmosome called Desmoglein 1 and break it up so that the skin cells become unstuck.
3. **What other names staphylococcal scalded skin syndrome is referred in children?**
   Staphylococcal scalded skin syndrome has also been called Ritter disease or Lyell disease when it appears in newborns or young.
4. **Who is at risk of staphylococcal scalded skin syndrome?**
   Mostly in children younger than 5 years, particularly neonates (newborn babies). SSSS lifelong protective antibodies against staphylococcal exotoxins are usually acquired during childhood which makes SSSS much less common in older children and adults. Lack of specific immunity to the toxins and an immature renal clearance system (toxins are primarily cleared from the body through the kidneys) makes neonates the most at risk.
5. **What are the other risk factors for staphylococcal scalded skin syndrome?**
   The other risk factors include: conditions producing immunocompromised states and chronic renal disease or renal failure.
6. **How a child gets staphylococcal scalded skin syndrome?**
   Staphylococcal scalded skin syndrome starts from a localized staphylococcal infection that is a producer of the two causative exotoxins (epidermolytic toxins A and B). An asymptomatic adult carrier (15–40% of healthy adults are carriers) of *Staphylococcus aureus* introduces the bacteria into the nursery.
7. **What are the signs and symptoms of staphylococcal scalded skin syndrome?**
   Staphylococcal scalded skin syndrome usually starts with fever, irritability, and widespread redness of the skin. Within 24–48 hours, fluid-filled blisters form. These rupture easily, leaving an area that looks like a burn or scald.
   Characteristics of the SSSS rash include:
   - Tissue paper-like wrinkling of the skin is followed by the appearance of large fluid-filled blisters (bullae) in the armpits, groin, and body orifices such as the nose and ears.
   - Rash spreads to other parts of the body including the arms, legs, and trunk. In newborns, lesions are often found in the diaper area or around the umbilical cord.
   - Top layer of skin begins peeling off in sheets, leaving exposed a moist, red and tender area. Nikolsky sign is positive (i.e., gentle strokes result in exfoliation).

- Other symptoms may include tender and painful areas around the infection site, weakness, and dehydration.

8. **How is staphylococcal scalded skin syndrome diagnosed?**
   The diagnosis of SSSS depends on the following:
   - History and physical examination
   - Tzanck smear
   - Skin biopsy, which shows intraepidermal cleavage at the granular layer
   - Bacterial culture from skin, blood, urine or umbilical cord sample (in a newborn baby).

9. **What are the treatment options for SSSS?**
   The best treatment plan for a pediatric patient is based on the following:
   - Age, overall health and medical history
   - Severity of the conditions
   - Response to therapies.

   Treatment of SSSS usually requires hospitalization, as intravenous antibiotics are generally necessary to eradicate the staphylococcal infection. A penicillinase-resistant, anti-staphylococcal antibiotic such as flucloxacillin is used. Other antibiotics include nafcillin, oxacillin, cephalosporin, and clindamycin. Vancomycin is used in infections suspected with methicillin-resistant staphylococcus aureus (MRSA). Depending on response to treatment, oral antibiotics can be substituted within several days. The patient may be discharged from hospital to continue treatment at home.

10. **How to prevent staphylococcal scalded skin syndrome?**
    If there is an outbreak of SSSS in either a neonatal care unit or childcare facility, the possibility of a staphylococcal carrier in the vicinity should be investigated. Identification of the healthcare worker, childcare worker, parent or visitor colonized or infected with *Staphylococcus aureus* is the key to managing the problem. Once identified, these individuals should be treated with oral antibiotics to eradicate the causative organism. To prevent further infections, these places should employ strict hand washing with antibacterial soaps or sanitizers.

    Corticosteroids slow down healing, and hence are not given to patients with SSSS.
    Other supportive treatments for SSSS include:
    - Paracetamol when necessary for fever and pain
    - Monitoring and maintaining fluid and electrolyte intake
    - Skin care (the skin is often very fragile). Petroleum jelly should be applied to keep the skin moisturized
    - Newborn babies affected by SSSS are usually kept in incubators.

    Although the outward signs of SSSS look bad, children generally recover well and healing is usually complete within 5–7 days after starting the treatment.

11. **What are the possible complications of ssss in a child?**
    The complications may include:
    - Loss of fluid causing dehydration and shock like a burn patient
    - Infection that gets worse
    - Scarring
    - Death.

Sturge–Weber Syndrome

Chapter 82

Ritesh Shah

> **CASE STUDY**
>
> A 14-month-old boy presented with recurrent right focal seizures which was started at 7 months of age. He has mild developmental delay. On examination, he has typical skin lesion over face (Fig. 1) and the neurological examination is normal.

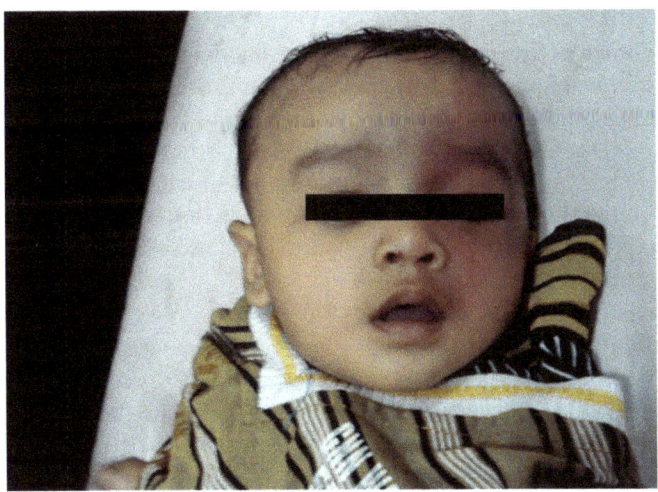

Fig. 1: Facial port wine stain.

1. **How will you describe skin lesion?**
   Facial port wine stains (Fig. 1) which are capillary malformation are characteristic skin lesion of Sturge-Weber syndrome (SWS). It is present at birth; usually unilateral, involving upper face and eyelid in ophthalmic and maxillary distribution of trigeminal nerve. It can also present over the lower face, trunk and mucosa of the mouth and pharynx.

2. **What is SWS?**
   Sturge-Weber syndrome is a sporadic vascular disorder that consists of facial, brain, and ophthalmic vascular malformation, and presents with port wine stain, leptomeningeal angioma, and glaucoma.

3. **What is the embryological basis of SWS?**
   Sturge–Weber syndrome is caused by the presence of residual embryonal blood vessels and its secondary effects are on the surrounding tissues. During development, a vascular plexus develops around cephalic portion of neural tube under ectoderm (which subsequently becomes facial skin) during the 6th week of gestation and regress at approximately 9th week. Failure of this regression results in residual vascular tissue forming angiomata of leptomeninges, face and ipsilateral eye.

4. **What is the common clinical presentation of SWS?**
   The syndrome should be suspected in any child with facial port wine stain at birth especially those involving the ophthalmic division of trigeminal nerve. Focal seizure (contralateral to the side of lesion) is present in up to 90% of the children before the age of 3 years. Refractory epilepsy develops in a significant number of cases (around 50%). Learning difficulty and developmental delay are common (50–60%). There will be headache in up to 60% due to vascular abnormalities and symptoms consistent with migraine. Hemiparesis and transient stroke like episodes may happen in 33% of cases. Glaucoma occurs in up to 30–70% of cases starting from infancy.

5. **What is the mechanism of seizure and stroke?**
   According to hypothesis, seizures result from cortical irritability caused by leptomeningeal angioma, resulting in regional hypoxia, ischemia, and gliosis. Associated cortical dysgenesis may also cause seizures. Hemiparesis and stroke-like events result from ischemia with venous occlusion and thrombosis due to venous congestion resulting from failure of cortical vein development.

6. **What is the choice of investigation once you suspect SWS?**
   Magnetic resonance imaging (MRI) brain with contrast is the preferred modality to look for leptomeningeal angioma ipsilateral to the side of facial port wine stain; sometimes white matter changes due to chronic hypoxia. Progressive cerebral atrophy ipsilateral to the angiomatosis with calcification is common. Calcification like tram–track pattern, mostly over parietal or parieto-occipital regions is better demonstrated on computed topography (CT) scan. Ophthalmic evaluation for glaucoma is also recommended at the time of diagnosis.

7. **What is the treatment of seizure in SWS?**
   Seizures should be treated with drugs effective against focal seizures. For those with early onset seizures and extensive cerebral angiomatosis refractory seizures are very common. After poly therapy, surgery in the form of hemisprectomy is a good option. Early hemispherectomy improves seizure control and promotes better intellectual development.

8. **What is the other treatment modalities used in patients with SWS?**
   Aspirin in the dose of 3–5 mg/kg/day is recommended to prevent stroke-like episodes. Recurrent thrombosis is a hypothetical mechanism for stroke-like episodes and neurological deterioration. Headache can be helped by standard anti-migarine agents. Laser therapy can be used for port wine stain. Regular ophthalmology review to monitor and manage glaucoma is required.

Systemic Lupus Erythematosus

Chapter 83

Anoop Verma

CASE STUDY

A 17-year-old female patient presented with fever for more than 7 days' duration with rash over face (Fig. 1) sparing nasolabial folds and weakness. An oral cavity examination reveals palatal rash and ulcers (Fig. 2). Antinuclear antibodies (ANA) titer and anti-double stranded deoxyribonucleic acid (anti-dsDNA) titer were positive.

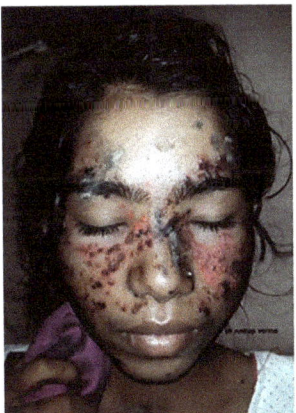 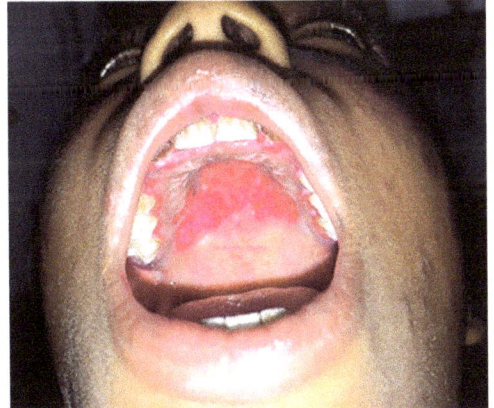

Fig. 1: Butterfly rash on face.   **Fig. 2:** Palatal rash and ulcers.

1. **What is systemic lupus erythematosus?**
   Systemic lupus erythematosus (SLE) is a chronic inflammatory autoimmune disorder of the connective tissue, primarily affecting the skin, joints, blood and kidneys, and follows a relapsing and remitting course. Here, antibodies are formed within the body, which target healthy body systems, causing inflammation and structural changes.
2. **Which factors contribute in the pathogenesis of SLE?**
   Systemic lupus erythematosus is an autoimmune disorder of unknown etiology, and associated with multiple factors in the development of the disease, like genetic, epigenetic, ethnic, immunoregulatory, hormonal and environmental factors. Immune disturbances, both innate and acquired, do occur in SLE.

3. **What are the peculiarities of a malar rash due to SLE?**

   There is classical malar rash or butterfly rash, characterized by an erythema over the cheeks and nasal bridge, but sparing the nasolabial folds, which is in contrast to the rash of dermatomyositis. It may be painful or pruritic and lasts for days and weeks.

4. **What are childhood-onset specific symptoms for SLE?**

   There are several statistically significant clinical symptoms commonly found in childhood-onset SLE, like malar rash, ulcers/mucocutaneous involvement, renal involvement, proteinuria, urinary cellular casts, seizures, thrombocytopenia, hemolytic anemia, fever and lymphadenopathy.

5. **What are the American College of Rheumatology Criteria for Diagnosis of SLE?**

   The American College of Rheumatology diagnostic criteria:

   As noted, lupus is a condition that is often difficult to diagnose due to the significant variation of symptoms among individuals. Based on that fact, the American College of Rheumatology (ACR) has developed 11 specific criteria for the diagnosis of lupus. In 2012, the Systemic Lupus International Collaborating Clinics (SLICC) group revised and validated

   > **BOX 1:** The American College of Rheumatology criteria for the diagnosis of SLE.
   >
   > A combination of 4 or more of the following 11 criteria, and at least 1 clinical and 1 immunologic criterion, in a patient's history indicates a diagnosis of SLE:
   > - Malar rash: Butterfly rash or facial erythema (red skin rash)
   > - Discoid rash
   > - Photosensitivity
   > - Oral or nasopharyngeal ulcerations
   > - Non-erosive arthritis
   > - Serositis (pleuritis or pericarditis)
   > - Renal disorder (persistent proteinuria or cellular casts)
   > - Neurological disorder (seizures or psychosis)
   > - Hematologic or blood disorder (hemolytic anemia, or leukopenia, or lymphopenia or thrombocytopenia; leukopenia and lymphopenia must be detected on two or more occasions; thrombocytopenia must be detected in the absence of drugs known to induce it)
   > - Immunologic disorder (anti-double stranded anti-DNA test; positive anti-Sm test; false-positive syphilis test)
   > - Positive ANA titer (in the absence of drugs known to induce it)
   >
   > *Source:* Petri M, Orbai AM, Alarcón GS, et al. Derivation and validation of the Systemic Lupus International Collaborating Clinics classification criteria for systemic lupus erythematosus. Arthritis Rheum. 2012;64(8):2677-86.

   the ACR lupus classification criteria. The SLICC classified a person as having lupus in the presence of biopsy-proven lupus nephritis with ANA or anti-DNA antibodies, or if 4 of the 11 diagnostic criteria, including at least 1 clinical and 1 immunologic criterion, have been satisfied (Box 1).

6. **What Are the EULAR recommendations for treating SLE?**

   The European League Against Rheumatism (EULAR) 2007, released recommendations for the treatment of SLE. In patients with SLE without major organ manifestations, glucocorticoids and antimalarial agents may be beneficial. Nonsteroidal anti-inflammatory drugs (NSAIDs) may be used for short periods in patients at low risk for complications from these drugs. Consider immunosuppressive agents (e.g., azathioprine, mycophenolate mofetil, methotrexate, etc.) in refractory cases or when steroid doses cannot be reduced to levels for long-term use.

Tuberculous Lymphadenitis with Sinus

Chapter 84

Abhay K Shah

CASE STUDY

An 18-month-old male child (full-term, delivered by normal vaginal hospital delivery, without any prenatal, natal or postnatal event, and unvaccinated) presented with low-grade fever off and on since 6 months, multiple neck swellings since 4 months followed by discharging sinus since 3 months. He was treated with multiple courses of antibiotics and has even undergone incision and drainage twice without much relief.

On examination, he was undernourished, pale, and cranky. There were multiple cervical glands bilateral, firm, matted, and adhered to underlying skin with sinus formation at places (Fig. 1). He was also having 2 cm palpable liver and 3 cm palpable spleen. There were no meningeal signs. The rest of clinical examination was normal.

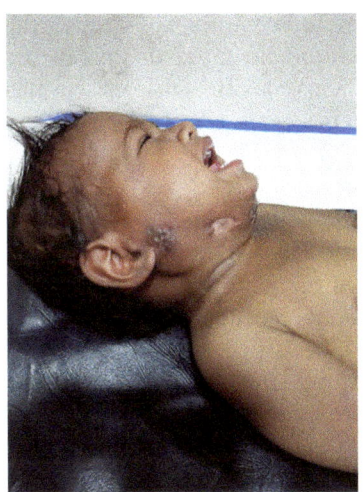

Fig. 1: Lymph node with sinus.

Clinical diagnosis: Tuberculosis (TB) lymphadenitis with sinus

Investigations

- Hemoglobin (Hb)—7.5
- Total count (TC)—6,800, P52, L 47, M1, E0
- Erythrocyte sedimentation rate (ESR)—70
- Serum glutamate-pyruvate transaminase (SGPT)—28
- Mantoux test (MT)—2 tuberculin unit (TU) 8 mm negative
- Chest X-ray (CXR)—nothing abnormal detected (NAD).

Excisional biopsy was performed. Histology was suggestive of caseating granulomatous lymphadenitis consistent with tuberculosis.

Ziehl–Neelsen (ZN) stain smear for acid fast bacilli—negative

A cartridge-based nucleic acid amplification test (CBNAAT)—*Mycobacterium tuberculosis* bacteria detected. Rifampicin resistance not detected

1. **What is generalized lymphadenopathy?**
   Generalized lymphadenopathy is abnormal enlargement of more than two non-contiguous lymph node regions.

2. **What are the characteristics of TB lymphadenitis?**
   Tuberculous lymphadenitis usually presents as a gradually increasing painless swelling of one or more lymph nodes of weeks to months' duration. Initially the nodes are firm, discrete and mobile. The overlying skin is free. Later, the nodes may become matted and the overlying skin inflamed. In a more advanced stage, the nodes may soften, leading to formation of abscesses and sinus tracts which may be difficult to heal. Unusually, large nodes may compress or invade the adjoining structures complicating the course of the disease.
   Intrathoracic nodes may compress one of the bronchus leading to atelectasis, lung infection, and bronchiectasis or thoracic duct leading to chylous effusion. Retroperitoneal nodes may lead to chylous ascites and chyluria. Sometimes, the cervical nodes may compress the trachea leading to extrathoracic upper airway obstruction. Some patients, especially those with extensive disease or a coexisting disease may have systemic symptoms, i.e., fever, weight loss, fatigue, and night sweats. Distressing cough may be a prominent symptom in mediastinal lymphadenitis.

3. **What are the differentials?**
   Tuberculous lymphadenitis needs to be differentiated from lymphadenopathy due to other causes. These include reactive hyperplasia, lymphoma, sarcoidosis, secondary carcinoma, generalized lymphadenopathy of human immunodeficiency virus (HIV), Kaposi sarcoma, lymphadenitis caused by Mycobacteria other than tuberculosis (MOTT), fungi and toxoplasmosis.
   In general, multiplicity, matting, sinus formation and caseation are features of tuberculous lymphadenitis but these are neither specific nor sensitive. In lymphoma, the nodes are rubbery in consistency and are seldom matted. In lymphadenopathy due to secondary carcinoma, the nodes are usually hard and fixed to the underlying structures or the overlying skin.

4. **How will you investigate/diagnose tuberculous lymphadenitis?**
   History of exposure to a person suffering from pulmonary tuberculosis is highly suggestive of tuberculosis in a given clinical setting.

Tuberculin test—A positive skin test seems to support the diagnosis but a negative test does not rule out TB. Skiagram chest should be obtained in all the patients suspected to be suffering from tuberculous lymphadenitis. It not only exclude any coexisting intrathoracic disease, but the presence of an active or healed pulmonary lesion acts as a supportive evidence for tuberculous lymphadenitis in cases where the diagnosis remains in doubt, i.e., a compatible biopsy but a negative culture.

Ultrasound examination of abdomen and computed tomography (CT) scan of the chest may be required in some patients. Enlarged lymph nodes may show hypodense areas with rim enhancement or calcification. It may also demonstrate the status of the adjoining structures. It may also help obtain the pathological specimens for cyto-histopathology and culture. Final diagnosis of tuberculous lymphadenitis requires demonstration of mycobacteria. Traditionally, excision biopsy is done to diagnose tuberculous lymphadenitis but fine-needle aspiration cytology (FNAC), a relatively less invasive, painless and outdoor procedure seems to have established itself as a safe, cheap and reliable procedure.

5. **What are the histological findings?**
   Typically, tuberculous lymph nodes show epithelioid cell granulomas, multinucleated giant cells and caseation necrosis. Caseating granulomas are seen in nearly all the biopsy specimens and 77% of the FNACs. So when FNAC is inconclusive, excisional biopsy is recommended. Cytology has a sensitivity of 77–98% with a specificity of 97–100%.

6. **Which tests are performed for confirmation of microbial diagnosis?**
   Specimen obtained after FNAC/biopsy are subjected to cytology, smear for acid-fast bacilli (AFB), culture for mycobacteria, culture for non-TB bacteria and CBNAAT.
   AFB smear is 100% specific but sensitivity is very low of 10–15%.
   CBNAAT has sensitivity of 35–56%.
   Culture yield is 20–50%

7. **How will you manage TB lymphadenitis?**
   As per the Indian Academy of Pediatrics-Revised National TB Control Program (IAP-RNTCP) guidelines, 2015, all cases of extrapulmonary TB, including TB lymphadenitis, should be treated with isoniazid (H), rifampicin (R), pyrazinamide (Z) and ethambutol (E) 2HRZE + 4HRE regimen.

8. **What will be the response to anti-tuberculosis therapy (ATT)?**
   With optimum therapy, there will be resolution of systemic symptoms and gradual decrease in size of the lymph nodes.
   In some cases, paradoxical enlargement of existing nodes with marked increase in constitutional features is noted due to immune reconstitution syndrome. Such children need symptomatic treatment, and very rarely, a short course of steroids.

9. **What about non-response to ATT?**
   This may be due to drug-resistant TB, immune-deficiency mainly HIV, or a faulty diagnosis. Ruling out alternative diagnosis is very important.

10. **How will you approach a suspected case of TB lymphadenitis?**
    Please check the algorithm Flowchart 1.

Flowchart 1: Algorithm for lymph node TB.

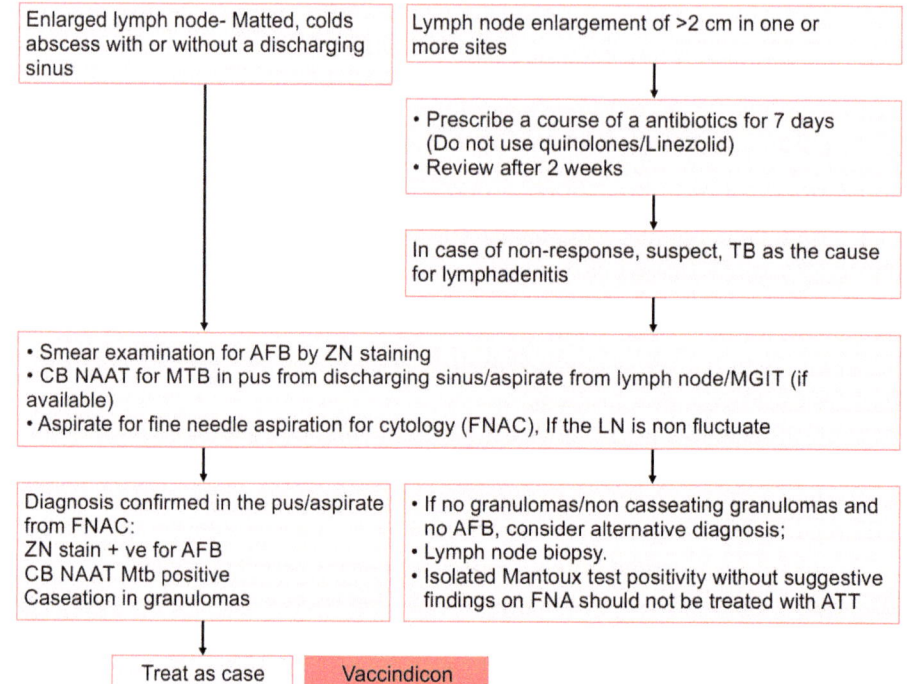

Torsion Testis

Chapter 85

Manish Jain

CASE STUDY

A 4-year-old child presented with history of acute onset of pain in groin of 12 hours duration with vomiting and altered gait. Ultrasonography (USG) showed torsion testis with altered echotexture of testis (Fig. 1).

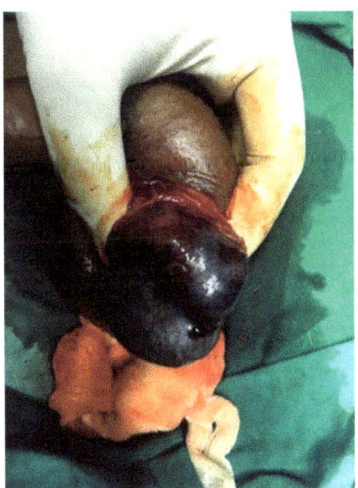

Fig. 1: Case of torsion testis.

1. **What is testicular torsion?**
   Testicular torsion refers to the torsion of the spermatic cord structures and subsequent loss of the blood supply to the ipsilateral testicle.
2. **What is the clinical importance of this condition?**
   This is an absolute emergency; early diagnosis and treatment are vital to save the testicle and preserve future fertility. The rate of testicular viability decreases significantly after 6 hours from onset of symptoms.

3. **What is the likely etiology for this condition?**
   With mature attachments, the tunica vaginalis is attached securely to the posterior lateral aspect of the testicle, and within it, the spermatic cord is not very mobile. If the attachment of the tunica vaginalis to the testicle is inappropriately high, the spermatic cord can rotate within it, which can lead to intravaginal torsion. This defect is referred to as the *bell clapper deformity*. This occurs in about 17% of males and is bilateral in 40%.

4. **What are the types of torsions?**
   Intravaginal torsion most commonly occurs in adolescents. It is thought that the increased weight of the testicle after puberty, as well as sudden contraction of the cremasteric muscles (which inserts in a spiral fashion into the spermatic cord), is the predisposing factor for acute torsion.
   By contrast, neonates more often have *extravaginal torsion*. This occurs because the tunica vaginalis is not yet secured to the gubernaculum, and therefore, the spermatic cord as well as the tunica vaginalis undergo torsion as a unit. Extravaginal torsion is not associated with bell clapper deformity.

5. **What is the role of color Doppler study?**
   This study definitely helps in establishing the vascularity of the affected testis but one cannot rely completely on this study for clinical or operative decisions.

6. **What is the standard line of management?**
   Surgical exploration, as early as possible even at the cost of negative exploration, remains the gold standard in suspected cases of testicular torsion. If color Doppler is equivocal or not providing any concrete information, surgical exploration should be planned without wasting much time.

7. **What do we do in surgical exploration?**
   We detorse the testis in confirmed cases of torsion and gangrene along with fixation of opposite testis. If no gangrene, we preserve the testis and fix it.

Trichobezoar

Chapter 86

Manish Jain

CASE STUDY

A 9-year-old girl presented with chronic pain abdomen and occasional vomiting. She is shy in nature and parents do give history of eating hair strands. Ultrasonography (USG) confirmed the presence of a hair ball in stomach (Fig. 1).

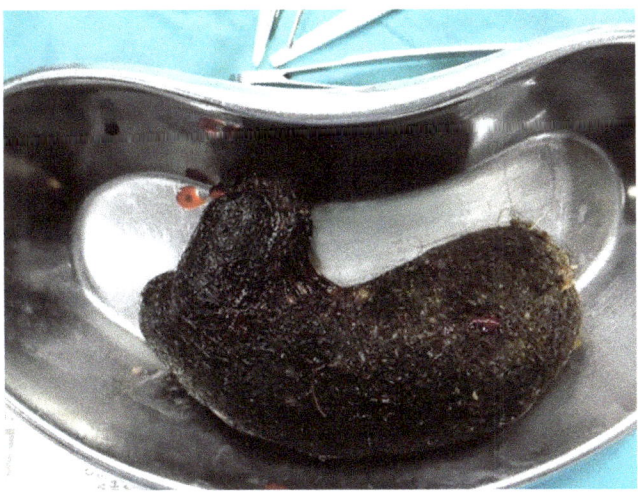

Fig. 1: Hair ball.

1. **What are trichobezoars?**
   Trichobezoars are bezoars [a mass found trapped in gastrointestinal (GI) system], consisting of hairs, usually located in the stomach, but may extend through the pylorus into the duodenum and small bowel (*Rapunzel syndrome*).
2. **What is its pathogenesis?**
   This rare condition is almost exclusively seen in young females. It is almost always associated with *trichotillomania and trichophagia* or other psychiatric disorders. Human

hair is resistant to digestion as well as peristalsis due to its smooth surface. Therefore, it accumulates between the mucosal folds of the stomach. Over a period of time, continuous ingestion of hair leads to the impaction of hair together with mucus and food, causing the formation of a trichobezoar. In most cases, the trichobezoar is confined within the stomach.

3. **Are there any other similar conditions?**
   Examples of other bezoars include phytobezoars (vegetable), lactobezoars (milk/curd) and miscellaneous balls (fungus, sand, paper, etc.).

4. **What can be the complications?**
   When not recognized, the trichobezoar continues to grow in size and weight due to the continued ingestion of hair. This increases the risk of severe complications, such as gastric mucosal erosion, ulceration and even perforation of the stomach or the small intestine. In addition, intussusception, obstructive jaundice, protein-losing enteropathy, pancreatitis and even death have been reported as complications of (unrecognized) trichobezoar in the literature.

5. **What is the treatment?**
   Surgical removal of hairball (laparotomy or laparoscopy) remains the treatment of choice, of course with management of associated psychological/psychiatric condition.

Tuberous Sclerosis

Chapter 87

Kewal Kishore Arora, Swati Mulye

CASE STUDY

A 4-year 6-month-old female child born of nonconsanguineous marriage presented with multiple left focal tonic daily seizures since past few months, refectory to multiple antieplictic drugs—sodium valporate, carbamazapin, clobazam, etc. She had past history of treatment refractory infantile spasms, and global developmental delay. She was exhibiting signs of autism. There was significant family history of elder sister with a single seizure well control on carbamazapin. She was a slow learner. Both girls had nodular pigmented facial legions on the nose and cheeks. Elder sister had small hypopigmented legions on the back to. The characteristic clinical features clinched the diagnosis of tuberous sclerosis (Figs. 1A and B).

The electroencephalogram (EEG) of index case was grossly abnormal and magnetic resonance imaging (MRI) brain conformed tubers. The index case was started on vigavatrin to which there was reasonable response in the form of more than 50% reduction in seizure frequency.

The ultrasonography of abdomen, 2D ECHO and X-ray of chest were done to look for tubers in kidney, heart, and lungs respectively, were normal.

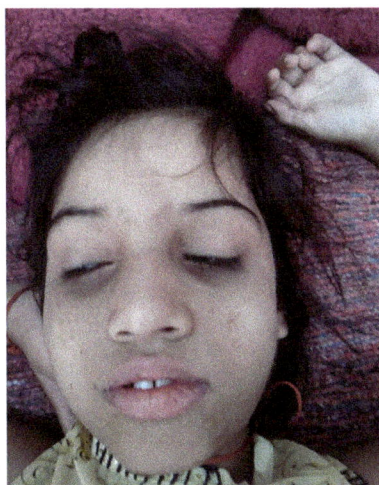

Fig. 1: Adenoma cebaceum in patient.

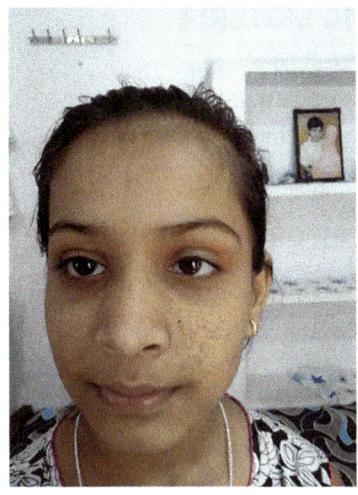

Fig 2: Adenoma sebaceum in sibling suggesting autosomal dominant transmission.

1. **What is tuberous sclerosis?**
   Tuberous sclerosis, also known as *tuberous sclerosis complex (TSC)* or *Bourneville disease*, is a neurocutaneous disorder (*phakomatosis*) characterized by the development of multiple benign tumors of the embryonic ectoderm (e.g. skin, eyes, and nervous system).

2. **What is the incidence of TSC?**
   It is estimated that 1/6,000 to 1/10,000 live births and 1/20,000 individuals in the population have a diagnosis of TSC.

3. **What are the main features of this disorder?**
   Tuberous sclerosis was classically described as presenting in childhood with a triad (Vogt triad) of:
   - Seizures: (absent in one-quarter of individuals)
   - Mental retardation: (up to half have normal intelligence)
   - Adenoma sebaceum: (only present in about three-quarters of patients).

4. **What is the underlying cause of TSC?**
   Spontaneous mutations account for 50–86% of cases, with the remainder inherited as an autosomal dominant condition. In the majority of such cases (80%) the mutation has been narrowed down to two tumor suppressor genes:
   - *TSC1*: Encoding hamartin, on chromosome 9q32-34
   - *TSC2*: Encoding tuberin, on chromosome 16p13.3 (accounts for most cases).

   Both of these genes have the function of suppressing tumor growth in the body. They also regulate cell growth through the inhibition of a specific protein called mammalian target of rapamycin (mTOR). If there is a mutation in either *TSC1* or *TSC2* gene, cell growth is not adequately regulated (suppressed) which results in the clinical manifestations of TSC.

5. **Are there any criteria for diagnosing TSC?**
   The full Vogt classical triad is only seen in a minority of patients (~30%).
   The tuberous sclerosis diagnostic criteria have been developed to aid the diagnosis of *tuberous sclerosis* and have most recently been updated in 2012 by the International Tuberous Sclerosis Complex Consensus Group.

GENETIC CRITERIA

The identification of either a *TSC1* or *TSC2* pathogenic mutation is sufficient to make a definite diagnosis of TSC. Of note, 10–25% of TSC patients have no mutation identified by conventional genetic testing, which does not exclude TSC or prevent the use of clinical diagnostic criteria to diagnose TSC.

CLINICAL CRITERIA

- Definitive TS complex: Either 2 major features or 1 major and 2 or more minor
- Possible TS complex: Either 1 major or more than or equal to 2 minor.

Major Features

- Angiofibromas (3 or more) or fibrous cephalic plaque
- Nontraumatic ungual or periungual fibroma (2 or more)
- Hypomelanotic macules (3 or more, at least 5 mm diameter)

- Shagreen patch
- Multiple retinal nodular hamartomas
- Cortical dysplasias (include tubers and cerebral white matter migration lines)
- Subependymal nodule
- Subependymal giant cell astrocytoma
- Cardiac rhabdomyoma
- Lymphangioleiomyomatosis (LAM)*
- Angiomyolipomas (AML) (2 or more)*.

Minor Features

- Dental enamel pits: 3 or more for the entire dentition
- Intraoral fibromas (2 or more)
- Nonrenal hamartomas
- Retinal achromic patch
- "Confetti" skin lesions
- Multiple renal cysts.

6. **At what age and with what symptoms and signs does TSC manifest?**

    Tuberous sclerosis complex can present at any age. In infants and children, it usually is identified as a cause of epilepsy, autism, or cardiac failure.

    Various organ systems are affected maximally at different points in life.
    - Cardiac involvement occurs during the intrauterine or neonatal period.
    - Rhabdomyomas tend to regress over time.
    - Epilepsy, autism, and developmental delays manifest themselves from infancy to adolescence.
    - Polycystic kidney disease usually is apparent in infancy or early childhood.
    - Angiomyolipoma may develop at any time from childhood into adult life.
    - Lymphangiomyomatosis typically presents in the third or fourth decade of life
    - Older persons may present with renal failure or pulmonary or cutaneous manifestations in the absence of prominent, or any, neurological symptoms.

7. **What investigations are done in a case of TSC?**

    This condition needs comprehensive and repeated tests for diagnosis as well as monitoring of new symptoms (Table 1).

TABLE 1: Recommendation for tuberous sclerosis complex.

Organ system/ Specialty area	Recommendation
Genetics	<ul><li>Obtain three-generation family history to assess for additional family members at risk of TSC</li><li>Offer genetic testing for family counseling or when TSC diagnosis is in question but cannot be clinically confirmed</li></ul>

Contd...

---

*A combination of the two following major features (LAM and angiomyolipomas) without other feature does not meet criteria for a definite diagnosis of TSC.

Contd...

Brain	• Perform magnetic resonance imaging (MRI) of the brain to assess for the presence of tubers, subependymal nodules (SEN), migrational defects, and subependymal giant cell astrocytoma (SEGA) • Evaluate for tuberous sclerosis complex (TSC)-associated neuropsychiatric disorder (TAND) • During infancy, educate parents to recognize infantile spasms, even if none have occurred at time of first diagnosis • Obtain baseline routine electroencephalogram (EEG). If abnormal, especially if features of TAND are also present, follow-up with a 24-hour video EEG to assess for subclinical seizure activity
Kidney	• Obtain MRI of the abdomen to assess for the presence of angiomyolipoma and renal cysts • Screen for hypertension by obtaining an accurate blood pressure • Evaluate renal function by determination of glomerular filtration rate (GFR)
Lung	• Perform baseline pulmonary function testing (pulmonary function testing and 6-minute walk test) and high-resolution computed tomography (HRCT) of chest, even if asymptomatic, in patients at risk of developing lymphangioleiomyomatosis (LAM), typically females 18 years or older. Adult males, if symptomatic, should also undergo testing • Provide counsel on smoking risks and estrogen use in adolescent and adult females
Skin	• Perform a detailed clinical dermatologic inspection/examination
Teeth	• Perform a detailed clinical dental inspection/examination
Heart	• Consider fetal echocardiography to detect individuals with high risk of heart failure after delivery when rhabdomyomas are identified via prenatal ultrasound • Obtain an echocardiogram in pediatric patients, especially if younger than 3 years of age • Obtain an electrocardiogram (ECG) in all ages to assess for underlying conduction defects
Eye	• Perform a complete ophthalmologic evaluation, including dilated fundoscopy, to assess for retinal lesions and visual field deficits

8. **What are the therapeutic interventions in the management of TSC?**
   There are a variety of therapeutic interventions available for TSC. They include various medications, surgical techniques, and interventional radiology procedures. Each therapeutic treatment options is based on:
   • The specific TSC organ manifestations
   • Age of the individual
   • Severity of symptoms
   • The risk and benefit of the treatment option.

   The main complication of TSC requiring long-term medical therapy is epilepsy. Antiepileptic medications are the mainstay of therapy for patients with TSC. Vigabatrin is the drug of first choice for children with TSC and infantile spasms. Topiramate, lamotrigine, valproate, and adrenocorticotropic hormone or steroids are also useful.

SURGICAL CARE

Surgical care for seizures in a patient with TSC can involve focal cortical resection or thermal ablation, corpus callosotomy, or vagus nerve stimulation.

TREATMENT OF SUBEPENDYMAL GIANT CELL ASTROCYTOMA

Patients with unilateral, single, gross total resectable subependymal giant cell astrocytoma (SEGA) without individual risk factors or other comorbidities preferentially may benefit from surgery, whereas patients with multisystem disease or multiple or infiltrating SEGA lesions that are not amenable to gross total resection may favor mTOR inhibitor treatment.

9. **What targeted therapies are available in TSC?**

    Although symptomatic treatment has been the mainstay of management of TSC patients, we are emabracing the era of targeted therapy. Evidence is accumulating to show that some mTOR inhibitors have become valuable additions to the armamaterium in the treatment of TSC. The mTOR inhibitors have been shown to be effective for facial angiofibromas, SEGAs, cardiac rhabdomyomas, and possibly epilepsy. Targeted therapy with mTOR inhibitors, such as rapamycin or everolimus, plays an important role in the management of TSC.

Tuberous Sclerosis Complex

Chapter 88

Ritesh Shah

CASE STUDY

A 9-month-old boy presented with sudden jerks. The jerks started 1 month before; they are more frequent in the mornings and they happen in clusters. In the last 1 month, the child was more irritable and regressed few achieved milestones. His general exam is showing skin changes as shown in Figure 1. His head size is 43 cm and neurological exam is normal.

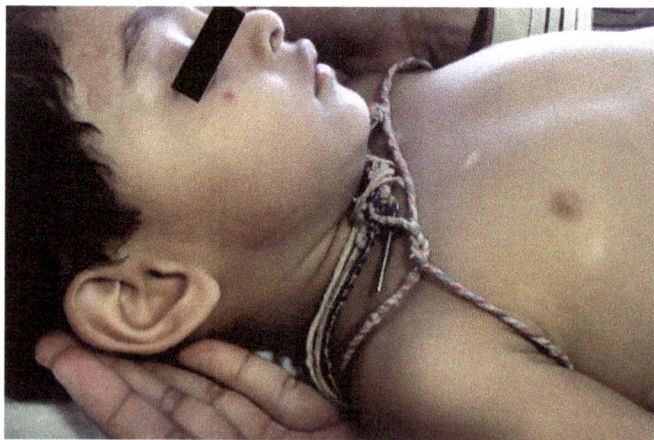

Fig. 1: Ash leaf macule and Shagreen patch.

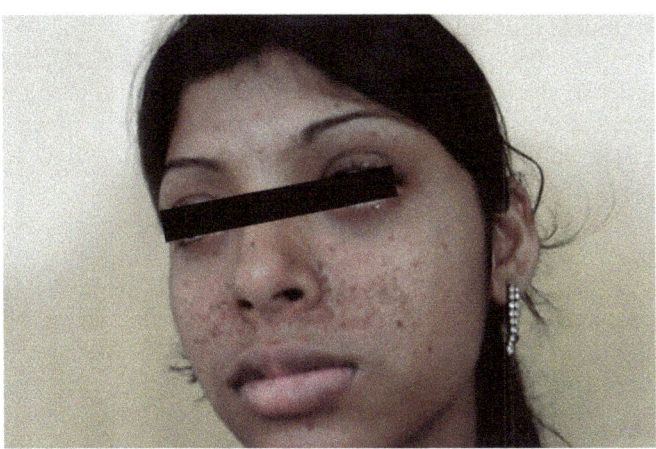

Fig. 2: Angiofibroma (adenoma sebaceum).

1. **What are the different types of seizures that present with jerks in infancy?**
   Myoclonic jerks, infantile spasm, and tonic seizures present as sudden jerks. They all have different causes and have different outcomes attached to it, so it is important to differentiate them clinically before proceeding for further work-up. Myoclonus is usually very brief (fraction of a second) shock-like movement, infantile spasm is little longer in duration which is of around 1 second and movement of head and shoulders (either flexor or extensor) and mostly in clusters and more on awakening, while tonic seizure is jerks lasting for few seconds with tonic phase.

2. **What are the different causes of infantile spasm?**
   The list could be endless but few common causes are perinatal injuries (hypoxia, hypoglycemia, infections, etc.), neurocutaneous syndromes [tuberous sclerosis complex (TSC), Sturge-Weber syndrome and many more], malformation of cortical development, neurometabolic disorders, genetic disorders and many more.

3. **How does Electroencephalography (EEG) correlate with infantile spasm?**
   Hypsarrhythmia is seen in many patients of infantile spasm. It consists of high-voltage slow waves, multifocal spikes and sharp waves, and suppression after burst of spikes. Modifications and variations of this pattern may occur.

4. **What is West syndrome?**
   It is a devastating age-specific epilepsy syndrome characterized by infantile spasm, neurodevelopmental impairments, and hypsarrhythmia on EEG. All of the above-mentioned causes can cause West syndrome.

5. **How to approach a child with West syndrome?**
   Initially for any child with infantile spasm, first on the basis of history and exam, make a possible clinical differential diagnosis, and then EEG should be the first investigation to confirm seizure type and then neuroimaging [preferably magnetic resonance imaging (MRI)] is to delineate probable cause of infantile spasm. If MRI is normal, then depending on case-to-case basis, further metabolic and genetic tests are required.

6. **What are the clinical manifestations of TSC?**
   Tuberous sclerosis complex most commonly presents with central nervous system (CNS) manifestations like seizures and developmental issues, and along with various skin manifestations. It can also present with other organ systems involvement like the heart, kidney, eyes, lungs, and bone.

7. **Can you describe CNS manifestations in detail?**
   Seizures present anytime during childhood commonly during infancy, and one-third of the patients present with infantile spasm along with other seizure types like focal seizures, tonic seizure, generalized tonic–clonic seizure (GTCS), and atypical absences. Intractable seizures are common with TSC. They can have cognitive impairment ranging from mild learning disabilities to severe intellectual disabilities.
   Behavioral abnormalities like ASD in 50% of the cases with attention-deficit/hyperactivity disorder (ADHD) in some. Adolescents and adults present with anxiety, depression and mood disorders. Subependymal giant cell astrocytoma (SEGA) can present with raised intracranial pressure (ICT) due to obstructive hydrocephalus.

8. **Describe the different skin findings.**
   Hypomelanotic patch (Fig. 1) (ash-leaf)—often at birth and more prominent during first several years of life. Oval- or leaf-shaped macules ranging from few millimeters to several centimeters in length and scattered over the trunk and limb. *Angiofibroma (adenoma sebaceum)(Fig. 2)*—appears between the age of 1 and 4 years, progress through childhood and adolescence, and typically pink or red papules appear in patches, or butterfly distribution on or around the nose, cheek and chin.
   Shagreen Patch (Fig. 1)—connective tissue hamartomas, roughened, raised lesion with orange peel consistency ranging from few millimeters to 1 cm and distributed asymmetrically on dorsal body surface, particularly on lumbosacral skin. It is usually present since birth and more easily identified as the child grows. *Subungual and periungual fibroma*—usually appears during adolescence and later and typically involves the toes more often than fingers.

9. **At initial diagnosis which other system screenings are recommended?**
   Screening of the kidney by ultrasonography (USG), and heart by echocardiography at the time of diagnosis. Later on in the course of disease, screening of the lungs and retina is indicated. In kidney, there are two types of lesions—angiomyolipoma in up to 80% and renal cyst in 20% of cases. Cardiac rhabdomyomas are detected in 50–60% of the cases with most detected prenatally, maximal at birth and early childhood. It undergoes spontaneous resolution during the first year of life. If symptomatic, it results in outflow tract obstruction or valvular dysfunction or arrhythmia by lesion affecting conductive system.

10. **What is the etiology of TSC?**
    Tuberous sclerosis complex is inherited in autosomal dominant (AD) manner with variable expression, and spontaneous genetic mutation occurs in 65% of the cases. The two genetic foci identified for TSC are *TSC1* and *TSC2*.
    TSC1 gene on Ch 9, encodes protein called hamartin and *TSC2* gene on Ch 16, encodes for protein tuberin. Both proteins bind to each other and work together, so mutation in either of the genes results in similar disease. *TSC1* and *TSC2* are tumor suppression genes, so loss of either tuberin or hamartin results in the formation of numerous benign tumors.

11. **How will you manage seizures of TSC?**
    Vigabatrin is the drug of choice if a patient presents with infantile spasm. Adrenocorticotrophic hormone is used if vigabatrin fails. For other seizure types, other anticonvulsants can be used as per any other patient with that particular seizure type. Medically refractory seizures can be treated with epilepsy surgery or ketogenic diet.

12. **What is the emerging treatment for TSC?**
    If you look at functions, hamartin and tuberin are components of mammalian target of rapamycin (mTOR) pathway. Protein mTOR is the master regulator of cell growth controlled by Rheb. In TSC, rheb is activated by protein complex formed by tuberin and hamartin. Once rheb is activated, protein synthesis machinery is turned on via mTOR and cell grows in size. So Everolimus—mTOR inhibitor is the new emerging treatment and it helps to slow down growth or reduces size of SEGA, and can be useful in refractory seizures and reduce volume of renal angiomyolipomas and lymphangiomyomatosis as well as facial angiofibroma.

13. **What are the standard follow-up recommendations for patients with TSC?**

Evaluation	Initial testing	Follow-up testing
Neuroimaging	At diagnosis	Every 1–3 years until age 20
Neuropsychological	At diagnosis	At school entry and as indicated
EEG	If seizure occurs	As indicated
Ophthalmic evaluation	At diagnosis	As indicated
ECG, ECHO	At diagnosis	As indicated
Renal USG	At diagnosis	Every 1–3 years, more frequently as indicated
Chest CT	At onset of adulthood	As indicated

14. **What is the risk in next pregnancy?**
    As it is autosomal dominant disorder, risk is 50% if one of the parents is affected which you can decide by either examining parents for skin changes or by gene sequencing for known mutation in index patients. In patients with de novo mutations, the risk is as per normal populations.

Hair Tuft at the Lumbosacral Spine

Chapter 89

Alok Gupta, Mohit Vhora

HYPERTRICHOSIS

Localized hypertrichosis is defined as the presence of a tuft of terminal hair in a patchy distribution. The most common location is in the midline over the lumbosacral region suggesting an underlying developmental defect.

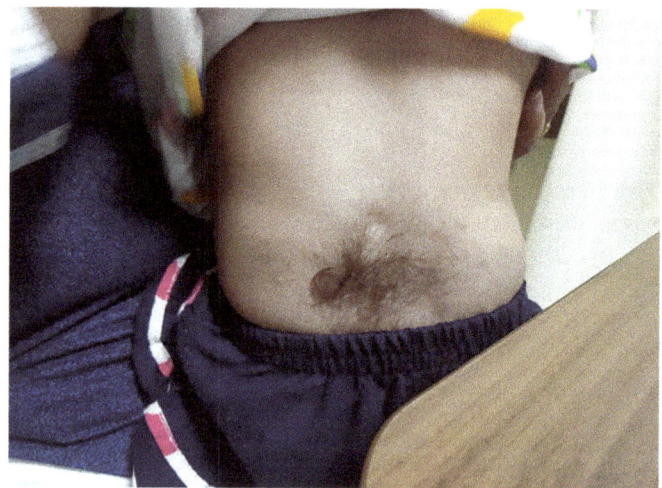

Fig. 1: Tuft of hair.

1. **What is the most common cause of tuft of hair present at LS spine since birth?**
   The most common association of this lesion is the spinal cord developmental defect where the spinal column does not close all the way down.
2. **Which is the most common type of spinal defect associated with this condition?**
   The spina bifida occulta is the most common type associated with this condition.
3. **What is the cause of a hair growth in the area of spina bifida occulta?**
   The ectodermal hair placode is initiated due to interactive hair signaling from mesoderm and activation of Wnt pathway.

4. **What are the different forms of spina bifida?**
   Spina bifida can occur in different forms, namely:
   - Spina bifida occulta
   - Meningocele
   - Meningomyelocele.

   Spina bifida occulta is the mildest form.

5. **What are the symptoms?**
   The symptoms can range from asymptomatic but with only hairy patch over skin at the back or a dimple at LS spine to serious symptoms including learning difficulties, incontinence and paralysis.

6. **What are the risk factors?**
   The risk factors for developing neural tube defects include:
   - Folate deficiency
   - Family history of neural tube defects
   - Medications like valproic acid during pregnancy
   - Uncontrolled diabetes
   - Hyperthermia in the early weeks of pregnancy.

7. **What are the investigations?**
   Magnetic resonance imaging (MRI) of LS spine is diagnostic. X-ray spine and ultrasonography (USG) of LS spine may give some clues.

8. **What are the treatment options available?**
   Reconstructive surgery is the only option.
   - For severe cases detected early on antenatal USG, fetal surgery, preferred lower segment cesarean section (LSCS) mode of delivery, and immediate postoperative surgery are the options

Turbinate Hypertrophy

Chapter 90

Jagdish Chinnappa

> **CASE STUDY**
>
> A 12-year-old boy has been brought with a history of poor sleep, snoring and mouth breathing since the last 3 years.

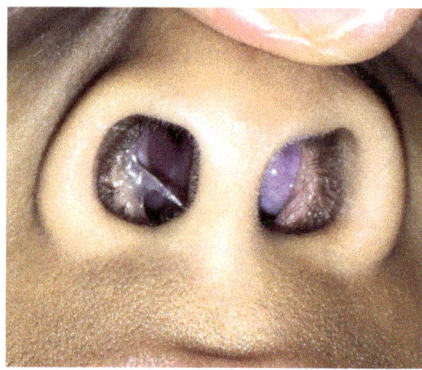

Fig. 1: Turbinate hypertrophy.

1. **What abnormalities are seen on nasal inspection?**
   The right side shows obstruction due to turbinate hypertrophy and discharge consistent with rhinitis (allergic or non-allergic) (Fig. 1).
   Left side shows a characteristic purple turbinate syndrome. The turbinate is pale and bluish, because of diminished airflow and vasoconstriction.
   This is a useful sign in the assessment of obstructive sleep apnea.

2. **How will you assess?**
   Assessment in this child will be comprehensive. Measurement of body mass index (BMI), assessment of craniofacial anomalies, allergy testing, imaging, nasal endoscopy and polysomnography are used in various combinations.

3. **What are the modalities of treatment?**
   Treatment could be medical or surgical depending on the abnormalities identified.
   Reduction of obesity, allergen avoidance, smoke-free homes, intranasal steroids, montelukast adenoidectomy and allergen desensitization. Some refractory cases may need noninvasive ventilation.

Chapter 91

Turner Syndrome

Alok Gupta, Mohit Vhora

CASE STUDY

A syndrome of defective gonadal development in phenotypic females associated with the karyotype 45, X (or 45, XO). Patients generally are of short stature with undifferentiated gonads (streak gonads), sexual infantilism, hypogonadism, webbing of the neck, cubitus valgus, elevated gonadotropins, decreased estradiol level in blood and congenital heart defects. Turner syndrome is a disorder caused by a partially or completely missing X chromosome. This condition affects only females.

1. **What is Turner syndrome?**
   Turner syndrome, named after Dr Henry H Turner, who first described it, is a genetic condition in which all or some portions of the X chromosome are missing. The lack of vital genes found on the X chromosome affects multiple organs in the body leading to medical problems seen in girls with Turner syndrome.
   One of the defining characteristics of Turner syndrome is that it affects the ovaries—the primary female gonads or sex glands. Abnormal development or premature insufficiency of the ovaries affects the glands' ability to produce monthly ovulation and estrogen. This can result in a variety of problems, including infertility, irregular or non-existent menstrual periods, early menopause and osteoporosis.
   The loss of X chromosome genes happens very early in fetal life. In fact, the pregnancy of many babies with Turner syndrome ends in miscarriage. The condition is one of the most common genetic conditions with an estimated 1 out every 2,500 girls born with Turner syndrome. This disorder affects all races and regions of the world equally. There are no known environmental risks for Turner syndrome. Parents who have had many unaffected children can still have a child with Turner syndrome later on.

2. **What are the signs and symptoms of Turner syndrome?**
   With Turner syndrome, certain alerting physical signs include:
   - *Short stature (Fig. 1):* The most common sign of Turner syndrome—the average height is 4 feet 8 inches

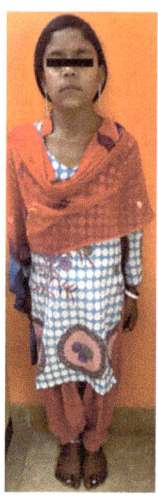

Fig. 1: Short stature (Dwarfism).

- *Undeveloped sex features:* Lack of breast development, delayed menstruation and undeveloped feminine body shape
- *Mouth and jaw abnormalities:* High-arched roof of mouth, crowded teeth and receding lower jaw
- Broad chest
- Droopy eyes
- Low-set ears
- *Webbed neck (Fig. 2):* Extra skin around the neck
- *Low hairline:* Hair extends down back of the neck toward the shoulders
- Fingernails and toenails that point slightly upward
- *Swollen hands and feet:* Usually present at birth.

The severity of health problems in Turner syndrome is variable and depends at least in part on the loss of gene activity from the missing X chromosome.

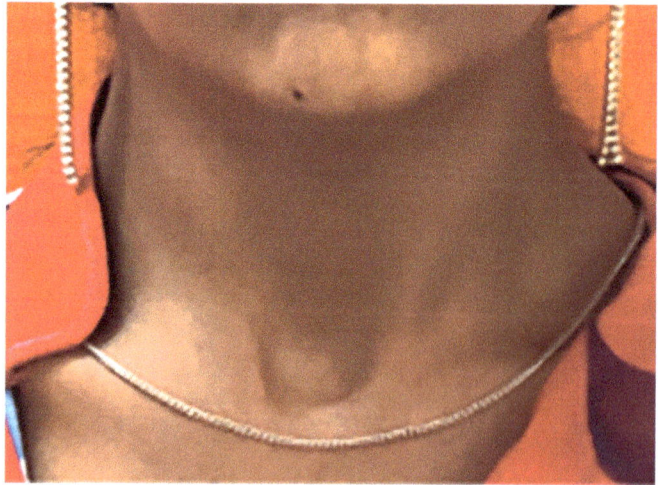

Fig. 2: Webbing of neck.

3. **What causes Turner syndrome?**

   Turner syndrome is caused by a defect of the second female sex chromosome. Turner syndrome occurs when part or all of an X chromosome is missing from most or all of the cells in a girl's body.

   A girl normally receives one X chromosome from each parent. The error that leads to the missing chromosome appears to happen during the formation of the egg or sperm.

   How is Turner syndrome diagnosed?

   The process of diagnosing Turner syndrome begins with a careful medical history. Unexplained short stature or delayed puberty may be the first clues in the diagnosis of Turner syndrome. Blood testing to check chromosomes is necessary to make a definite diagnosis. The test used to diagnose Turner syndrome is known as a karyotype. A karyotype is a blood test that produces an image of the chromosomes.

   Turner syndrome can also be diagnosed during pregnancy by testing the cells in the amniotic fluid. Newborns may be diagnosed after heart problems are detected or after certain physical features, such as swollen hands and feet or webbed skin on the neck, are noticed. Other characteristics, like wide spaced nipples or low-set ears, may also lead to a suspicion of Turner syndrome. Some girls may be diagnosed as teenagers because of a slow growth rate or a lack of puberty-related changes. Still others may be diagnosed as adults when they have difficulty becoming pregnant.

3. **What are the complications of Turner syndrome?**

   Following are the medical conditions that are commonly associated with Turner syndrome:
   - Infertility
   - Heart problems
   - Kidney problems
   - Hypothyroidism
   - Ear and hearing problems
   - Celiac disease.

4. **Is Turner syndrome inherited?**

   Turner syndrome is usually not inherited, but it is genetic. It is caused by a random error that leads to a missing X chromosome in the sperm or egg of a parent. Very few pregnancies in which the fetus has Turner syndrome result in live births. Mostly ends in early pregnancy loss.

   Most women with Turner syndrome cannot get pregnant naturally. In one study, as many as 40% of women with Turner syndrome got pregnant using donated eggs. However, pregnant women with Turner syndrome are at increased risk for high blood pressure during pregnancy, which can result in complications, including preterm birth and fetal growth restriction.

5. **Can Turner syndrome be prevented?**

   Turner syndrome cannot be prevented. It is a genetic problem that is caused by a random error that leads to a missing X chromosome in the sperm or egg of a parent. There is nothing the father or mother can do to prevent the error from occurring. However, there are many options for treatment.

6. **Is Turner syndrome considered a disability?**

   Turner syndrome is not considered a disability, although it can cause certain learning challenges, including problems learning mathematics and with memory. Most girls and women with Turner syndrome lead a normal, healthy and productive life with proper medical care.

7. **Will the girl mature normally?**
   Most girls with Turner syndrome do not mature typically. They may not develop breasts or start getting a period. Estrogen treatment can replace hormones that the body does not naturally produce, spurring development and preventing osteoporosis.

8. **Will she have problems in school?**
   Some girls with Turner syndrome have difficulty with arithmetic, visual memory and visuospatial skills (such as determining the relative positions of objects in space). They may also have some trouble understanding non-verbal communication (body language and facial expression) and interacting with peers.

9. **What care will she need as she grows up?**
   Girls and women with Turner syndrome usually require care from a variety of specialists throughout their lives.

10. **Will she be able to have a normal sex life as an adult?**
    Women with Turner syndrome can enjoy normal sex lives.

11. **Will she be able to have children?**
    Most women with Turner syndrome cannot get pregnant naturally. Those who can are at risk for blood-pressure-related complications, which can lead to premature birth or fetal growth restriction. Pregnancy also is associated with increased risk for maternal complications, including aortic dissection and rupture. This happens about 2% of the time.

12. **How is Turner syndrome treated?**
    Turner syndrome is first treated with human growth hormone. When a girl reaches puberty, she will then begin estrogen replacement therapy (ERT).
    The primary purpose of growth hormone is to regain height in girls with Turner syndrome. Without growth hormone treatment, the average height of an adult woman with Turner syndrome is 4 feet 8 inches. If treatment starts early and is maintained, it is possible for girls with Turner syndrome to reach a normal height.
    Like growth hormone, ERT is a standard treatment for Turner syndrome. The purpose of estrogen therapy is twofold—to prompt the body into beginning puberty and to maintain healthy sexual development and functioning throughout adulthood.
    Early ovarian insufficiency is common in people with Turner syndrome. If the ovaries are unable to produce sex hormones, such as estrogen, then healthy sexual development would not occur. Fortunately, ERT effectively replaces these hormones if the body cannot make them itself. ERT can help start the secondary sexual development that normally begins at puberty (around age 12). This includes breast development and the development of wider hips. Healthcare providers may prescribe a combination of estrogen and progesterone to girls who have not started menstruating by age of 15. ERT also provides protection against bone loss.
    Regular health checks and access to a wide variety of specialists are important to care for the various health problems that can result from Turner syndrome. These include ear infections, high blood pressure and thyroid problems.

Umbilical Hernia

Chapter 92

Aniruddh Shah, Amar Shah

CASE STUDY

A 1-year-old girl has a swelling over the umbilicus since birth. The swelling was initially small and gradually, persistently and painlessly increased in size. The swelling increases in size on crying and straining, and reduces when the child is sleeping or playing.
On examination, the child has a midline swelling over the umbilicus which is soft and painless. The contents reduce with a gurgle and the defect admits the tip of the index finger.

1. **What are umbilical hernias?**

    Umbilical hernia is seen in 5% of children. The umbilical cord is attached to the area of the umbilicus in the intrauterine life. This area has a defect in the abdominal wall which closes after birth and forms the umbilicus (belly button). When this defect does not close spontaneously, the intestines may bulge through it when the child cries or strains, and is called an umbilical hernia (Fig. 1). Umbilical hernias are more common among African-American children than Caucasian children. In addition, low birth weight and premature infants are more likely to have umbilical hernias.

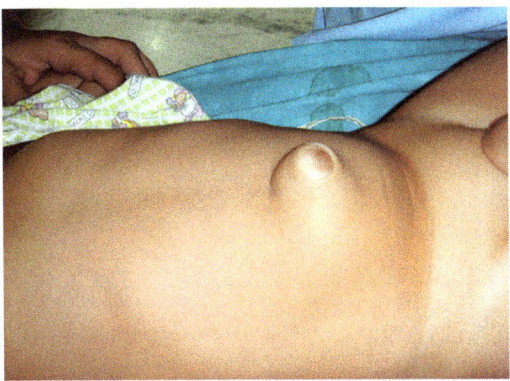

Fig. 1: Swelling over umbilicus.

2. **When is surgery required for umbilical hernias?**
   Umbilical hernias normally resolve spontaneously by the age of 2 years. If the size does not reduce after 2 years, then surgery is advisable. In hernias where the size of the defects are reducing and do not admit the tip of the index finger by 2 years of age, there is a chance that the umbilical hernia may reduce spontaneously. In these cases, waiting for a further period of 2 years may be advised.
3. **When is early surgery required for umbilical hernias?**
   In children with large umbilical hernias or children with hypothyroidism or connective tissue disorders, early surgery is indicated. The family should be explained about the possibility of a recurrence in such cases.
4. **Does umbilical hernia get obstructed?**
   The chance of umbilical hernias getting obstructed are very less.
5. **When is early surgery required?**
   Many a times, the hernia may not be located at the umbilicus, but around it. These are called paraumbilical hernias. Paraumbilical hernias do not resolve spontaneously. They also have a chance of the intestine getting obstructed in the defect. Hence, early surgery is advisable in cases of paraumbilical hernias unlike umbilical hernia.
6. **Does umbilical hernia repair require a mesh?**
   No, mesh repairs are not required in umbilical hernias. The repair is an anatomical repair of the defect.
7. **How to differentiate between umbilical and paraumbilical hernias?**
   In umbilical hernias, the umbilical cicatrix (scar) would be facing perpendicular to the child's abdominal wall. In paraumbilical hernias, the umbilical cicatrix would be facing either caudally (supraumbilical hernia) or cranially (infraumbilical hernia). Also the defect on palpation would be around the umbilicus. Ultrasound scan may also be helpful to assist and confirm the clinical suspicion.
8. **Can any non-surgical options be tried?**
   Application of coins (Fig. 2) or belts does not help in cure of umbilical hernias.

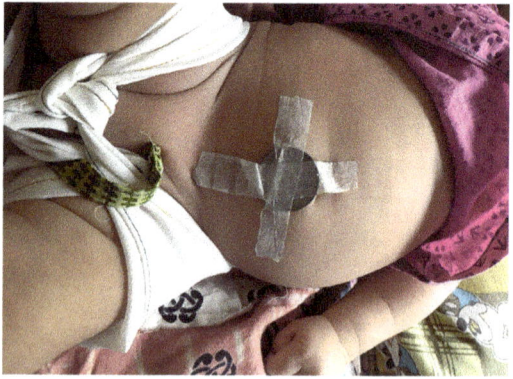

Fig. 2: Coin pressed over umbilicus.

Urticaria Multiforme

Chapter 93

Ashok Kapse, Himanshu P Tadvi

CASE STUDY

A 7-year-old male child presented with annular polycyclic erythematous lesions over the last 3 days. Lesions were evanescent and intensely pruritic. Child had distinct periorbital edema (Figs. 1A to C).

Child was afebrile but had history of fever 10 days before and was treated with amoxicillin. Child was treated with hydroxizine and ranitidine wherein he improved over the next 2 days.

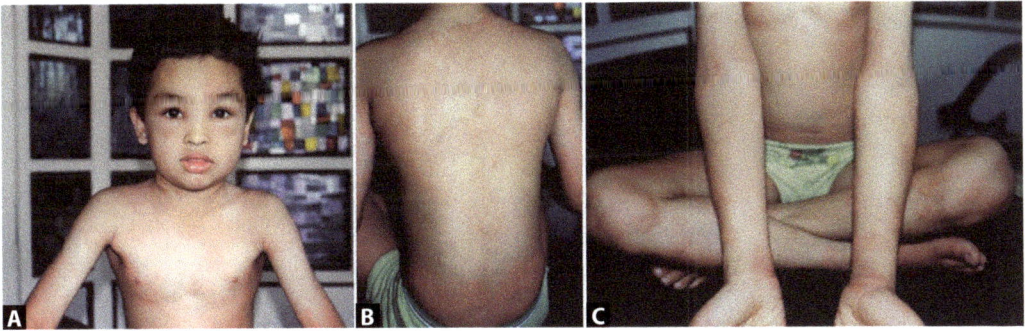

Figs. 1A to C: A 7-year-old male child presented with annular polycyclic erythematous lesions.

1. **What is urticaria multiforme?**
   It is an acute urticaria with characteristic annular, arcuate and polycyclic intensely pruritic lesions, and is the manifestation of benign cutaneous hypersensitivity reaction.
   Lesions of urticaria multiforme are characteristically evanescent; initially lesions appear as small urticarial macules, papules or plaques, but they soon expand to form annular, arcuate and polycyclic wheals that subsequently fade within hours.
   Reaction is predominantly mediated by histamine and characterized by transient cutaneous erythema and dermal edema. It may be immunoglobulin E dependent or independent.

2. **What are the other important cutaneous findings?**
   Angioedema of the face, hands and feet is often associated in affected patients. Dermatographism (the production of transient erythema and edema "wheal and flare") at sites of skin trauma is commonly inducible. Dermatographism may be apparent in linear or geometric patterns.

3. **What are the systemic findings?**
   A short duration fever (1–3 days) with or without other symptoms is commonly observed along with concomitant diarrhea or cough may occur. Six months to five years is the common age of presentation; patients are non-toxic and playful in appearance.
   History of an antecedent viral or bacterial infection or recent use of a systemic medication, often an antibiotic (amoxicillin, cephalosporin or macrolide) is commonly obtained.
4. **How long the disease lasts?**
   The eruption is self-limited, and episodes usually resolve within 8–10 days.
5. **What are the common differentials?**
   The commonest differentials are erythema multiforme and serum sickness like reaction.
6. **How to differentiate urticaria multiforme from erythema multiforme?**
   In some of the cases, lesions may display a dusky, ecchymotic, hemorrhagic hue, which has been reported to occur more commonly in infants with acute urticaria.
   This dusky hemorrhagic hue creates confusion between urticaria multiforme and erythema multiforme. Lesions of urticaria multiforme have a fleeting nature, they usually last for few minutes to few hours as opposed lesions of erythema multiforme lasts for days together, and moreover, lesions of urticaria multiforme swiftly clear with anti-histaminics.
7. **What is the Treatment of Urticaria Multiforme?**
   Administration of systemic antihistamines benefits patients with urticaria multiforme. Combination H1 antihistamine (e.g., diphenhydramine) and an H2 antihistamine (e.g., ranitidine) is desirable. Severe cases may need systemic corticosteroids.

Vesicoureteric Reflux

Chapter 94

Fagun Shah

CASE STUDY 1

A 2-year-old male child presented with recurrent history of fever without focus and failure to thrive. The current evaluation showed plenty of white blood cells (WBCs) in urine confirmed to be urinary tract infection (UTI) on culture examination. Ultrasonography (USG) showed mild dilatation of right renal pelvis. After control of infection, micturating cystourethrogram (MCUG) was done which revealed Grade 3 reflux on right side.

UTI is the third most common cause of infection in children below 5 years of age. Rapid evaluation and treatment of UTI in this age group is very important to prevent renal parenchymal damage and renal scars that eventually may lead to chronic kidney disease and hypertension.

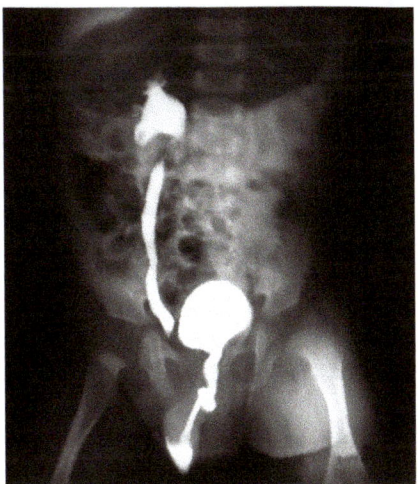

Fig. 1: Right side VUR Grade three.

1. **What are the symptoms of UTI in younger children?**
   The classical symptoms of UTI like dysuria, loin pain, etc. may be absent in younger children below 2 years. They usually present with non-specific symptoms like failure to

thrive, recurrent episodes of fever without focus, loose stools, sepsis, etc. High index of suspicion is required to diagnose UTI in these patients. All children with fever without focus not responding after 2 days should undergo at least a urine microscopy examination.

2. **How to Confirm UTI?**
The gold standard for diagnosis of UTI is urine culture and sensitivity. The urine for culture has to be collected before commencing antibiotics.

3. **What is Vesicoureteric Reflux?**
Vesicoureteric reflux (VUR), as the name suggests, is reflux of urine from bladder to the ureters and renal pelvis. It could be primary or secondary to increased bladder pressures. It is found in 40–50% of infants and 30–50% of children. VUR is diagnosed by MCUG and grades determined using International Reflux Grading system.

CASE STUDY 2

Eighteen months female child had recurrent episodes of UTI. USG showed bilateral hydronephrosis and hydroureter. MCUD showed bilateral reflux—Grade 4 on right side (reflux extending up to renal pelvis with dilatation of ureters, and renal pelvis and tortuosity of ureter) and Grade 5 reflux on left side (significant dilatation of renal pelvis and ureters, diameter of ureter almost as an intestine).

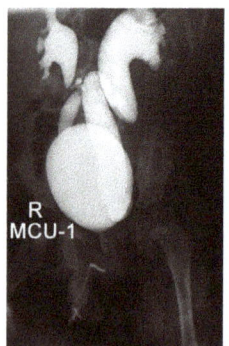
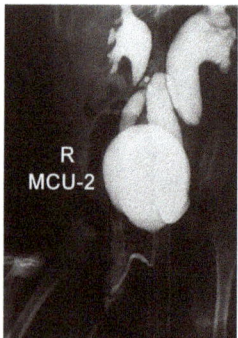
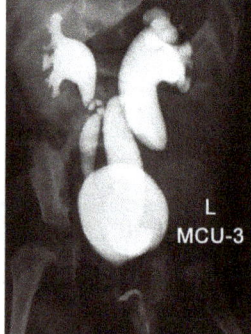
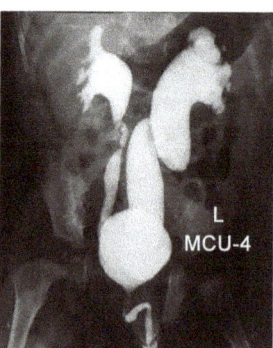

Fig. 2: VUR grade 5 on left side, grade 4 right side.

4. **Does VUR Cause Renal Damage?**
Intrauterine high grades of primary reflux may prevent normal development of kidneys and there might be renal hypoplasia or dysplasia. Postnatally, VUR *per se* does not lead to renal damage. However, it is a risk factor for recurrent UTI episodes especially in children below 5 years. The recurrent UTI episodes may lead to renal scarring if not managed prudently in time.

5. **How is VUR Managed?**
The conventional therapy of VUR includes antibiotic chemoprophylaxis. Surgical intervention is reserved for children with high grades of reflux with breakthrough UTI despite chemoprophylaxis.

This is a dimercaptosuccinic acid scan (DMSA) of child with right Grade 3 reflux and recurrent UTI. The right side kidney is reduced in size with irregular margins suggestive of renal scars and areas of decreased uptake of nuclear dye.

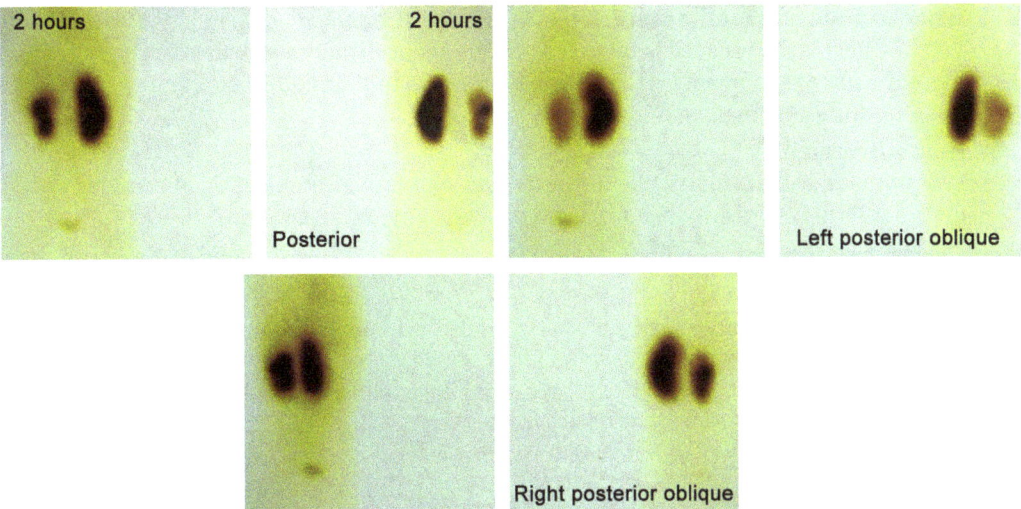

Fig. 3: DMSA scan pictures.

6. **What is DMSA scan?**

   It is a nuclear scan done to evaluate cortical function of kidneys (Fig. 3). It detects renal scars secondary to UTI and evaluates differential cortical function. It can also detect hypoplasia/dysplasia.

7. **What are the imaging studies required in the evaluation of child with UTI?**

   All children with UTI irrespective of age should have USG done for evaluation of kidney sizes, renal pelvis dilatation, ureteric dilatation, bladder contour and post void residue. Other imaging studies involve DMSA and MCUG. The Indian Society of Pediatric Nephrology has laid guidelines for these studies in children.

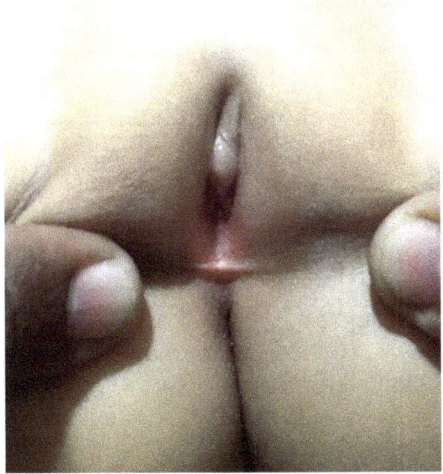

Fig. 4: Labial synchiae.

Picture shows a tight vulval synechiae (labial adhesion)(Fig. 4) in female with recurrent UTI.

8. **What is important for the detection of vulvul synechiae?**

   Vulvul synechiae may cause pooling of urine in vagina, urinary stasis and urinary retention, thereby causing recurrent UTI. It is very imperative to thoroughly examine genitals, anal opening and spine in all patients of UTI.

9. **How is it treated?**

   Symptomatic Labial adhesions may be treated with topical application of estrogen cream for 2–4 weeks. Severe adhesions may necessitate surgical separation.

CASE STUDY 3

Eight years old female child with recurrent UTI, significant post void residue on USG and constipation. The child also had a history of increased urinary frequency, urgency and urge incontinence.

MCUG done in view of recurrent UTI showed left Grade 3 reflux with thick trabeculated bladder (Fig. 5), left para vesicoureteral diverticulum and dilated bladder outlet.

This represents bowel bladder dysfunction (BBD) due to overactive detrusor and problems with bladder emptying.

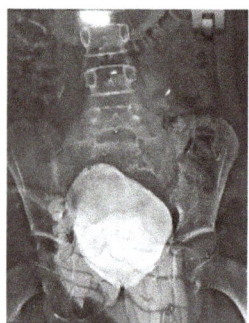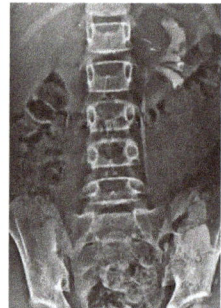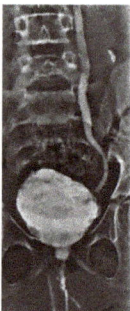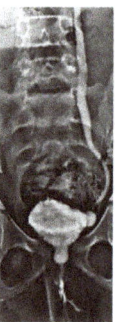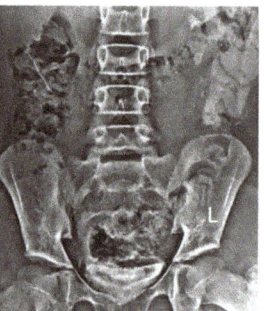

Fig. 5: Thick trabeculated bladder, VUR grade 3 left sided.

10. **What is BBD?**

    In the presence of intact neuronal pathways, problems with either bladder filling (overactive detrusor) or bladder emptying constitute BBD. Constipation is present up to the tune of 80% in such patients.

11. **What are the symptoms of BBD?**

    Urgency, frequency, urge incontinence, voiding postures, constipation, recurrent UTI, persistence of VUR or secondary VUR, small capacity bladder, significant post void residue, etc.

12. **How to evaluate these patients?**

    Apart from proper history and a thorough examination of abdomen, bladder, back, spine and genitals, a strict voiding diary is a must. A good ultrasound especially to look for full bladder volume and post void residue is very important. If indicated, MCUG is required as well. In severe cases and suspected spinal dysraphism, magnetic resonance imaging (MRI) spine and urodynamic study for detailed evaluation of bladder function are also required.

13. **How to treat these patients?**

    Basic principles of treatment include good counseling, behavioral therapy, timed voiding, treatment of constipation and pharmacological therapy like anticholinergics or alpha blockers. Consultation with a pediatric nephrologist may be required for proper evaluation and management.

All children with recurrent UTI without reflux or persistence of reflux at an older age should always be evaluated for BBD.

CASE STUDY 4

Eight years old child with recurrent UTI with urinary retention and intermittent urinary incontinence (Fig 6). The MCUG shows right Grade 4 reflux, thick trabeculated bladder and an inverted pine tree appearance suggestive of detrusor sphincter dyssynergia causing high pressure system and secondary reflux. The child was operated for meningomyelocele and has tethered cord. *This is not a BBD* but the child is having spinal dysraphism. These children benefit from anticholinergics and clean intermittent catheterization.

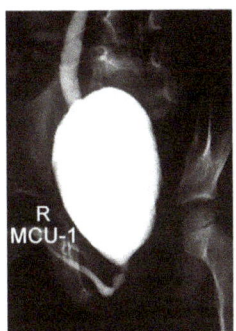
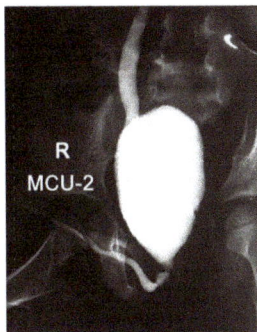
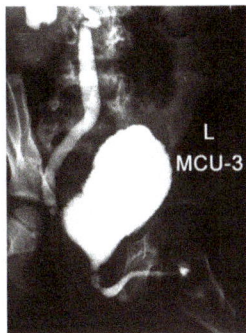
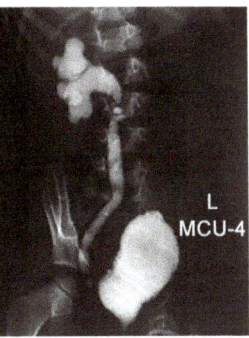

Fig. 6: Thick trabeculated bladder with inverted pine tree appearance.

CASE STUDY 5

A 1-day-old male child was brought with difficulty of passing urine, poor stream. Examination showed palpable bladder. USG showed left gross hydronephrosis and hydroureter with thick trabeculated bladder and suspicion of bladder outlet obstruction. MCUG showed a dilated posterior urethra with thick trabeculated bladder and left Grade 5 reflux in a child with posterior urethral valves (PUV)(Fig. 7).

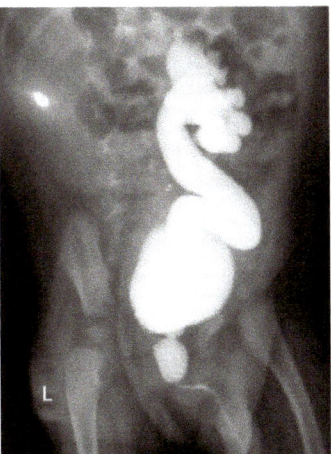

Fig. 7: PUV with dilated posterior urethral valves.

14. **What Is PUV?**

    A PUV is an obstructing membrane in the posterior male urethra as a result of abnormal in utero development. It is the most common cause of bladder outlet obstruction in male newborns.

15. **How to manage PUV?**

    PUV is a urological emergency and has to be dealt with immediately after birth. All patients with PUV need to be catheterized to allow bladder outlet. Primary management includes correction of electrolyte and blood gas anomalies.

    The primary intervention includes ablation of valves.

16. **What are the consequences of PUV?**

    These children develop significant bladder issues due to high pressure system, recurrent UTIs and renal parenchymal damage if not managed meticulously. Long-term follow-up of child is mandatory, and a multidisciplinary approach comprising pediatrician, pediatric nephrologist and pediatric surgeon is required in management.

Varicella Zoster

Chapter 95

Anoop Verma

CASE STUDY

A 7-year-old patient presented with the vesicular rash in the right mandibular nerve dermatome (Fig. 1). Diagnosis is obvious, child has Herpes zoster.

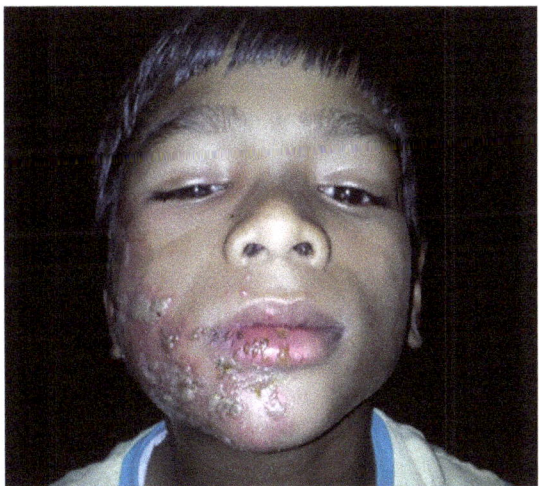

Fig. 1: Vesicular eruption over right mandibular nerve.

1. **What is herpes zoster (Shingles)?**
   Herpes zoster is caused by varicella zoster virus (VZV) which is an exclusively human neurotropic herpes virus that causes varicella (chickenpox) during primary infection, after which the virus becomes latent in cranial nerve, dorsal root and autonomic ganglia along the entire neuraxis. Years later, the virus may reactivate to cause herpes zoster (Shingles), an extremely painful vesicular skin rash confined to one or more sensory dermatomes.
2. **How the patient presents in herpes zoster (Shingles)?**
   The patient presents with prodromal sensory phenomena along one or more adjacent dermatomes lasting 1–10 days (average, 48 hours), which usually are noted as pain or,

less commonly, itching or paresthesias. The pain in prodromal period before the onset of cutaneous findings has been believed to represent the spread of VZV particles along sensory nerves, but around 10% of patients report the simultaneous onset of pain and rash.

3. **What are the complications of herpes zoster?**
   In children, VZV infection may involve facial nerve leading to *facial palsy*. *Zoster sine herpete* refers to a condition in which dermatomal distribution pain occurs in the absence of an antecedent rash, more frequently in children than adults. *Ramsay Hunt syndrome* (herpes zoster oticus) which is a *triad* of ipsilateral facial paralysis, ear pain and vesicles on the face, on the ear or in the ear is the typical presentation. Patients are at increased risk of *arterial ischemic stroke* and may precipitate a childhood arterial ischemic stroke.

4. **What is glossopharyngeal zoster and vagal zoster?**
   Glossopharyngeal zoster (herpes pharyngis) and vagal zoster (herpes laryngis) involve the jugular and petrosal ganglia, which are adjacent and often involved in some combination; however, individual involvement of both ganglia has been observed. Painful vesicular rash typically involves the palate, posterior tongue, epiglottis, tonsillar pillars, and occasionally, the external ear. A unilateral distribution can distinguish this variation of zoster from herpes simplex and herpangina.

5. **What is herpes occipiticollaris?**
   Herpes occipiticollaris involves the posterior scalp, the nuchal area, portions of the ear and portions of the lower mandible and anterior neck. The vertebral nerves C2 and C3 often are involved together. Branches of these two vertebral nerves communicate with CN VII and CN X, sometimes causing symptoms related to these cranial nerves as well.

6. **What is bilateral herpes zoster?**
   Rarely, herpes zoster manifests bilaterally. Bilateral presentations should always raise concern for disseminated disease (immunocompromise) or for alternate diagnosis, specifically for herpes simplex.

7. **What is the role of antiviral therapy in the treatment of herpes zoster (Shingles)?**
   The earlier antiviral medications are started, the more effective they are in shortening the duration of zoster and in preventing or decreasing the severity of postherpetic neuralgia (PHN). Ideally, therapy should be initiated within 72 hours of symptom onset.

Cardiac Causes of Stridor and Dysphagia

Chapter 96

Ritesh Sukharamwala, Chintan Bhatt

CASE STUDY 1

A-20-day-old neonate was admitted in the intensive care unit (ICU) with the complaints of breathing and feeding difficulty. The baby was intubated in view of severe respiratory distress. On clinical examination, the child had significant subcostal retraction with normal looking chest X-ray. On careful evaluation, right sided aortic arch was suspected on chest X-ray. Hence, as there was no significant respiratory disease which can be attributed to clinical symptoms, two-dimensional (2D) echocardiography was ordered. Echocardiography showed normal size heart with aberrant left subclavian artery with right aortic arch. Anatomy was confirmed on computed tomography (CT) scan with contrast which showed significant compression of both bronchus and esophagus. The child was advised for urgent surgery.

Figure 1 shows aberrant sub-clavian artery with right arch (red arrow) and Figure 2 shows with significant external compression of both bronchi and esophagus.

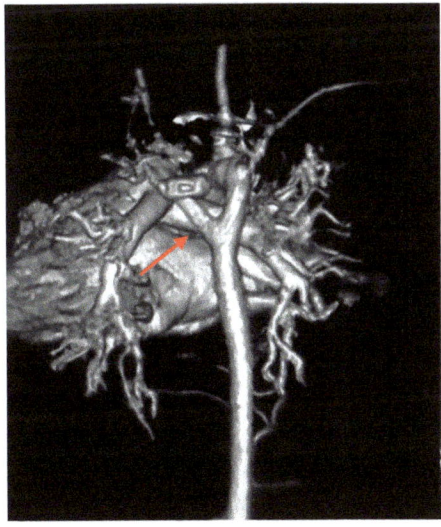

Fig. 1: Right sided aortic arch with aberrant left subclavian artery.

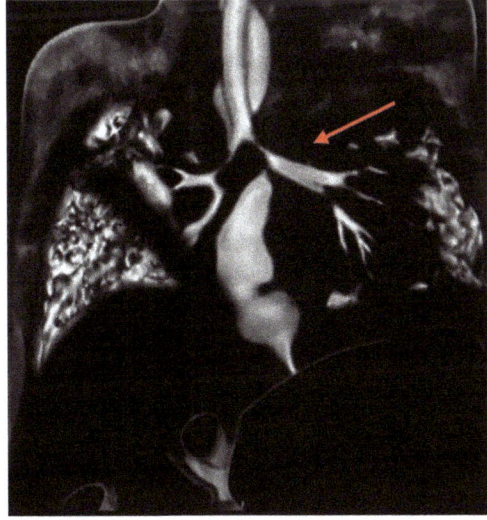

Fig. 2: External compression of both bronchi and esophagus.

CASE STUDY 2

A 3-month-old baby weighing 3.5 kg, failure to thrive (FTT) was being treated for lower respiratory tract infection (LRTI) and was admitted three times in 3 months. On general examination, the patient had respiratory distress and inspiratory stridor, which was more evident in awake state. Stridor was considered due to trachea-bronchomalacia. In view of recurrent LRTI and FTT, the baby was referred for cardiac opinion. On 2D echocardiography, the baby was found to have anomalous origin of left pulmonary artery (LPA) distally from right pulmonary artery (RPA) encircling the trachea producing compression symptoms (LPA sling). CT scan was done, which confirmed the same. The child improved after surgery.

Figure 3 shows significant sternal in drawing due to upper airway compression.

Figure 4 shows CT scan showing LPA sling: LPA arises distally from RPA and encircles trachea to compress airway from right and posterior aspects.

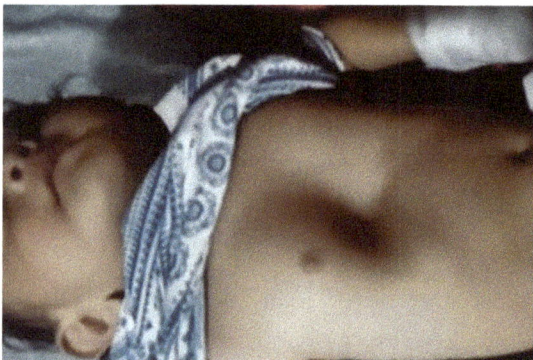

Fig. 3: Significant sternal indrawing due to upper airway compression.

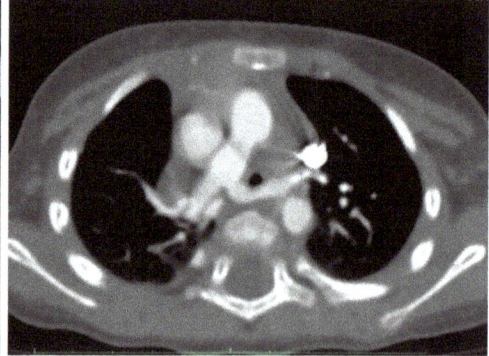

Fig. 4: LPA arising distally from RPA and encircles trachea to compress airway from right and posterior aspects.

1. **What is vascular ring (VR)?**
   It is the presence of vascular structure that completely or partially surrounds the trachea and esophagus. Ring can be formed by a patent vessel, an atretic vessel or its remnants (i.e., arterial ligaments). VR or sling can compress trachea and esophagus causing respiratory- or feeding-related symptoms.
   In one of the surgical studies, it was found that double aortic arch is the most common anomaly causing symptoms (40–50 %). Most children with VR present with compression symptoms in the first few months of life and require surgery within the first year of life.

2. **What are the different types of VR?**
   VRs are classified into two main types:
   - Complete (double aortic arch—Figures 5 and 6) and right arch with aberrant left subclavian artery (Figs. 1 and 2)
   - Incomplete (pulmonary slings, left arch with aberrant right subclavian artery)

   Figure 5 shows computed tomography scan of three-dimensional reconstructed double aortic arch and Figure 6 shows compression produced by both aortic arches on airway and esophagus (shown by arrows).

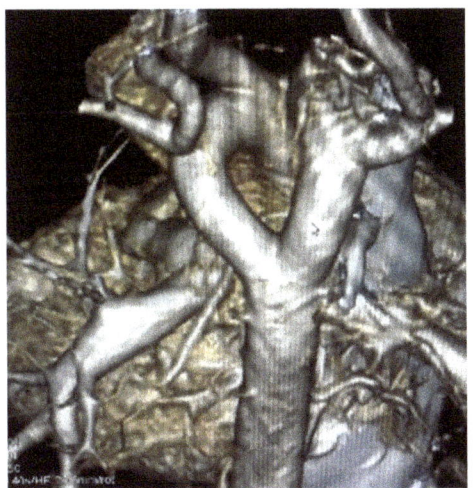

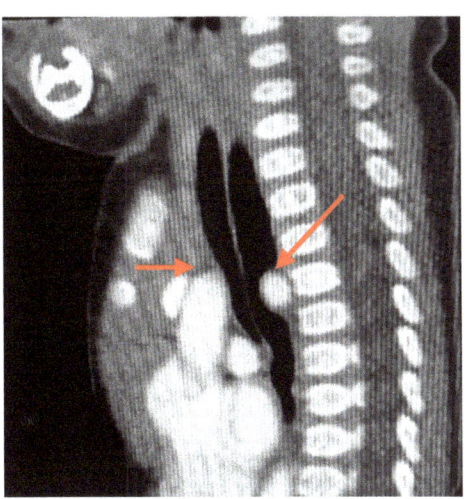

Fig. 5: CT scan 3 D reconstruction of double aortic arch showing both right and left limb of arch.

Fig. 6: External compression of esophagus and airway as shown by red arrows.

3. **What is pulmonary sling?**
   Normally main pulmonary artery (MPA) bifurcates in LPA and RPA, but when LPA arises distally from RPA and courses behind the esophagus and trachea compressing them causing symptoms is known as pulmonary sling. In this case, true ring is absent so it falls in the category of incomplete VR.

4. **When to suspect VRs in clinical practice?**
   Most of the patients have upper respiratory difficulty in the form of stridor and persistent cough during early infancy period. Few of them have feeding difficulty. Patients with vascular sling are more symptomatic during the first few weeks of life in the form of severe wheezing episodes, coughing and cyanotic episodes.

5. **What are investigations to be done to diagnose VR?**
   - Chest X-ray will provide important clue regarding indentation of tracheal air column and sidedness of arch
   - Barium swallow was historically considered gold standard for assessment of esophageal external compression
   - Echocardiography will identify most of the VRs and slings except few in which one of the ring components is atretic. It will also help in identifying associated congenital heart disease, which will have significant impact in overall management.
   - Currently, MRI and multislice CT scan are considered most important investigations in the therapeutic point of view. CT scan is better than MRI as it is less time-consuming and provides excellent details of vascular structures.

6. **How to treat VR?**
   - Symptomatic VRs need surgical treatment as early as possible. Earlier, bronchoscopy was advocated in many of these patients, but now it not necessary and babies can be directly taken for surgery after proper anatomical assessment.
   - In asymptomatic patients, surgery is indicated if there is associated congenital cardiac disease which warrants open heart surgery. Postoperatively most of the babies have normal outcome and it allows proper tracheal growth.

Waardenburg Syndrome

Chapter 97

Narayanappa D, Rashmi Nagaraj

CASE STUDY 1

A 5-year-old girl, born to second degree consanguineously married couple, presented to the outpatient department (OPD) with history of hearing loss since birth and inability to speak. She was diagnosed to have sensorineural hearing loss and referred to us for cochlear implant. She had normal development in gross motor, fine motor and social adaptive domains. On examination, she had anterior forelock (premature graying of anterior hair), heterochromia iridis, more specifically bilateral isohypochromia iridis (pale blue eyes), hypertelorism (dystopia canthorum), synophrys, broad and upturned nasal tip, short philtrum and absence of frontonasal angle. She also was found to have profound bilateral sensorineural hearing loss, syndactyly of middle and ring fingers on the left hand and an achromic nevus over the right leg and also scattered hypopigmented patches over the face. Eye examination did not reveal cataract or an abnormal fundus. She did not have any musculoskeletal abnormalities and spine was normal. She has a younger male sibling who is normal. None of the other family members had similar features. Genetic studies could not be done due to financial constraints. A diagnosis of Waardenburg syndrome (overlap of both Type I and Type II) was made based on clinical criteria (Fig. 1).

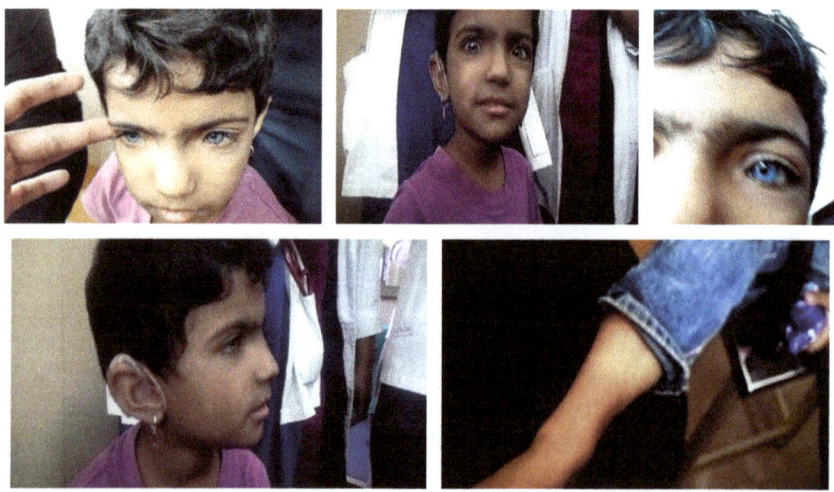

Fig. 1: A case of Waardenburg syndrome (overlap of both Type I and Type II).

Waardenburg Syndrome

CASE STUDY 1

An 8-year-old girl born to non-consanguineous couple, was admitted in our pediatric ward for dengue fever. Her past history and records revealed that she had undergone surgery for Hirschsprung's disease in the newborn period. She had been evaluated for hearing as her language milestones were delayed, and was reported to have profound sensorineural hearing loss on the right side. Her clinical features as shown in Figure 2 are characterized by heterochromia iridis, more specifically bilateral isohypochromia iridis (pale blue eyes), hypertelorism (dystopia canthorum), short philtrum and absence of frontonasal angle and left-sided microtia. She also had ichthyosis, which is unusual in this condition. In view of the above features along with Hirschsprung's disease, a diagnosis of Waardenburg-Shah syndrome (Type IV) was made. Genetic testing could not be done in this child also due to the same reason as case 1.

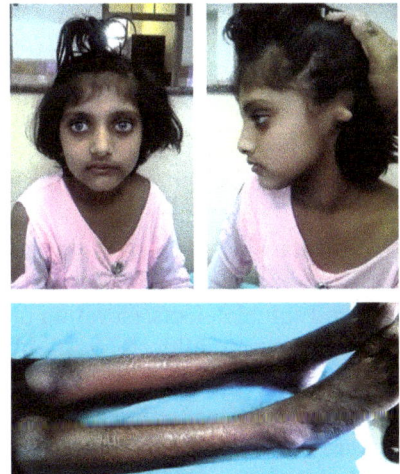

Fig. 2: A case of Waardenburg-Shah syndrome (Type IV).

1. **What is Waardenburg syndrome?**
   Waardenburg syndrome is a group of genetic conditions that can cause hearing loss and changes in coloring (pigmentation) of the hair, skin and eyes. It is the auditory–pigmentary complex disorder with features characterized by failure of proper melanocyte differentiation affecting skin, hair, eyes or stria vascularis of cochlea.
2. **What is its frequency?**
   Waardenburg syndrome affects an estimated 1 in 40,000 people. It accounts for 2–5% of all cases of congenital hearing loss. Types I and II are the most common forms of Waardenburg syndrome, while Types III and IV are rare.
3. **What are the most frequent clinical signs of waardenburg syndrome?**
   Sensorineural hearing loss, affecting about 60% of the patients; heterochromia of the iris; hypoplastic blue eyes; white streak; premature gray hair; leucoderma; high nasal root and hyperplasia of the medial portion of the eyebrows (synophrys).
4. **What are the types of Waardenburg syndrome?**
   There are four recognized types of Waardenburg syndrome, distinguished by their physical characteristics and sometimes by their genetic cause.

Type I patients have epicanthus, increasing the distance of the internal medial corners of the eyes (canthorum dystopia), iris isocromia with bright blue color or heterochromia of iris, white hair streak (poliosis) that can appear at any age, confluent eyebrows (sinophrys) and changes in skin pigmentation.

Type II differs from Type I by not having canthorum dystopia. In addition, hearing loss occurs more often in people with Type II than in those with Type I.

Type III (also called Klein-Waardenburg syndrome) includes abnormalities of the arms and hands, microcephaly and mental disabilities, in addition to hearing loss and changes in pigmentation.

Type IV (also known as Waardenburg-Shah syndrome) has signs and symptoms of both Waardenburg syndrome and Hirschsprung disease.

5. **What are the characteristic eye abnormalities in WS?**
   Iris pigmentary abnormality:
   - Two eyes of different color
   - Iris bicolor/segmental heterochromia—an eye with two different colors
   - Characteristic brilliant blue (sapphire) iris (alternatively described as "Waardenburg blue eye," sky-blue eyes, or hypopigmented iris)

   Dystopia canthorum: Lateral displacement of inner canthi, with a reduction of visible sclera medially.

6. **What are the other congenital disorders associated with Waardenburg syndrome?**
   Waardenburg syndrome has also been associated with a variety of other congenital disorders, such as intestinal and spinal defects, elevation of the scapula, and cleft lip and palate, congenital heart defects, abnormalities of vestibular function and low anterior hairline.

7. **What are the diagnostic criteria for Waardenburg syndrome?**
   Diagnostic criteria for WS were established by Farrer et al. in 1992.
   - **Major criteria**: Congenital sensorineural hearing loss, hair hypopigmentation, abnormal pigmentation of the iris (complete or partial heterochromia), telecanthus, first-degree relatives affected.
   - **Minor criteria**: Gray hair before the age of 30, synophrys, skin hypopigmentation, high nasal root or large and hypoplastic nose wing.

   The diagnosis is given by the presence of two major criteria or one major and two minor.

8. **What are the inheritance patterns in WS?**
   Waardenburg syndrome is usually inherited in an autosomal dominant pattern, which means one copy of the altered gene in each cell is sufficient to cause the disorder. In most cases, an affected person has one parent with the condition.

   A small percentage of cases result from new mutations in the gene; these cases occur in people with no history of the disorder in their family.

   Some cases of Waardenburg syndrome, Type II and Type IV, seem to have an autosomal recessive pattern of inheritance, which means both copies of the gene in each cell have mutations.

   Most often, the parents of an individual with an autosomal recessive condition carrying one copy of the mutated gene each do not show signs and symptoms of the condition.

9. **Which are the genes associated with Waardenburg syndrome (WS)?**
   According to the current medical literature, six genes are associated with WS:
   - *PAX3* (encoding the paired box 3 transcription factor)
   - *MITF* (microphthalmia-associated transcription factor)
   - *EDN3* (endothelin 3)
   - *EDNRB* (endothelin receptor type B)
   - *SOX10* (encoding the SRY Box10 transcription factor)
   - *SNAI2* (snail homolog 2)

10. **What is the treatment approach in WS?**
    The treatment approach should be multidisciplinary involving pediatrician, ophthalmologist, otorhinolaryngologist and genetic counselor. Early diagnosis allows efficient audiological approach improving quality of life.
    Also, early intervention has major impact on the patient's quality of life. Genetic counseling and multidisciplinary patient approach is crucial.
    Some studies have shown effective results in the treatment of WS with cochlear implants, as well as excellent prognosis with proper hearing rehabilitation.

11. **What is the role of a pediatrician in treating children with WS?**
    The primary pediatricians coming across a child with blue eyes and white forelock of hair must get the child's hearing tested at the first instance, if not already done. An early diagnosis and improvement of hearing impairment with timely intervention and speech therapy are most important for psychological and intellectual development of these children.

Index

Page numbers followed by *b* refer to box, *f* refer to figure, *fc* refer to flowchart, and *t* refer to table.

A

Abdomen
  and limbs 228*f*
  and thighs 146*f*
Abdominal
  surgeries 155
  ultrasound 38
  wall and gluteal muscle 202
Abundant sunshine 221
Acanthosis nigricans 1, 19
  case of 1
  causes of 2
  characteristic of 2
  complications of 3
  diagnoses of 2
  laboratory investigations 2
  pathophysiology of 2
  predilection of 3
  prognosis of 3
  skin biopsy in 3
  treatment of 3
  types of 3
Acid-base disorders 241
Acid-fast bacilli 273
Activated partial thromboplastin time 146
Acyclovir 146, 150
Adenoma
  cebaceum 279*f*
  sebaceum 285*f*, 286
Adolescent gynecomastia 4, 5
  case of 4*f*
  causes of 5
  differential diagnosis of 5
  final diagnosis 6
  prevalence rate of 5
Adrenal crisis 39
Adrenal glands 70
Adrenocorticotropic hormone 282
Aerophilic Streptococcus 202
Airway foreign bodies 122
Aldolase deficiency 53
Alginate 135
Allergy testing 290

Allogenic bone marrow transplantation 53
Alopecia totalis 221, 222*f*
American College of Rheumatology 270
Amiloride 241
Amniotic band syndrome 7, 8, 11
  associated with 11
  body involved in 11
  causes 8
  clinical manifestations of 8
  complications of 12
  diagnosed 9
  different degrees of severity of 9
  different types of 8
  differential diagnoses 9
  epidemiology of 11
  etiologies of 11
  examples of 7*f*
  management of 10
  manifestations in 0
  medical treatments available for 12
  mode of inheritance 8
  pathophysiology of 11
  presence of 8
  prognosis of 10, 12
  risk of recurrence of 10
  surgical treatments available for 12
  ultrasonography useful in 12
Amoxicillin 262, 263
Anal position index 16
  calculation of 17*f*
  using 15
Anal-fourchette distance 16
Anaplasma phagocytophilum 243
Anemia type 1
  clinical features 52
  differential diagnosis 53
  etiology 52
Aneuploidy 41
Angioedema of the face 297
Angiofibroma 285*f*, 286
Angiomyolipoma 281, 286
Anhidrotic ectodermal dysplasia 89

Ankyloglossia 13
   case of 13f
   children 14
   clinical implications 13
   clinical issues 14
   treatment 14
Annular
   atresia 49
   non-itchy erythematous rash 107f
   polycyclic erythematous lesions 297
Anogenital 16
Antacids like aluminum hydroxide 135
Antenatal
   corticosteroid therapy 42
   diagnosis 24
   fetal surgical intervention 44
Antibiotic
   empirical choice of 145
   prophylaxis 177
Anti-double stranded anti-DNA test 270
Antiepileptic medications 279, 282
Anti-gastric parietal cells 79
Antihistaminics-hydroxyzine 125
Anti-leishmanial drugs 228
Anti-migarine agents 268
Anti-phospholipid antibodies 207
Antiplatelet medications 28
Antipyretic and analgesic 162
Antistaphylolysin 125
Antistreptolysin 125
Anti-tuberculosis therapy 273
Antiviral therapy, role of 306
Anus, anteriorly displaced 15, 15f
   in females 16
   in males 16
Anxiety 286
Aorta with vegetation 174f
Aortic root 174
Aplasia of brain 72
Aplastic anemia 116
Aqueductal
   gliosis 63
   stenosis 63
Arachnoid space 63
Arcus juvenilis 104
Arnold Chiari malformation type 2 250
Arterial
   blood gas 42
   ischemic stroke 306
   lesions 172

Arthritis 142
Arthrogryposis multiplex congenita 45
Ascitis 209
Ash leaf macule 284f
Ataxia telangiectasia 18
   associated with 24
   clinical signs of 19
   differential diagnosis 25
   inheritance pattern 24
   life expectancy in 25
   manifestations of 20
   recommendations for 25
   sites of telangiectasia 20
   treating children 25
   treatment approach 24
   types of 20
Atretic ear canal 188f
Atrial septal defect 116, 176
Autosomal dominant
   disorder 287
   pattern 312
Autosomal recessive disorder 52
Azithromycin 247

B

Bacillus Calmette-Guérin immunization 82
Baclofen 135
Bacteroids 202
Balanoposthitis undergo circumcision 226
Ballooning of prepuce front view 225f
Band obstruction 49
Barrier agents like sucralfate 135
Bartter's syndrome 241
Basal
   cisterns 63
   ganglia 195
Bazin's disease 112
Beau's line 162
Behcet's disease 111
Benazol 156
Benzathine penicillin 258f
Berinert 155
Bernard-Soulier syndrome 26-28
Beta-carotene levels 30
Bile stasis 70
Biopsy, indications of 211
Blackish hyperpigmentation 204f
Bleeding
   diathesis 207
   tendencies 138

Blockade of vessels 195
Blood culture sensitivity report 175
Blood neutrophils level 137
Blood samples 157f
Body mass index, measurement of 290
Bone deformities, severe 237f
Bone marrow 51, 164
    examination of 136
Bones, stunting and deformed 238f
Bony pathologies in thalassemia 140
Bourneville disease 280
Bowel bladder dysfunction 302
    symptoms of 302
Brachial plexus birth palsy 99
    types of 99
Brachioradialis 87
Branchio oto renal syndrome 188
Breastfeeding 17
Bronchi 307
Bronchopulmonary sequestration 41
Bronchoscopy, role of 122
Brown black spots 217f
Brownie nose 205
Bulbar conjunctiva 18f
Butterfly rash on face 269
Buttocks, eruptions on 161f

C

Café au lait 217f
    macules 216
    spot 116, 217
Calcineurin inhibitors like cyclosporine 211
Calcipenic rickets 220, 221
Calcitriol therapy 223
Calcium channel blockers 196
Campylobacter 114
Canthaxanthin 31
Canthorum dystopia 312
Caput quadratum 219f
Carbamazepine 279
Cardiac
    abnormalities 172
    causes
        dysphagia 307
        of stridor 307
        rhabdomyoma 281, 286
    valve repair 177
    valvulopathy, develop 177
Cardiomegaly with narrow pedicle 58f

Cardiothoracic ratio 56
    on chest X-ray 56
Carotene 30
Carotenemia 29, 30
    cause hypervitaminosis A 31
    diagnosis 31
    etiology 31
    treated 31
    yellow discoloration 31
Cartridge-based nucleic acid amplification test 272
Cast in maximally corrected position 46f
Cat-scratch
    disease 111
    fever 114
Causative agent 262
Cavernous lymphangioma 186
Cavernous sinus thrombosis 198
Cavities diagnosed 76
Celiac disease 293
Central nervous system 70, 149, 172
Central scolex 213f
Cephalosporins 263
Cerebrospinal fluid 63, 249
CHARGE syndrome 188
Chediak-Higashi syndrome 138
Cheilitis 260f
Chest X-rays in congenital heart disease 56
Chiari malformation 63, 64f
Chik sign 205
Child abuse 126, 127
    by step mother 128
    different forms of 128
    forms and types of 129
    magnitude of 129
Child and mother, bowing of legs in 222
Child in pavlik harness 47f
Child sexual abuse 130
    characteristics of 130
    consequences of 132
    response to 131
    types of 130
Child underwent computed tomography 121f
Child Welfare Committee 131
Child with phimosis
    non-surgical options for 226
    surgical options for 226
Chlamydia 114
Chloramphenicol 247
Cholecystectomy for cholelithiasis 53

Choledochal cyst 34
   complications of 35
   investigation of choice of 35
   symptoms of 34
   treatment of choice for 35
   useful in managing 35
Chorioretinitis 72
Christ-Siemens-Touraine syndrome 90
Chromatin bridges 52f
Chromosomal instability 117
Chronic gingival bleeding 28
Chronic meningitis 70
Chronic mononuclear interstitial pneumonitis 70
Cicatricial skin lesions 72
Ciliary body necrosis 70
Cimetidine 135
Ciniryze 155
Cisapride and domperidone 135
Clarithromycin 247
Clindamycin 263
Clobazam 279
Clostridium 202
Cloxacillin 145
Coarctation of aorta 58
Coccidioidomycosis 111
Coccyx-fourchette distance 16
Cochlea, stria vascularis of 311
Cochlear hemorrhage 70
Coin pressed over umbilicus 296
Collagen tissue disease 79
Collapsed distal bowel 50
Collapsed lung 93f
Colonic polyp 32
   case of 32f
   present 33
Colorectal cancer, risk of developing 33
Common bile duct, massive dilatation of 34
Common renal tubular, problems of 241
Compensatory marrow hyperplasia 139
Complete blood count 107, 125, 142
Congenital adrenocortical hyperplasia 36
   cases of 37f
Congenital cardiac anomalies 41
Congenital diaphragmatic hernia 40, 41
Congenital dislocation of knee 45
Congenital duodenal atresia, types of 48
Congenital dyserythropoietic anemia 52
Congenital esotropia 54
   case of 54f
   caused 55
   hereditary 55

Congenital glaucoma, bilateral 68f
Congenital heart disease 57, 116
Congenital hydrocephalus, case of 62
Congenital hypothyroidism
   causes of 66
   differentiate causes 67
   early treatment 67
Congenital lupus 205
Congenital neutropenia, severe 117
Congenital rubella syndrome 68, 69
Congenital sensorineural hearing loss 312
Congenital varicella syndrome 71-73
Conjunctivitis 105
Connective tissue hamartomas 286
Cookie test 102
Corneal arcus 104
Cornelia de Lange syndrome 41
Cortical
   cytomegaly 70
   dysplasias 281
   thinning 216
Corticosteroids 142
Corticotropin-releasing hormone
   diagnosed 38
   excessive secretion of 38
   manage, case of 39
   types of 38
Coxiellaburnetti 243
Coxsackievirus 162
Coxsackievirus A4 84
Craniofacial anomalies 290
Crohn's disease 114
Cupping and fraying of radius and ulna 219f
Cushingoid features 210, 210f
Cutaneous fungal infection 125
Cyanosis and dyspnea 42
Cyclosporine 211
Cyclosporine A 114
Cyclosporine for resistant, cases of 80
Cystic
   hygromas 187
   lymphangioma 186
   selling in neck 186f
Cysticidal 215
Cysticidal drugs contraindications of 215

D

Dandy-Walker malformation 64
Dandy-Walker syndrome 63
Darier disease 149

Deep carious primary 1st molar 75
Deep venous thrombosis 203
Defect of iodide organification 67
Defect repaired 44
Deflazacort 88
Deltoid 87
Dental caries 74, 76
   cause 74
   implications in 77
   increased risk of 77
   prevention of 77
   responsible for 74
Dental enamel pits 281
Dental procedures 155
Dental sepsis 125
Deoxyribonucleic acid 146, 194
Depression 286
Dermatitis
   herpetiformis 78
   herpetiformis, case of 78
Dermatographic urticaria 125
Dermatographism 297
Desquamating rash 81
Desquamating rash 81*f*
   cause of 84
   clinical signs compatible with 82
   complications of 84
   diagnostic criteria for 82
   differential diagnosis of 82
   incomplete 82
Diamond blackfan anemia 117
Diet 135
Diffuse erythema 262
Diffuse erythroderma 82
Dilated left atrial 189
Dilated right pulmonary artery 60
Dilated stomach and duodenum 48
Diloxanide furuoate 145
Dimercaptosuccinic acid scan 300, 301*f*
Dinitrophenol 31
Diphenhydromine 125
Direct immunofluorescence 79
Disease transmitted 105
Disseminated intravascular coagulation 207, 235
Double aortic arch 309*f*
Double bubble appearance 48
Doudeno-denostomy 50
Down's syndrome 188
Doxycycline 247

Drug reaction 82
Drugs like aspirin 196
Duchenne muscular dystrophy 85
   case of 85
   clinical features of 87
   diagnose 87
   etiology of 86*f*
   incidence of 86
   manifest in females 86
Duodenal atresia 50*f*
Duodenal obstruction types of 48
Duodeno-duodenostomy 50
Duodenum 277
Dwarfism 292*f*
Dyselectrolytemia 211
Dyskeratosis congenita 117
Dysplasia of hip, developmental 45
Dystopia canthorum 312

E

Ear and hearing problems 293
Ectodermal dysplasia 89
   x-linked 89
Ectropion 184*f*
Eczema herpeticum 149
Edema
   lower limb 200*f*
   uvula with pharyngitis 261*f*
Ehler-Danlos syndrome 10
Ehrlichia 243
Electroencephalogram 282
Electrolytes and blood gases 49
Empyema
   progressive increase in 97*f*
   thoracis 92, 98
Enamel and dentin 75
Endothelial necrosis 70
Enterobacteriaceae 202
Enterococcus 202
Enzyme deficiency 140, 158
Enzyme-linked immunosorbent assay 246
Epidermal growth factor receptor 2
Epidermal nevus 223
Epidermolytic toxins 265
Epstein-Barr virus 114
Erb's palsy 99
   clinical presentation 100
   differential diagnoses 100

Erythema
  induratum 112
  infectiosum 105
    case of 105
    treatment of 106
  multiforme 107-109, 298
    causative agents for 109
    characteristic of 109
    conditions for 109
    considerations for 109
    diagnosing 109
    hallmark character of 108
    lesions features of 108
    pathogenesis of 109
    prognosis of 109
  nodosum 2, 110-114
    case of 110, 113
    clinical manifestations of 111
    diagnose 111
    differential diagnoses of 114
    epidemiology of 111
    etiology of 111
    findings of 114
    pathogenesis of 111
    recurrent 114
    treatment of choice for 112
Erythematous rash 256f
Erythroid hyperplasia 51
Erythromycin 135
Erythropoiesis in dermis 70
Esophageal chair 135
Esophagus 307
  and airway 309f
Estrogen
  replacement therapy 294
  treatment 294
Ethambutol 273
European League Against Rheumatism 270
Exanthema, stages of 106
Exanthematic necrolysis 109
Extensive eczema herpeticum 150
Extracorporeal membrane oxygenation 42
Extramedullary hematopoiesis 70
Exudative tonsillitis 260f
Eyebrows, absent 89f
Eyelids, swelling of 154f

F

Face, yellow discoloration of 9f
Facial
  hemangioma 172
  look during recovery 210f
  port wine stain 267
Failure to thrive 308
Familial glucocorticoid deficiency 205
Famotidine 135
Fanconi anemia 115, 117
  genes 115
  inherited 117
  patient 117
Fasting lipid profile 156
Febrile urticaria 123, 124f
  differential diagnosis for 125
  etiology of 125
Fetal growth restriction 293
Fetal medicine 44
Fetoscopic endoluminal tracheal occlusion 44
Fiber optic transillumination 76
Fibrin and immunoglobulin m 142
Fibrin degradation products 206
Fibroblast growth factor receptor 2
Fibropurulent stage 98
Fibrosis 70
Fine-needle aspiration cytology 273
Fissures on the skin 185
Flaccid wrist elbow persistent 101
Flat gluteal cleft 253
Flucloxacillin 266
Focal seizure in children, causes of 213
Folate deficiency 289
Foley's to drain urine 255
Foramen of magendie 63
Forehead hematoma 126
Forehead swelling 126f
Foreign body 121f
  bronchus, diagnostic features of 122
  in bronchus 118
  X-ray 118f
Forensic examination 131
Fourniers gangrene 202
Fracture humerus 128, 128f
Frank nephritis 142
Fresh frozen plasma 146, 206, 236
Fryns syndrome 41
Fully corrected knee 47f
Fungal sepsis 205

G

Gangrene of digits 245
Gangrene of ear lobe 245f
Gas gangrene 203

Gastroesophageal reflux disease 133
   clinical presentations 134
   diagnosed 134
   dye study 133
   treated 134
Gastrointestinal disorders 114
Gene therapy 164
Generalized tonic-clonic seizure 286
Genetic disorders 285
Genetic transmission pattern of 27
Genital herpes present 149
Gentle strokes 265
Genu varus 219f
Germinal centers 70
Giant platelets on peripheral smear 27
Giemsa staining 227
Glomerular filtration rate 237, 282
Glossopharyngeal zoster 306
Glucocorticoids 39
Glucose-6-phosphate dehydrogenase 51
   deficiency 53
Gluten-free diet 79
Glutii 87
Glycoprotein 26
Goldenhar syndrome 188
Gower's maneuver 87
Gower's sign 85
Griscelli syndrome 136, 138
   diagnosis of 136
   inheritance pattern 137
   names of 137
   signs and symptoms of 137
Grocott's methenamine silver stains 199
Group A *Streptococcus* 202, 262

H

Hair ball 277
Hair growth, cause of 288
Hair on end appearance 139, 139f
Hair shaft medulla 137f
Hair tuft 288
Hamartin 286
Hand, eruptions on 161f
Hand-foot-mouth disease 160
Hands and feet, swollen 292
Heart problems 293
Helicobacter pylori 125
Hematoma 127
Hemoglobin abnormal 159
Hemolytic anemia 270

Hemolytic disease of newborn 53
Hemorrhage bullae 207
Henderson-Patterson inclusion bodies 104
Henoch-Schonlein purpura 141
   causative agents 142
   complications of 142
   epidemiology of 141
   features of 142
   symptoms 142
   treatment options 142
   type of disease 141
Hepatic
   abscess 143-144
      clinical signs and symptoms 143
      complications of 145
      in right lobe of liver 145f
   giant cell transformation 70
Hepatitis B 114
Hereditary
   angioedema 154
      causes attacks 155
      management of 155
      signs and symptoms of 155
   elliptocytosis 53
   methemoglobinemia 157
   spherocytosis 53, 140
Herpes labialis 147, 148
Herpes occipiticollaris 306
Herpes simplex infection 146
Herpes simplex virus 107, 249
   clinical manifestations of 147
   in immunocompromised patients 149
   infection present 147
   infections caused 147
   types of 147
Herpes zoster 151, 305
   bilateral 306
   clinical features of 152
   complications of 306
   diagnose 152
   disseminated 152
   in later life 153
   infection 151
   treat 153, 306
Herpetic whitlow 148
Heterochromatin pattern 52
Hiatus hernia 133
Hidrotic ectodermal dysplasia 89
Hirschsprung's disease 311, 312
   surgery for 311

Histiocytic reaction 70
Histoplasmosis 111
Horner's syndrome 101
Horseshoe 116
Host immunity 147
Human chorionic gonadotropin 169
Human immunodeficiency virus 114, 152, 202
Human leukocyte antigen 53
Hunter's disease 163, 163f
   diagnosis 164
   treatment possibilities 164
Hydranencephaly 64
Hydrocele 165
   cases of bilateral 167
   causes 166
   clinical features 166
   communicating 166
   developing contralateral 167
   differ from hernia 167
   encysted 167
   encysted cord 166
   noncommunicating 166
   treatment required 166
   tunica vaginalis 165
Hydrocephalus 63, 64, 65
Hydrochloroquine 114
Hypercalciuria 239
Hypercholesteremia 209
Hyperextended knees 45
Hyperinflated, right lung 119f
Hyperkeratotic skin 183f
Hypernatremic dehydration 185
Hyperphosphatemia 221
Hyperpigmentation 205
Hyperpigmented basal melanocytes 138f
Hyperthermia 289
Hypertrichosis 288
Hypoalbuminemia 209
Hypoallergic formula 135
Hypohidrotic ectodermal dysplasia 90
   diagnose 90
   features of hidrotic 91
   inheritance pattern in 90
   management options for 91
   pattern of hidrotic 91
   signs 90
   symptoms of 90
   treat 91
   variants of 91
Hypomelanotic patch 286
Hypopigmentary immunodeficiency syndrome 138
Hypopigmentation 72, 137
Hypopigmented
   eyebrows 136
   hairs 138
   patches 228, 310
   silvery hairs 137f
Hypospadias 168, 226
   child with 169
   distal 169f
   mid 169f
   proximal penile 169
   surgery 169
   types of 168
Hypothyroidism 293

I

Ibuprofen 112
Ichthyosis 182
   clinical features of 183
   complications 185
   diagnosis 184
   different types of 183
   histological finding 184
   risk to life 185
Idiopathic focal epilepsy 213
Idiopathic nephrotic syndrome 209
Idiopathic purpura fulminans 235
Idiopathic thrombocytopenic purpura 26, 127
Idursulfase 164
Illness, course of 106
Immobilized after birth 101
Immune thrombocytopenic purpura 243
Immunization against rubella 70
Immunize child on steroids 211
Immunodeficiency disorders 152
Immunofluorescence, indicates immunoglobulin A 142
Immunofluorescent assay 246
Immunologic disorder 270
Immunological abnormalities 23
Immunomodulatory agents 125
Immunosuppressant role of 142
Immunosuppressive therapy 152
Indian Academy of Pediatrics-revised National TB Control Program 273
Indomethacin 112

Infantile hemangioma 171, 172
  classified 172
  complications 172
  course of 172
  risk factors for 172
Infantile spasm 285
  different causes of 285
Infective endocarditis 174
  cardiac complications in 177
  clinical grounds 176
  clinically suspected 176
  diagnosis of 176
  in newborn infants 176
  incidence of 176
Inflammatory bowel disease 111
Influenza vaccination 125
Infraspinatus 87
Infraumbilical hernia 296
Inherited autosomal dominant disease 155
Inherited bone marrow failure syndromes 117
Intact interatrial septum 189
Intercostal drainage 98
International Tuberous Sclerosis Complex
    Consensus group 280
Interstitial nephritis 70
Intracranial pressure 286
Intrahepatic biliary radicals 34
Intraintestinal injections of steroids 112
Intraoral fibromas 281
Intrauterine growth restriction 240
Iodides 111
Iridocyclitis 70
Iris isocromia 312
Iron deficiency anemia 140, 178
  common causes 179
  management of 179
  symptoms of 178
  treatment of 181
  types of 181
Irreversible pulpitis 76
Isohypochromia iridis, bilateral 310, 311
Isoniazid 273
Itchy wheal 124f

J

Jaundice 31
Jerks in infancy 285
Juvenile polyp
  histopathology of typical 33
  characteristic features of 33

K

Kala azar medical research centre 227
Kala-azar 228
Kawasaki disease 82
Keratolytic agents 91, 184
Kidney
  function test 49
  injury, acute 211
  problems 293
Klebsiella 202
Klein-Waardenburg syndrome 312
Klinefelter's syndrome 5
Koch's 211
Koilonychia 179f
Kostmann syndrome 117

L

Labial synchiae 301f
Lactobezoars 278
Lactophenol cotton blue staining 199
Lamellar ichthyosis 182, 183
Lamellar ichthyosis treatment of 184
Lamotrigine 282
Lansoprazole 135
Large hepatic abscesses 145
Large volume abscess 145
Larsen's syndrome 45
Laser therapy 268
Lax lower esophageal sphincter 133
Leishman-Donavani bodies 227
Leishmaniasis 114
Leishmanin skin test 228
Lemierre syndrome 202
Lesions, development of 79
Leukemia 111
Leukopenia 270
Liberal application of emollients 91
Life threatening 149
Lifelong gluten-free diet 79
Limp right upper limb 231
Lipidized dermal 104
Lips, swelling of 154f
Lisch nodules 216
Liver abscess 143
  diagnostic tests 144
  etiologic organisms for 143
  pathogenesis of 144
  predisposing factors for 143
Liver function test 49, 125, 136

Liver herniation 42
Liver, right lobe of 144
Lobular disarray 70
Low serum levels of immunoglobulins 24
Lower segment cesarean section 206, 289
Ludwigs angina 202
Lumbosacral spine 288
Lung-to-head ratio 42
Lycopenemia 31
Lyell disease 265
Lymph node tuberculosis, algorithm for 274
Lymph node with sinus 271f
Lymphangio-hemangiomas 186
Lymphangioleiomyomatosis 281, 282
Lymphangioma 186
    classified 187
    common sites of 187
    natural progress of 187
    simplex 186
    treatment options for 187
    types of 186
Lymphogranuloma venereum 111
Lymphopenia 23, 270

M

Macrolides 263
Maculopapular 82
Magnesium hydroxide 135
Magnetic resonance imaging 23
Main pulmonary artery 61, 309
Malar flush 190f, 191
Malformation of cortical development 285
Malformed osteoid 70
Maternal active rubella infection 69
Mediastinal shift 40f
Megakaryocytic thrombocytopenia 117
Megaloblastosis 51
Meningocele 289
Meningomyelocele 289
Menorrhagia 27, 28
Menstrual bleeding 27
Mepacrine 31
Metabolic derangements 238
Metallic foreign body 119
Metaphyseal dysostosis 223
Methemoglobin
    diagnosed 159
    manifestations of 159
    treatment of 159

Methemoglobinemia 158
    etiopathogenesis of 158
    manifestations of 158
    pathophysiology of 158
Methicillin-resistant *Staphylococcus aureus* 145, 266
Microarray analysis 42
Microcephaly 72
Microphthalmia 70, 72
Microtia with congenital canal atresia 188
Micturating cystourethrogram 299
Miescher's radial granulomas 111
Miltefosine 230
Ministry of Women and Child Development 129
Mitral stenosis 189
    indicated in work-up of 191
    investigations 190
    medical treatment for 191
    prognosis of 192
    role of ECG in 191
    signs of 191
    symptoms of 191
    treated 192
Mitral valve 175f
Molecular confirmation 199
Molluscum contagiosum 104, 193, 193f
    clinical differential diagnoses of 194
    common sites of 194
    commonest age of 193
    diagnostic investigations of 194
    from chickenpox 194
    hallmark character of 193
    in immunosuppressed patient 194
    predisposing factors for 194
    prognosis of 194
    responsible for 194
    therapeutic considerations 194
Monitor blood pressure 156
Mood disorders 286
Motilin receptor agonist 135
Moyamoya disease 195
    causes 196
    diagnostic modality for 196
    symptoms of 195
Mucormycosis 197, 198, 198f, 199
    clinical differential diagnosis 197
    clinical forms of 198
    despite early treatment 200
    histological features of 199
    mucormycosis 197
    treatment of 200

Mucus membrane involvement 108
Multidisciplinary approach 131
Multiorgan failure 207
Multiple pterygium syndrome 187
Multiple retinal nodular hamartomas 281
Multiple small nodules 227f
Muscle
    aches 105
    biopsy 88
    calves 87
Muscular dystrophy 86, 87
Mutans streptococci 76
Mycophenolate mofetil 211
Mycoplasma 114
    immunoglobulin 107
Myelodysplastic syndrome 116
Myeloid leukemia, acute 111
Myocarditis 70

N

Nafcillin 266
Nagayama spots 248
Naproxen 112
Naraka's grade 1-2 101
Narakas grading 100
Nasal inspection 290
Nasogastric tube 43
National Commission for the Protection of Child
    Rights 131
Necrotic purpura 206f
Necrotic rash 245
Necrotizing
    cellulitis 201
    fasciitis 202
        clinical manifestations of 202
        diagnosis of 202
        differential diagnosis of 203
        organisms causing 202
        pathogenesis of 202
        treatment modalities of 203
        types of 202
    myositis 201
    soft tissue infections, types of 201
Neonatal
    brachial plexus palsy 99, 101
    chikungunya 205
        feature of 205
        manifestations of 205
    ebstein anomaly 58
    herpes infection 149, 150

herpes patterns of 150
intensive care unit 71, 187
post-pyrexial hyperpigmentation 204
purpura 69
    fulminans 206, 235
skin rash, differential diagnoses of 205
transmission of chikungunya 205
Nephrocalcinosis 239
Nephrotic syndrome 142, 208-209
    clinical classifications of 211
    complications of 211
    drugs used for treatment 211
Nerve conduction velocity 101
Nerve grafting 102
Nerve injuries, types of 100
Nerve transfer 102
Neural tube defects 41, 289
Neuroblastoma 140
Neurocutaneous syndrome 216, 285
Neurocysticercosis 212
    characteristic features of 214
    diagnostic study for 214
    different stages of 214
    differentiate 214
    prognosis in 215
    treat 214
    treat seizures in 214
    types of 213
Neurofibromatosis 216
    complications of 218
    hallmark character of 216
    mode of transmission 218
    pathogenesis of 218
    role of oncogene 218
    single entity 217
    treatment of 218
Neurofibromin 218
Neurometabolic disorders 285
Newborn babies 265
Nicotinic acid 104
Nikolsky sign 265
Nissan fundoplication 135
Non-communicating hydrocephalus 63
Noninvasive positive pressure ventilation 88
Nonrenal hamartomas 281
Nonspecific inflammatory cell infiltrate 199
Nonsteroidal anti-inflammatory drugs 112, 114,
    202, 270
Noonan's syndrome 187
Nutritional rickets 219

O

Obstructive hydrocephalus 63
Ocular lubrication 91
Oligemic lungs 60
Omega-3-fatty acids 104
Omeprazole 135
Optic atrophy 72
Oral cavity 74
Otoscope 55
Outpatient department 89, 310

P

Palatal erythema 259f
Palatal fungal growth 197
Palatal mucormycosis symptoms of 198
Palatal rash and ulcers 269
Pale tongue 178f
Pallister-Killian syndrome 41
Palms, discoloration on 30f
Palpable purpura 142, 245
Pancreato-biliary anomalies 35
Pancytopenia 136, 228
Pandora's box, opening of 128
Paracetamol 266
Paranasal sinuses 198f
Parathyroid hormone 220
Paraumbilical hernias 296
Parenchymal necrosis 70
Parietal pleura, peeling of 95f
Paromomycin 145
Partial oculocutaneous albinism 138
Partial pressure of oxygen 42
Partial thromboplastin time with kaolin 206
Pastia's lines 262
Patent ductus arteriosus 41, 70, 116
Paternal uncle 127
Patterson's classification 11
Pemphigus 149
Pena-Shokeir syndrome 187
Penicillin-Allergic children 262
Peptosteptococcus 202
Percutaneous catheter drainage 145
Perilesional edema 212f
Perinatal infections 150
Perinatal injuries 285
Perineural spaces 198
Perioral pallor 260f
Periorbital
  ecchymosis 127f
  edema 209f

Peripheral nerve sheaths 216
Peritoneal cavity opened 43
Periungual fibroma 286
Petechiae 142
  rash 244
Phagocytic immunodeficiency, severe 138
Phimosis 225, 226
  complications 226
  need medical attention 226
  physiological 225
Phosphate
  binders 238
  levels stimulate parathyroid hormone 238
  supplementation 223, 239
Phosphofructokinase deficiency 53
Phosphopenic rickets 220, 222, 223
Phrenic nerve palsy 101
Phytobezoars 278
Picric acid 31
Plasma protein C1 inhibitor 155
Platelet flow cytometry 26
Pleural cavity 42, 43
Pneumococcal vaccination 88
Pneumonia 97f
Polycystic kidney disease 281
Polymerase chain reaction 88, 146, 199, 205, 227, 246, 249
Polymicrobial type 202
Polymorphous erythematous papular lesions 108
Polyp in children, type of 32
Polyphasic motor unit 88
Poor mineralization of osteoid 70
Positive points in clinical examination 4
Post kala-azar dermal leishmaniasis 227
  cause 229
  characteristic of 229
  diagnosing 229
  features of 229
  hallmark character of 229
  treatment of 230
Postherpetic neuralgia, severity of 306
Post-thoracoscopic decortication 94f
Potassium iodide 114
Preamble 126
Predinoslone 142
Prenatal chorionic villi sampling 88
Preputial skin retraction 225
Preterm birth 293
Prokinetics like metoclopramide 135
Prominent calf muscle 85

Proteinuria 209
Proton-pump inhibitors 135
Proximal duodenum 50
Pseudomeningocele 101
Psittacosis 111
Psychiatric disorders 277
Pulled elbow 231
    reduction of 232
    technique for reduction of 233f
Pulmonary
    artery, right 308
    artery stenosis 70
    blood flow 60
    hypoplasia 41
    oligemia 58, 59
        on X-ray 59f
    plethora
        on X-ray 59f
        with cardiomegaly 60
    sling 309
    stenosis 57
Pulp of primary 1st molar 75f
Punctate erythema 256f
Purpura fulminans 234
    causes of 235
    clinical features of 207
    complications of neonatal 207
    diagnose 235
    etiology of 207
    forms of 235
    lesion appear 235
    management of neonatal 207
    management protocol of 235
    pathophysiology of 207
    prenatal diagnosis of 207
    prognosis in 207, 236
    types of 207
Purpuric rashes 141f
Pus, suctioning and removal of 94
Pyoderma gangrenosum 203
Pyomyositis 203
Pyrazinamide 273
Pyruvate kinase deficiency 53
Pyruvate kinase levels 51

Q

Quinacrine 31

R

Rachitic rosary 219f
Ramsay Hunt syndrome 306

Ranitidine 135
Rapamycin, mammalian target of 280
Rapunzel syndrome 277
Rash on sole 244
Rash, recurrence of 106
Recessive mucopolysaccharidosis 163
Rectal fissures 202
Rectal polyp 32
Reflux-inducing foods 135
Refractory infantile spasms 279
Regional sensory ganglions 147
Reifenstein's syndrome 5
Renal
    cyst 286
    damage 300
    function test 209
    osteodystrophy 237
        cause rickets 239
        diagnose 239
        primary treatment for 239
    tubular
        acidosis, case of 240
        disorder 240, 241
        functions 238
        problem 241
Residual
    damage 100
    defects 177
Respiratory distress induces reflux 133
Respiratory failure 207
Retinal achromic patch 281
Retinal colobomas 55
Retinoblastomas 55
Retinoids 184
Retinopathy of prematurity 55
Rheumatic
    fever prophylaxis 192
    heart disease 189
        prevalence of 191
Rhinocerebral 198
Rhinoorbitocerebral 198
Rickets, signs of 222
Rickettsial
    diseases 242
        classification of 243
        types of 242
    fever 242
        complications of 246
        epidemiology of 243
        etiology 242

history of 242
method of transmission 242
treatment of 247
infection 242
diagnosis of 246
rash characteristics of 243
Rifampicin 273
Ring
constriction 12f
enhancing lesion 213
Ritter disease 265
Robert's syndrome 187
Rochalimaea quintana 243
Rocky mountain spotted fever 242
Roseola infantum 248
clinical manifestations of 248
complications of 249
etiology 248
incubation period 248
mode of transmission 248
prognosis of 249
treatment of 249

S

Sabouraud's dextrose agar 199, 199f
Sacral agenesis 253, 254
clinical features 253
etiology 254
important features 254
treatment 255
Sacral dimple indicate 250
Saffron 31
Salicylic acid 184
Saliva 77
Salmonella 114
Salt-wasting form 38
Sandifer syndrome 134
Sandpaper rash 260f
Sarcoidosis 111
Scapula suggest root avulsion 101
Scarlet fever 82, 259
alternative drugs 263
associated complications 262
causative organism of 257
complications of 257
diagnoses of 257-258, 262
duration of treatment 263
hallmark feature of 261
sufferers from 257
symptoms and signs of 257
treat 258, 262

Sclerosants 187
like bleomycin 187
Screening of the kidney by ultrasonography 286
Serositis 270
Serum
alpha-fetoprotein 156
concentration of adrenal precursors 39
creatinine 241
for herpes simplex virus 146
glutamic oxaloacetic transaminase 88
glutamic pyruvic transaminase 88
parathormone levels 220
Sexual offences 130
Sexually transmitted disease 131
Shagreen patch 281, 284f, 286
Shingles 305
Short stature 292f
Sick newborn care unit 250
Sickle cell disease 140
Sign in hydrocephalus 63
Sinusitis upper respiratory tract infection 125
Skin hypopigmentation 312
Skin necrosis with hemorrhagic blebs 234f
Skin peeling 256f
Skin rash treated 263
Slapped cheek rash 106
Smegma 225
Sodium valporate 279
Sole, discoloration on 30
Soles, eruptions on 160f
Sparse hair 19
Special Juvenile Police Unit 131
Sphenoid dysplasia 216
Spina bifida 250, 251
complications of 251
different forms of 289
differential diagnoses of 251
epidemiology of 251
etiology of 251
management of 251
occulta 288-289
pathophysiology of 251
prognosis of 252
studies used in 251
symptoms 289
types of 251
Spinal defect, common type of 288
Spinal dysraphism 303
Splenomegaly 51f
Spotted fever group 243
Stanazolol 156

Staphylococcal scalded skin syndrome 264, 265
   blisterous lesions 264
   causes 265
   complications of 266
   diagnosed 266
   investigations 265
   risk factors for 265
   risk of 265
   signs and symptoms of 265
Staphylococci 125
Staphylococcus aureus 174, 202
State Commissions for the Protection of Child Rights 131
Stem cell transplantation 164
Steroids 215
Stevens-Johnson syndrome 109
Strawberry tongue 259f, 261f
Streeter dysplasia 11
Streptococcus 114
Streptococcus pyogens 202
Sturge-Weber syndrome 267, 285
   common clinical presentation of 268
   embryological basis of 268
   seizure and stroke 268
   treatment of seizure in 268
Subclavian artery
   left 307
   right 308
Subependymal giant cell astrocytoma 282-283, 286
   treatment of 283
Subependymal nodule 281, 282
Suboptimal breast enlargement 39
Sulfonamide 111, 114
Suppress calcitriol synthesis 223
Supraumbilical hernia 296
Sural nerve cable grafting 102
Swachman Diamond syndrome 117
Sweet syndrome 111
Synophrys 18f
Synpneumonic effusion 93f
Syphilis 114
Systemic diseases 31
Systemic lupus erythematosus 269
   diagnosis of 270
   malar rash due to 270
   pathogenesis of 269
   symptoms for 270
Systemic Lupus International Collaborating Clinics group 270
Systemic toxicity 203

T

Tacrolimus 211
Taenia solium 213
Tale-tell X-ray features 57
Tazarotene 184
Telecanthus 312
Tenexamic acid 156
Testosterone 169
Tetracycline 247
Tetralogy of Fallot 58
Thalassemia major 53, 140
Thiazides 241
Thoracic diameter 59
Thoracoscope 94f
Thoracoscopic decortication 97
Thrombocytopenia 270
   absent radii 117
Thromboembolic phenomenon 211
Thymic shadow 57
   on chest X-ray 56
Thyroid-stimulating hormone 79
Tissue plasminogen activator 236
Tomisaku Kawasaki 84
Tongue tie 13
Tooth decay 76
Topiramate 282
Torsion testis 275
   case of 275
   clinical importance of 275
   etiology for 276
   management 276
   surgical exploration 276
   types of 276
Toxic epidermonecrolysis 109
Trabeculated bladder 303f
Transesophageal echo 174
Transglutaminase deficiency in skin biopsy 184
Transitional group 243
Transthoracic diameter 56
Treacher-Collins syndrome 188
Trichobezoar 277
Trichobezoar
   complications 278
   pathogenesis 277
   treatment 278
Trichophagia 277
Trichotillomania 277
Triosephosphate isomerase deficiency 53
Tuberculoma 214

Tuberculous lymphadenitis 272-273
    diagnose 272
    investigate/diagnose 272
    investigations 272
    microbial diagnosis 273
    suspected case of 273
    with sinus 271
Tuberous sclerosis 279
    clinical criteria 280
    complex 281, 282, 284-285
    complex clinical manifestations of 286
    complex etiology of 286
    complex manage seizures of 287
    complex manifestations in 286
    complex treatment for 287
    criteria for diagnosing 280
    diagnosis of 279
    genetic criteria 280
    incidence of 280
    investigations 281
    management of 282
    minor features 281
    surgical care 282
    underlying cause of 280
Tuft of hair 288
Tumor necrosis factor-alpha 111
Turbinate hypertrophy 290, 290f
    modalities of treatment 290
Turner's syndrome 41, 86, 187, 291, 293-294
    causes 293
    complications of 293
    inherited 293
    signs and symptoms of 291
Typhus group 243

U

Ulcerative colitis 114
Ulcers on tongue 160f
Umbilical
    cicatrix 296
    hernia 295
        early surgery 296
        surgery required for 296
Umbilicus, swelling over 295
Upper airway compression 308
Urethral valves, posterior 303
Urinary tract infection 125, 299
    confirm 300
    evaluation of 301
    symptoms of 299

Urticaria
    facilitia 125
    multiforme 297
    multiforme treatment of 298
    pathophysiology of 124

V

Vagal zoster 306
Valproate 282
    acid during pregnancy 289
Vancomycin 145
Varicella
    vaccine 153
    zoster virus 84, 305
Vascular ring 308
    clinical practice 309
    diagnose 309
    different types of 308
    treat 309
Vasculitis with calcification 70
Vein of galen malformation 63
Venous blood gas 241
Ventricular septal defect 70, 57, 116
Ventricular system 63
Vesico-bullous eruption 151
Vesicoureteric reflux 226, 299
Vesicular rash 204f
Vigabatrin 282
Viral infections 205
Virtual bronchoscopy 121f
Visceral pleura, removal of 95f
Visual memory 294
Visuospatial skills 294
Vitamin
    C deficiency 127
    D sources of 221
    D supplementation 223
Vulvul synechiae detection of 302

W

Waardenburg syndrome 310, 312
    affects 311
    case of 310
    clinical signs of 311
    common forms of 311
    diagnosis of 310
    diagnostic criteria for 312
    inheritance patterns in 312
    types of 311

Walls of small vessels 142
Warning signs 130
Webbed neck 292
Webbing of neck 292f
Wedge-shaped feature 253
West syndrome 285
Whipple disease 111
Widened wrist 219f
Wilson's disease 222

X

X chromosome 86, 293
X chromosome genes 291
X linked recessive condition 117
Xanthomas 103f
    causes 104
Xanthomatosis, eruptive 103
X-linked
    dominant hypophosphatemia 222
    hypohidrotic ectodermal dysplasia 90
$Xp21$ gene leads 86
X-ray abdomen 49
X-ray normal 92f

Y

Yersinia 111, 114, 125

Z

Ziehl-Neelsen stain 272
Zoster sine herpete 306

EU GSPR Authorised Reprsentative
Logos Europe, 9 rue Nicolas Poussin
1700, La Rochelle, France
Phone: +33 (0) 6 67 93 73 78
E-mail: contact@logoseurope.eu

www.ingramcontent.com/pod-product-compliance
Ingram Content Group UK Ltd.
Pitfield, Milton Keynes, MK11 3LW, UK
UKHW050429150426

5217IPUK00019B/1310